MEDICINAL CHEMISTRY
The Role of Organic Chemistry in Drug Research

MEDICINAL CHEMISTRY
The Role of Organic Chemistry in Drug Research

Edited by

S. M. ROBERTS
Department of Microbiological Chemistry
Glaxo Group Research Ltd.
Greenford, Middlesex, England

B. J. PRICE
Chemistry Division
Glaxo Group Research Ltd.
Greenford, Middlesex, England

1985

ACADEMIC PRESS

Harcourt Brace Jovanovich, Publishers

London   Orlando   San Diego   New York
Austin   Montreal   Sydney   Tokyo   Toronto

ACADEMIC PRESS INC. (LONDON) LTD.
24–28 Oval Road
LONDON NW1 7DX

United States Edition published by
ACADEMIC PRESS, INC.
Orlando, Florida 32887

BRITISH LIBRARY CATALOGUING IN PUBLICATION DATA
Medicinal chemistry : the role of organic chemistry
    in drug research.
    1. Drugs   2. Chemistry, Medical and
    pharmaceutical
    I. Roberts, S.M.   II. Price, B.J.
    615'.3   RS403

    ISBN 0-12-589730-8

LIBRARY OF CONGRESS CATALOGING-IN-PUBLICATION DATA
Main entry under title:

Medicinal chemistry.

    Includes index.
    1. Chemistry, Pharmaceutical—Addresses, essays,
lectures.   2. Drugs—Research—Addresses, essays,
lectures.   I. Roberts, Stanley M.   II. Price, B. J.
(Barry J.)   [DNLM: 1. Pharmacology. QV 38 M4795]
RS410.M43   1985   615'.7   85-11233
ISBN 0-12-589730-8 (alk. paper)

PRINTED IN THE UNITED STATES OF AMERICA

85 86 87 88   9 8 7 6 5 4 3 2 1

Contents

10. Steroid Contraceptives
F. J. Zeelen

11. Injectable Cephalosporin Antibiotics: Cephalothin to Ceftazidime
C. E. Newall

12. Clavulanic Acid and Related Compounds: Inhibitors of β-Lactamase Enzymes
A. G. Brown

13. Ketoconazole and the Treatment of Fungal Diseases
J. Heeres

14. Oxamniquine: A Drug for the Tropics
H. C. Richards

Contributors

Numbers in parentheses indicate the pages on which the authors' contributions begin.

A. G. Brown (227), Beecham Pharmaceuticals Research Division, Chemotherapeutic Centre, Betchworth, Surrey RH3 7AJ, England

M. G. Davis (27), Division of Biological and Environmental Sciences, The Hatfield Polytechnic, Hatfield, Hertfordshire, England

J. Elks (167), 83 The Ridgeway, London NW11 8PL, England

C. R. Ganellin (93), Smith Kline & French Research Ltd., The Frythe, Welwyn, Hertfordshire AL6 9AR, England

J. Heeres (249), Department of Chemistry, Janssen Pharmaceutica, B-2340 Beerse, Belgium

J. W. Lewis (119), Pharmaceutical Division, Reckitt & Colman, Kingston-upon-Hull, England

L. H. C. Lunts (49), Glaxo Group Research Ltd., Ware, Hertfordshire SG12 0DJ, England

B. G. Main (69), Chemistry Department, ICI Pharmaceuticals Division, Macclesfield, Cheshire, England

C. E. Newall (209), Department of Microbiological Chemistry, Glaxo Group Research Ltd., Greenford, Middlesex UB6 0HE, England

G. H. Phillipps (167), Department of Medicinal Chemistry, Glaxo Group Research Ltd., Greenford, Middlesex UB6 0HE, England

H. C. Richards (271), Pfizer Central Research, Sandwich, Kent CT13 9NJ, England

S. M. Roberts (1), Department of Microbiological Chemistry, Glaxo Group Research Ltd., Greenford, Middlesex UB6 0HE, England

J. B. Stenlake (143), Department of Pharmacy, University of Strathclyde, Glasgow G1 1XW, Scotland

H. Tucker (69), Chemistry Department, ICI Pharmaceuticals Division, Macclesfield, Cheshire, England

B. Walker (19), Her Majesty's Inspectorate, Department of Education and Science, London SE1 7PH, England

F. J. Zeelen (189), Organon Scientific Development Group, 5340 BH Oss, The Netherlands

Preface

Compared to the long-established natural sciences, medicinal chemistry is in its infancy. However, our understanding of the interaction of drug substances with receptors and enzymes in the human body has improved considerably over the past 20 years. This knowledge is fundamental to the search for new and improved treatments of common ailments and diseases carried out in academic laboratories and in the pharmaceutical industry. Chemists play a key role in pharmaceutical research; they are required to synthesise, purify and analyse novel compounds for biological testing. The preparation of a selected compound is *relatively* straightforward: with the wealth of chemical literature available, a chemist should be able to construct any thermodynamically stable molecule (though, depending on the complexity of the molecule, the task may take many man-months to complete and a number of seemingly reasonable routes might fail due to unforeseen and unexpected courses being taken by the reactions). The real difficulty is in deciding what to make. Which fundamental molecular framework will have the desired biological action? What are the optimum positions for substituents on the basic skeleton to maximize activity? Using chemistry, we must also try to understand the aetiology of the disease in order to be in a position to suggest molecules that might correct the underlying malfunction.

This book is designed to help chemists with little or no knowledge of the drug industry to begin to understand how some of the currently important and widely used drug substances were discovered. The text assumes a basic knowledge of organic chemistry; a background in biology, biochemistry or pharmacology would be useful but is by no means essential. Helpful inexpensive paperback books can be consulted as aids to the understanding of the workings of the human body (*1*) and to explain in more detail the nature and function of receptors (*2*). Standard biochemistry texts (*3*) expound upon the nature of enzymes.

Two of the chapters introducing enzymes and receptors were written by members of a team from Hatfield Polytechnic which has many years experience in teaching the fundamental principles of biology to chemists. The other chapters, which describe the discovery of a variety of therapeutic agents, were written by chemists who are experts in the different areas of drug research.

Four chapters deal with drug substances discovered as a result of studies in receptorology. The structure of the naturally occurring neurotransmitter was known in each case, namely, noradrenaline (Chapters 4 and 5), histamine (Chapter 6) and acetylcholine (Chapter 8), and it was necessary to modify these small molecules to provide selective agonists (e.g., noradrenaline β_2 receptor stimulants) or antagonists (e.g., noradrenaline β receptor blockers, histamine H_2 receptor antagonists and antagonists of the acetylcholine receptor at the neuromuscular junction) and hence to provide useful drug substances.

Chapter 7 describes the development of the potent painkiller buprenorphine. In this example, morphine was used as a template since the latter substance has the desired analgesic activity although its usefulness in the clinic is diminished by its well-known and undesirable side effects.

Two chapters describe drugs that have been designed from natural hormones. Anti-inflammatory steroids (Chapter 9) were designed and prepared on the basis of the structure and action of cortisone, while the fascinating story of the birth of the contraceptive pill (Chapter 10) starts with an appreciation of the roles of progesterone and the estrogens in fertility.

The historic work of Fleming led to the discovery of penicillin, the first of the β-lactam antibacterials. In the 1960s the structure of another antibiotic produced by a fungus was found to contain a β-lactam ring; this naturally occurring material, cephalosporin C, has been modified to produce powerful broad-spectrum antibacterial agents (Chapter 11). However, the effectiveness of the ''semisynthetic'' penicillins, derived by modification of Fleming's original production process, was diminished by the development of resistant bacterial strains. The origin of this resistance and the way it has been overcome, initially through the screening of many different fungal broths, is elegantly described in Chapter 12.

Anti-bacterial chemotherapy is well advanced compared to anti-fungal chemotherapy. There are several reasons for this state of affairs, the most important being that the fungi are higher organisms than the bacteria and thus do not differ as markedly from the host (man). However, fungal cells differ from mammalian cells in the composition of the cell membranes. In particular, the steroid components in the cell membranes are different, and this fact can be utilised by the medicinal chemist. Compounds which block the synthesis of steroids that are important to fungi but not to *Homo sapiens* afford useful anti-fungal agents (Chapter 13).

The final chapter tells the story of oxamniquine, a powerful anti-schistosomal agent. In this case, a pragmatic approach was taken: worms were treated with chemical compounds to find which structural types were toxic to the trematodes. The structures of the active compounds were refined in a thoughtful way to provide the clinically useful drug.

An underlying theme can be distilled from this volume: that the medicinal chemist is becoming expert at modifying the structure of a known biologically active molecule in order to accentuate a particular aspect of its activity, eventually to provide a safe medicine. This is not a simple process in any case, and in some cases it can be soul destroying. For instance, the importance of prostaglandins *in vivo* has been recognised for a long time; the structures of the prostaglandins were elucidated 20 years ago, but the prospect of obtaining a drug based on a modified prostaglandin structure is only just in sight.

Over the next 20 years it will probably become increasingly common to find drugs designed *de novo*. As enzymes become available in quantity and in a pure state, powerful techniques such as X-ray crystallography, computer graphics and molecular mechanics will allow the medicinal chemist to predict structures that will fit and interact with the "active site" on the surface of the enzyme. This research will provide a useful end product if the enzyme is involved in the critical path of a key biological process. If the enzyme is peculiar to a bacterium, a fungus or a virus, then blocking the active site will lead to non-viability of the pathogen. If the enzyme is one of our own, then an ability to modulate the process handled by a key enzyme can be beneficial (e.g., inhibition of renin or angiotensin-converting enzyme and the control of blood pressure).

In the area of receptorology, it is clear that other neurotransmitters and associated receptors will be found. These new receptors, and indeed sub-classes of established receptors, will provide the chemist with new objectives involving the synthesis of novel compounds to block or activate these macromolecules.

Before a medicinal chemist can have a major impact on any area of enzymology or receptorology, the biology of the relevant system in health and in disease must be understood. In cancer and rheumatism little is known about the key factors controlling the onset and maintenance of the condition. Much more biology-based research is needed before serious drug design can begin.

It is hoped that this book will whet the appetite of the reader. More information on the compounds described in the following chapters will be found in detailed medicinal chemistry texts (4). Other tomes review the different drugs available for particular disease states (5). We have restricted discussion to drugs which are well known, well established and widely used. In an attempt to emphasize the basic discoveries which led to breakthroughs in chemotherapy and medicinal chemistry, we have neglected many of the finer points of the science (*inter alia* drug absorption, drug metabolism, drug formulation and the use of pro-drugs).

Finally, we thank all the contributing authors for combining scientific accuracy with a highly readable text, Miss Roz Atkinson and Mr. Dinos Santafianos for help in finalizing the script and Mrs. Sue Davies for expert assistance in the preparation of the typescript.

B. J. Price
S. M. Roberts

REFERENCES

1. P. Lewis and D. Rubenstein, "The Human Body." Hamlyn, Feltham, England, 1970.
2. Z. L. Kruk and C. J. Pycock, "Neurotransmitters and Drugs." Croom Helm, London, 1979.

3. L. Stryer, "Biochemistry," 2nd Ed. Freeman, San Francisco, 1981; H. R. Mahler and E. H. Cordes, "Biological Chemistry." Harper & Row, New York, 1971; G. Zubay, "Biochemistry." Addison-Wesley, Reading, Massachusetts, 1983; *see also* M. Dixon and L. C. Webb, "Enzymes," 2nd Ed. Longman, London, 1971.
4. M. E. Wolff, ed., "The Basis of Medicinal Chemistry: Burger's Medicinal Chemistry," Parts 1–3, 4th Ed. Wiley, New York, 1980; L. S. Goodman and A. Gilman, eds, "The Pharmacological Basis of Therapeutics," 6th Ed. Macmillan, New York, 1980.
5. A. Wade and J. E. F. Reynolds, eds, "Martindale: The Extra Pharmacopoeia," 27th Ed. The Pharmaceutical Press, London, 1977, and other pharmacopoeias cited in the preface therein.

Glossary

Actinomycetes	non-acid-fast bacteria, some varieties used in the production of antibodies
Adipose	of or related to fat
Agonist	a drug that can interact with receptors (specific sites in certain cells) and initiate a drug response (e.g., acetylcholine)
Allosteric control	alteration of enzyme's activity by molecules non-competitively bound to sites other than the active or catalytic site of the enzyme
Angina	a spasmodic, oppressive, severe pain
Antacid	an agent which reduces the acidity of gastric juice or other secretions
Antagonist	a drug that opposes the effect of another by physiological or chemical action or by a competitive mechanism for the same receptor sites
Apnoea	the cessation or suspension of breathing
Arrhythmia	irregularity, especially of the heart beat
Atria	upper chambers of the heart
Autonomic	independent, self-controlling
Biliary	relating to bile and the bile ducts
Carcinoma	a malignant tumour causing eventual death (i.e., cancer)
Catecholamines	amine compounds which have sympathomimetic activity and are concerned with nervous transmission and many metabolic activities
Chromatin	the portion of the cell nucleus, easily stained by dyes, consisting of nucleic acids and proteins
Cytoplasm	the substance of a cell surrounding the nucleus, carrying structures within which most of the cell's life processes take place
Cytosol	the soluble portion of the cytoplasm after all particles (e.g., mitochondria, endoplasmic reticular components) are removed
Denaturation	modification of the enzyme's biological structure (secondary and tertiary) due to extremes of pH or temperature, organic solvents, high salt concentrations, oxidation or reduction
Disseminated	widely distributed throughout an organ, tissue or the body
Dopaminergic	neurotransmitting action by the substance dopamine
Endometrium	mucosal layer lining the cavity of the uterus, its structure changes with age or with menstrual cycle
Flexor	muscle that flexes a joint

Ganglia	(plural of ganglion) collection of nerve cell bodies located outside the brain and spinal cord
Hypophysis	the pituitary gland, important to growth, maturity and reproduction
Infarction	formation of a dead area of tissue caused by an obstruction of the artery supplying the area
Intravenous infusion	introduction of a fluid into a vein
Isoenzyme	one of a group of enzymes which catalyses the same chemical reaction but which has different physical properties
Juxtaposition	a side-by-side position
Lumen	the interior space of a tubular structure
Mitochondria	organelles present in nearly all living cells, generating energy by the formation of ATP (adenosine triphosphate)
Neuropsychiatry	the study of both organic and functional diseases of the nervous system
Obstetrics	a branch of medicine concerned principally with the care of women and their offspring during and after gestation
Osmolarity	the osmotic concentration of a solution expressed as moles of the dissolved substance per litre of solution
Parietal	pertaining to the wall of a cavity
Pellagra	a condition caused by vitamin deficiency, marked by skin lesions, gastrointestinal disturbances and nervous disorders
Pernicious anaemia	deficiency of vitamin B_{12} resulting in degeneration of posterior/lateral columns of the spinal cord
Potency	an expression of drug activity (i.e., the dose required to produce a specific effect of given intensity as compared to a standard of reference)
Proteolytic enzymes	enzymes which hydrolyse (break down) proteins into simpler, more soluble forms
Psoriasis	chronic inflammatory skin disease characterised by red patches covered with silvery scales
Psychotomimetic	producing symptoms that resemble those of psychosis, a severe mental illness (i.e., loss of contact with reality, regressive behaviour, delusions)
Purine	fundamental part of organic compounds found in nature (e.g., uric acid compounds, adenine, guanine and xanthines)
Secretagogue	a substance promoting secretion (e.g., in the stomach)
Serum	clear fluid of blood, devoid of fibrinogen and cells
Spheroplast	cell surrounded solely by its limiting membrane
Sympathomimetic	producing effects similar to those caused by stimulation of the sympathetic nervous system
Systemic	relating to or affecting the whole body
Thymic	relating to the thymus gland
Urticaria	a skin condition (e.g., rash)

Vagus	tenth cranial nerve
Vascular	consisting of, or provided with, vessels
Viscera	(plural of viscus) large internal organs, especially in the abdomen

CHAPTER 1

Introduction to Enzymes, Receptors, and the Action of Drugs

S. M. ROBERTS

Department of Microbiological Chemistry
Glaxo Group Research Ltd.
Greenford, England

I. COMMUNICATION BETWEEN CELLS: THE ROLES OF RECEPTORS AND ENZYMES

Some species of animals are composed of a single independent cell (the protozoa) while mammals are multicellular organisms. In between these two extremes there are life forms of varying complexity. All these organisms use cell(s) to compartmentalize various chemical reactions in order to use available materials for energy and the maintenance of life's processes.

Cells of different life forms have different characteristics (Fig. 1) and, indeed, different cells from the same organism can be distinguished readily. For example, mammalian cells come in all shapes and sizes: compare the spheroidal leucocyte (the white blood cell), the flat epithelial cells found near the surface of membranes, and the nerve cell shown in Fig. 2.

The cells are organised such that chemical transformations can be accomplished efficiently, the rate of these transformations being controlled by Nature's catalysts—enzymes. Enzymes are high molecular weight compounds which catalyse anabolic (synthesis) and catabolic (degradation) reactions. The trivial name of the enzyme often gives a guide to its role (a more comprehensive list of enzyme activities is contained in Chap. 3):

1

$$RCO_2R^1 \xrightarrow[H_2O]{\substack{\text{esterase} \\ \text{enzyme}}} RCO_2H + R^1OH \qquad (1)$$

$$\underset{\substack{| \\ OH}}{RCHR^1} \xrightarrow[\substack{A^+ \quad AH + H^+}]{\substack{\text{dehydrogenase} \\ \text{enzyme}}} RCOR^1 \qquad (2)$$

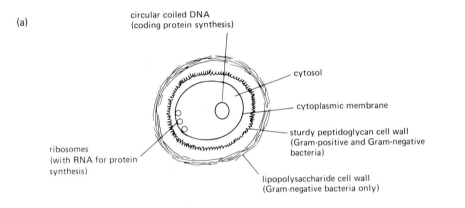

$$\xrightarrow[H_2O]{\substack{\text{phospho-diesterase} \\ \text{enzyme}}} \underset{\substack{| \qquad | \\ OPO_3H \quad OH}}{RCH—CH_2—CHR^1} \qquad (3)$$

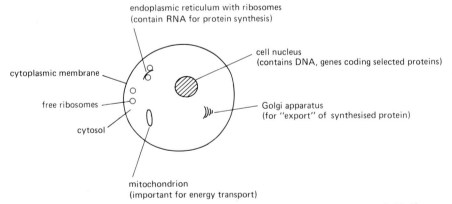

(a)

circular coiled DNA
(coding protein synthesis)

cytosol

cytoplasmic membrane

sturdy peptidoglycan cell wall
(Gram-positive and Gram-negative
bacteria)

ribosomes
(with RNA for protein
synthesis)

lipopolysaccharide cell wall
(Gram-negative bacteria only)

(b)

endoplasmic reticulum with ribosomes
(contain RNA for protein synthesis)

cell nucleus
(contains DNA, genes coding selected proteins)

cytoplasmic membrane

free ribosomes

cytosol

Golgi apparatus
(for "export" of synthesised protein)

mitochondrion
(important for energy transport)

Fig. 1   A prokaryotic bacterial cell (a) and a eukaryotic (possessing a nucleus) human cell (b). Not all the substructures that may occur in a cell are represented.

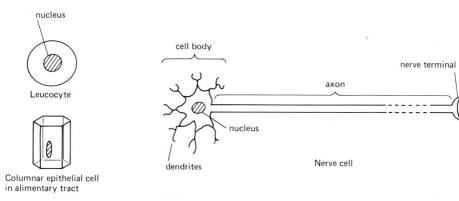

Fig. 2   Shapes and sizes of mammalian cells.

In order to coordinate their activities the different cells in multicellular organisms need to communicate and this correspondence is accomplished mainly by small chemical molecules. For example, on receiving the appropriate signal, nerve terminals release a substance such as acetylcholine (**1**), noradrenaline (**2**), or dopamine (**3**) and these substances, known as neurotransmitters, can interact with the appropriate receptors.

$$CH_3COOCH_2CH_2\overset{+}{N}(CH_3)_3$$

(**1**)

(**2**)   R = H
(**6**)   R = CH$_3$

(**3**)

The receptors lie on the surface of the cells adjacent to the terminal (Fig. 3). The interaction of a neurotransmitter (agonist*) with its receptor usually effects a change in conformation of the macromolecular receptor and possibly the surrounding membrane, leading to either activation of an enzyme within the cell (Fig. 4), and/or movement of ions into or out of the cell (Fig. 5).

One specific example of the process diagrammatically illustrated in Fig. 4 is given by noradrenaline, which will act on a receptor (see later) to activate the intracellular enzyme adenylate cyclase to produce cyclic adenosine 3′,5′-mono-

---

*Agonist is a name coined by Gaddum in 1937 and is now used to describe all physiological mediators and drugs which mimic their action by activating the same cellular reactions.

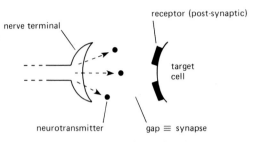

Fig. 3   A neuro-effector junction.

phosphate (**5**) (cyclic AMP) from adenosine triphosphate (ATP) (**4**) as shown in Eq. (4). Cyclic AMP initiates a cascade of other enzyme activations leading to the observed biological response. Cyclic AMP is inactivated by a phospho-diesterase enzyme.

An example of the process represented in Fig. 5 is the interaction of acetyl-choline at its receptor which causes a series of events resulting in a movement of sodium ions into the cell. Figures 4 and 5 illustrate that receptor occupation may

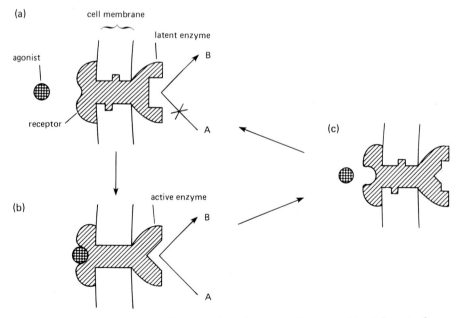

Fig. 4   Activation of an enzyme by occupation of a receptor by an agonist. (a) Receptor free, enzyme inactive. (b) Receptor occupied, enzyme triggered into action (allosteric activation of enzyme). (c) Agonist leaves receptor surface, and enzyme quickly returns to inactive form.

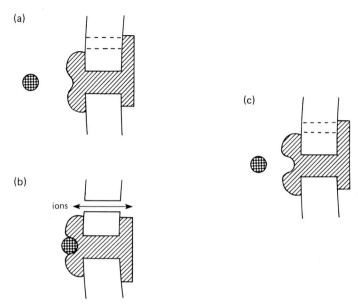

Fig. 5 Opening of an ion-channel by the occupation of a receptor by an agonist. (a) Receptor free, channel closed. (b) Receptor occupied, channel opened, ion migration rapidly takes place down the concentration gradient. (c) Channel closes, neurotransmitter diffuses away. Difference in metal ion (e.g., Na^+) concentration across the membrane is re-established by exergonic metal-ion pump.

result in an effect (e.g., enzyme activity) that will last for the life-time of the occupation, or the effect (e.g., ion movement) may be triggered and will not reoccur until disengagement of the agonist, repriming of the system and re-engagement of the agonist and the receptor.

Note that if a neurotransmitter remains in the synaptic cleft, disengagement/reengagement will continue and the receptor will continue to be fired: this

$$\xrightarrow[\substack{+H_2O \\ -H^+}]{\text{phosphodiesterase}}$$

(structure of adenosine monophosphate with NH_2 purine base, $^-O-\overset{O}{\overset{\|}{P}}OCH_2$, O^-, and OH OH on the ribose)

$$CH_3COOCH_2CH_2\overset{+}{N}(CH_3)_3 \xrightarrow[H_2O]{\text{acetylcholinesterase}} CH_3CO_2H + HOCH_2CH_2\overset{+}{N}(CH_3)_3 \quad (5)$$

$$HO-\text{(catechol ring)}-CHCH_2NH_2 \xrightarrow[\substack{R\overset{+}{S}R' \\ | \\ Me}]{\text{COMT}} {}_{\substack{RSR' \\ + \\ H^+}} \quad HO-\text{(ring)}-CHCH_2NH_2 \quad (6)$$

with HO and OH substituents on the left, and H_3CO, OH on the right.

will carry on until the chemical diffuses away from the site. To allow a faster return to the resting state after the neurotransmitter has ceased to be released from the nerve terminal, an enzyme is usually present which will convert the neurotransmitter into an inactive substance. For example, acetylcholine is deactivated by an esterase [Eq. (5)] while noradrenaline is rendered inactive by methylation of one of the phenolic groups [Eq. (6)] through the enzyme catechol O-methyltransferase (COMT).* These examples illustrate that enzymes are not always contained within cells. Equally, not all chemical messengers are released from nerve terminals to act on adjacent terminals before being degraded. For example, adrenaline (6), noradrenaline (2), and various steroids are released into the circulation from endocrine glands. Local hormones or autocoids are released from cells, and travel through extra-cellular fluid to act on end organs. The three types of intracellular communication processes are shown in Fig. 6.

It is important to understand that while enzymes and receptors are both composed of amino-acids condensed into high molecular weight polypeptide chains, and can be associated with ions and small molecules, there the likeness ends. One of the major differences is that enzymes catalyse bond-making and bond-breaking reactions while the receptors release the substrate unchanged.

In the normal healthy state, all cells are communicating, synthesising and

*Some neurotransmitters are removed by reabsorption into the presynaptic terminal, and indeed the majority of the noradrenaline released from a nerve terminal is removed from the synapse by this method.

(a)

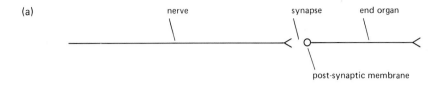

(b)

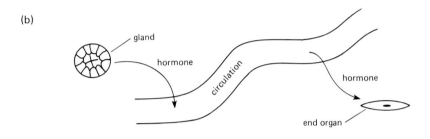

(c)

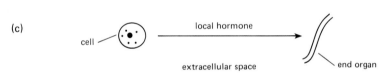

Fig. 6 Intercellular communication processes. (a) Nerve releases a neurotransmitter substance, e.g., acetylcholine, which diffuses across a synapse to act upon a post-synaptic membrane. (b) Endocrine gland releases a hormone, e.g., steroid, which is distributed throughout the body by the circulatory system. (c) Local hormone (autacoid) is released by cells and diffuses through the extracellular space to act locally, e.g., histamine released from mast cell or cells in the stomach.

degrading molecules, and changing ion concentrations for the overall well-being of the organism. As a result of disease, damage or degeneration, cellular activities may become impaired and the correct dynamic equilibrium must then be reinstated by the means of a suitable drug.

It may be desirable to amplify the effect of a neurotransmitter: this can be accomplished by

1. Increasing the concentration of the natural neurotransmitter by (a) direct supplementation through introduction of the substance into the body or (b) inhibition of enzymes that degrade the transmitter.
2. Using a more potent and/or less readily metabolised surrogate of the natural substance (an unnatural agonist).

Alternatively it may be prudent to decrease the effect of a particular neuro-

transmitter at a given receptor. This can be done using an antagonist substance,*
i.e., an unnatural compound which will bind strongly to a receptor without
eliciting a response and which will prevent access to the receptor by the neurotransmitter.

Similarly, certain enzyme substrates and specific or highly selective enzyme
inhibitors can provide useful drug substances.

Before amplifying these points, the central control of cell communication and
a more detailed consideration of certain neurotransmitters and receptors is
warranted.

II.   NEUROTRANSMITTERS, RECEPTORS, AND THE NERVOUS SYSTEM

In complex organisms such as man there are a considerable number of receptors and a multitude of different enzymes. Actions are coordinated by the central
nervous system (CNS) (the brain and spinal cord) and some actions come as a
result of sensory input (sight, sounds, touch, blood glucose levels, etc.). Output
from the CNS is directed towards the autonomic nervous system (the sympathetic
and parasympathetic functions) and nerves associated with voluntary motor functions as illustrated in Fig. 7. Voluntary motor function deals with the controlled
movement of muscles (skeletal muscle) and the associated limbs; some of the
actions involving the parasympathetic and sympathetic nerves are listed in Fig. 8
and the effects on selected organs from the two systems are listed in Table I. In
short, the sympathetic and parasympathetic systems operate in a complementary
fashion. In response to a particular external influence, enhanced stimulation of
the sympathetic nervous system occurs and leads to preparation for "fight or
flight" (Fig. 9). In the relaxed state (Fig. 10), stimulation of the parasympathetic
nervous system predominates and deals with secretion and voidance of materials
from the body.

Some important neuro-junctions and the associated neurotransmitters in the
nervous system are shown in Fig. 11.

Note that the acetylcholine receptors are divided into two categories: the
classification is based on the actions of two drugs of plant origin.† The receptors

---

*An antagonist diminishes or abolishes the effects of its corresponding agonist. Two types of
antagonist are known: a competitive antagonist competes with the agonist for the active site of the
receptor while a noncompetitive antagonist binds at a different site than that of the agonist. In the
former situation the effect of an antagonist decreases in the presence of increasing concentrations of
agonist while in the latter situation the effect of the antagonist is independent of agonist concentration.

†The sub-division of the various receptors is based on agonist and/or antagonist actions of substances not normally found in the mammalian system.

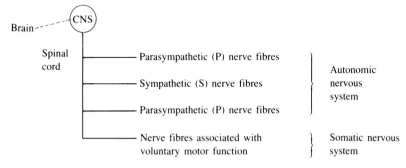

Fig. 7   The peripheral nervous system.

which are activated by muscarine are termed muscarinic receptors, and those activated by binding nicotine are called nicotinic receptors. Thus nicotine and muscarine mimic the action of acetylcholine at two different distinct receptors. The effects on various end-organs on stimulation of the appropriate acetylcholine receptor are listed in Table II. Inhibition of the action of acetylcholine at the neuro-muscular junction leads to muscle relaxation (Chap. 8).

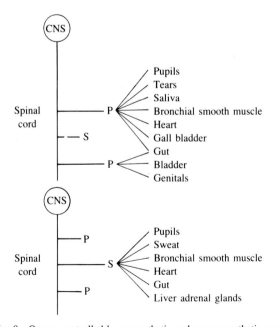

Fig. 8   Organs controlled by sympathetic and parasympathetic nerves.

TABLE I

Response to Activation of Sympathetic and Parasympathetic Nervous Systems

Organ	Response to activation of nerve	
	Sympathetic	Parasympathetic
Pupil	Dilation	Constriction
Bronchi	Dilation	Constriction
Heart	↑ Acceleration	↓ Slowing
Digestive tract	↓ Slowing	↑ Increase
Sphincters of gut	Constriction	Relaxation
Bladder	Relaxation	Contraction Emptying
Blood vessels	Constriction	
Glands of alimentary canal— salivary, gut, pancreas		↑ Increase in activity

Noradrenaline and adrenaline stimulate adrenoceptors. When noradrenaline is released from a pre-synaptic nerve terminal it crosses the synaptic cleft and initiates a response in the post-synaptic tissue by combining with one of two types of receptor called α-adrenoceptors and β-adrenoceptors.* The type of receptor found post-synaptically to noradrenergic nerves in the sympathetic system depends on the type of tissue; classification of adrenoceptors in different tissues is again based on the ability of agonists to initiate responses and antagonists to prevent responses. A further subclassification of β-adrenoceptors has been made: in man the majority of β-adrenoceptors in the heart are called β_1-adrenoceptors and these are distinct from other β-adrenoceptors (dubbed β_2-adrenoceptors*) found elsewhere in the periphery (outside the CNS). Many tissues have a mixed population of β_1- and β_2-receptors. Noradrenaline and adrenaline have different effects on α- and β-receptors; noradrenaline is potent at stimulating α-receptors but is less potent at activating β-receptors while adrenaline elicits activity from both α- and β-receptors at about the same level.

Some important sites of α- and β-adrenergic receptors are given in Table III.

Note that activation of α-receptors generally results in a stimulatant response (except in the gut) while activation of β-receptors leads to an inhibitory response, namely, relaxation of muscle (except in the heart). Blocking of α- and β-receptors causes, *inter alia,* relaxation of peripheral blood vessels and slowing of the heart, respectively, and can have beneficial effects in the treatment of angina and

*The sub-division of the various receptors is based on agonist and/or antagonist actions of substances not normally found in the mammalian system.

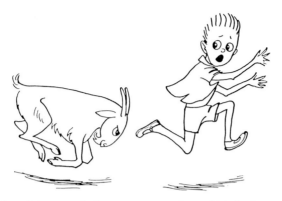

Fig. 9   Stimulation of the sympathetic nervous system due to *fright* leads to preparation of the system for *fight* or *flight:* increase in heart rate, dilation of bronchi, dilation of pupils, constriction of peripheral blood vessels (pallor), etc.   (From B.L.A.T. Booklet "Action of Drugs", Centre for Health and Medical Education, London.)

hypertension (Chap. 5), while β_2-stimulants can alleviate mild to moderate asthmatic attacks by relaxation of bronchiolar muscle and widening of airways (Chap. 4).

Some peptides act as neurotransmitters. For example, receptors for the enkephalins (**7**) have been demonstrated within the CNS. It is believed that morphine (**8**) and the other opiates exert their analgesic action by interaction with these receptors. Thus morphine (**8**), heroin (**9**), and codeine (**10**) can be consid-

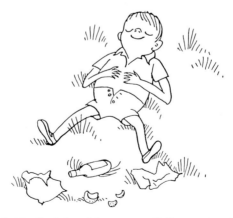

Fig. 10   In the relaxed state stimulation of the parasympathetic nervous system is predominant and leads to (*inter alia*) slowing of the heart and increase in the activity of the gastro-intestinal tract. (From B.L.A.T. Booklet "Action of Drugs", Centre for Health and Medical Education, London.)

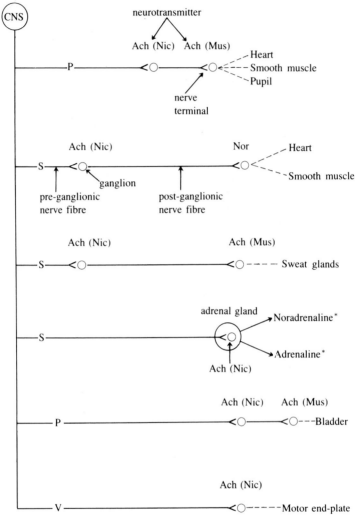

Fig. 11 Neurotransmitters in the peripheral nervous system. Asterisk indicates release into the circulation to act on distant receptors in the periphery. S, sympathetic nervous system; P, parasympathetic nervous system; V, voluntary motor function.

ered to be agonists at the enkephalin receptor while buprenorphin is a partial agonist, i.e., it has mixed agonist and antagonist properties (see Chap. 2 for fuller explanation). Opiate receptor blockers (antagonists), e.g., nalorphine, are also known (see Chap. 7).

Histamine (11) is not a neurotransmitter but it does occur in several tissues in the body. It is stored in mast cells and platelets and is released from these sites in

TABLE II

Situation of Some Acetylcholine-controlled Neuro-junctions

Organ	Type of receptor	Control by voluntary motor (VM), parasympathetic (P), or sympathetic (S) nervous system	Effect of agonist
Heart	Mus	P	Slowing rate of contraction, decreasing force of contraction
Eye	Mus	P	Constriction of pupil
Sweat glands	Mus	S	Activation
Gastro-intestinal smooth muscle	Mus	P	Increase in tone, increase in contractions and peristalsis
Adrenal gland	Nic	S	Release of adrenaline and noradrenaline
Bladder	Mus	P	Contraction
Skeletal muscle	Nic	VM	Muscle contraction
CNS	Mus and Nic	—	Various

response to stimuli such as allergic reactions and injury. Two types of histamine receptor, termed H_1 and H_2, have been identified: they differ in sensitivity to various unnatural agonists and antagonists. Bronchiolar smooth muscle has H_1 receptors: activation by histamine causes contraction of the muscle and bronchoconstriction. The actions of histamine on vascular smooth muscle are complex, species dependent, and mediated by both H_1 and H_2 receptors, while gastric acid secretion from parietal cells is stimulated by mucosally released

TABLE III

Important Adrenaline and Noradrenaline Receptors

Organ	Major adrenoceptor present	Effect of stimulation
Eye	α	Pupillary dilation
Blood vessels (periphery including skin)	α	Constriction
Gastro-intestinal tract	$\alpha + \beta$	Relaxation
Heart	β_1	Tachycardia (speeding of the heart) Increased force of contraction
Small intestine	β_1	Relaxation
Blood vessels (skeletal muscle)	β_2	Relaxation (vasodilation)
Bronchioles (lung)	β_2	Relaxation (bronchodilation)

H-Tyr-Gly-Gly-Phe-Met-OH   Methionine enkephalin
H-Tyr-Gly-Gly-Phe-Leu-OH   Leucine enkephalin

(7)

(8) $R^1 = R^2 = H$ (11)
(9) $R^1 = R^2 = COCH_3$
(10) $R^1 = CH_3; R^2 = H$

histamine acting at H_2 receptors. H_2 receptor blockers are useful in the treatment of conditions in which there is excess acid secretion in the stomach, especially in gastric ulceration (see Chap. 6).

It is noteworthy that all the previously mentioned neurotransmitters, i.e., acetylcholine, noradrenaline, enkephalins, and dopamine, as well as histamine and adrenaline, have receptors in the CNS. Interaction with these receptors will elicit a response and if interaction of a potential drug substance with peripheral receptors (e.g., at the neuromuscular junction, on bronchiolar smooth muscle, in parietal cells, in heart muscle, on blood vessels etc.) is beneficial then it is often necessary to ensure that the compound does not cross the "blood–brain barrier" to cause unwanted side effects through interaction with receptors in the CNS.

III.   ENZYMES AND ENZYME INHIBITORS

The active centres of enzymes are similar in many ways to the active sites of receptors, and enzyme inhibitors are identical in principle with receptor blockers. Simple inhibitors derange the active centre by engaging it directly (isosteric inhibition) or by inducing a conformational change affecting the active site through binding to a distant site (allosteric inhibition). Unnatural substrates for an enzyme which are slowly processed are also effective inhibitors of the physiological enzyme action provided that they have a substantially greater affinity than the natural substrate for the enzyme centre. Substantial inhibition of a key enzyme-controlled process in an organism will generally lead to the demise of the organism. If the enzyme in question is peculiar to a bacterium, fungus, or worm that has invaded the mammalian host then inhibition will erradicate the pathogen and leave the host unharmed (see Chaps. 11–14).

IV. OTHER TYPES OF BIO-ACTIVE MOLECULES

Not all drugs act on discrete receptors or at active sites of particular enzymes. Others, such as some general or local anaesthetics, act by forming mono-molecular layers on membranes, thereby modifying transport across the membrane. Some drugs have a stabilising or a labilising effect on the membranes of cells. Yet others, such as antacids or some diuretics, produce their effects by means of their physicochemical properties. Many steroid drugs and hormones (Chaps. 9 and 10) must first pass into cells, becoming associated with a specific cytoplasm (cytosol) fraction which facilitates their transport into the cell nucleus where the function of the DNA, and ultimately protein synthesis, becomes modified.

V. FACTORS INFLUENCING DRUG ACTION

The aim of administering a drug is to get it to the right place in the right concentration and for the right period of time. Except for topical treatments (e.g., application of an anti-inflammatory steroid to the skin or lungs) humans are usually dosed by a route which is remote from the intended site of action. Thus there will generally be a certain latent period before the action of the drug is initiated. This latent period will depend upon the route of administration, the formulation of the compound, and the mode of distribution. The duration and intensity of action will, in turn, depend on the relative rates of arrival at and removal from the site of action. These rates depend primarily on the distribution, metabolism and excretion of the drug. The overall chronology of events between drug administration and elimination is summarised in Fig. 12.

Some drugs (prodrugs) will not exert pharmacological activity until they have undergone biotransformation within the body. For example the penicillin ester pivampicillin (12) is well absorbed when taken by mouth unlike the parent acid; the ester must be de-esterified by a blood-borne esterase enzyme before anti-bacterial activity is exhibited.

$$NH_2$$
$$PhCHCON \quad S \quad CH_3$$
$$CH_3$$
$$O \quad N$$
$$CO_2CH_2OCOC(CH_3)_3$$

(**12**)

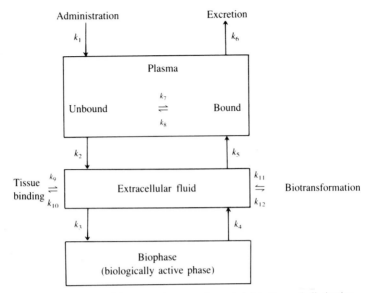

Fig. 12   Summary of the events between drug administration and elimination.

Having succeeded in getting a drug into the biophase, binding to the appropriate site of an enzyme or receptor must take place. The binding of the small drug molecule to the macromolecule involves many complementary forces (electrostatic forces, hydrogen bonding, hydrophobic bonding, van der Waals forces).

Electrostatic attraction, for example between the quaternary ammonium group of acetylcholine analogues and a carboxylate residue in the macromolecule, is a

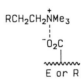

powerful binding and stabilizing influence. Ion–dipole and dipole–dipole interactions are of less importance. Hydrophobic bonding is also very important and leads to good binding mainly due to the increase in entropy of the system ($\Delta G = \Delta H - T\Delta S$) through displacement of water molecules from "uncomfortable" quasi-crystalline arrangements adjacent to the hydrocarbon surfaces to a less ordered, more favourable situation (Fig. 13). On the other hand the gain in free energy through hydrogen-bonding between enzyme or receptor and drug molecule is not as significant as may be imagined at first sight.

For example the phenol moiety forming the part-structure of the drug molecule

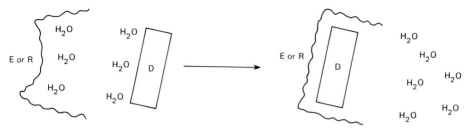

Fig. 13　Approach of hydrophobic faces of a drug molecule (D) and a receptor (R) or enzyme (E).

D—C_6H_4OH can be nicely accommodated at the active site of an enzyme (E) or receptor (R) as shown in Fig. 14a: strong hydrogen bonds are formed and good binding takes place. However, the hydrogen bonds between the drug and the enzyme or receptor can only be formed at the expense of the hydrogen bonds between the separate entities and associated water molecules (Fig, 14b). Hence the net gain in energy through hydrogen bonding between the drug and macromolecule is marginal. Note that a closely related drug substance D—C_6H_5 lacking the phenolic hydroxy group would displace the water molecule(s) from the surface of the macromolecule without forming the compensating hydrogen bonds (Fig. 14c): in this case binding would be less secure.

The pharmacokinetic profile of a drug will vary from species to species and be influenced by many factors such as the route of administration, formulation, age, sex, disease, diet, environmental influences and other drugs.

Clearly the design of a drug molecule is hampered by the transient and changing nature of pharmacological receptors, accessability to target enzymes or other

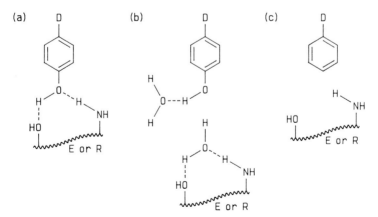

Fig. 14　Changes in hydrogen-bonding that take place on approach of a drug to the surface of an enzyme (E) or receptor (R).

intended sites of action, and other undesirable and toxic effects. In addition, development of a therapeutic agent from a drug is fraught with difficulties as the ideal structure to fit an enzyme or a receptor may not be suitable to allow a molecule to run the gauntlet between administration and elimination at a rate and concentration which is clinically convenient.

It can be appreciated that a drug molecule has somewhat greater difficulty in travelling to its intended site of action than, for example, a natural neurotransmitter which is released close to the appropriate receptor. The localised release and rapid disposal of these small molecules means that a complex organism can operate with the minimum number of different neurotransmitters: when an active substance such as histamine and adrenaline is released into a large part of the system many different effects are seen due to the stimulation of receptors at many sites. Drugs can be regarded to be more closely analogous to hormones and local hormones (autacoids) in that they are widely distributed in the body. All these molecules are sterically more bulky and possess more functional groups: the extra features within the molecules restrict binding to relatively few receptors or enzymes.

Before moving on to describe the case histories of drugs that act through interaction with specific enzymes or receptors, a more detailed account of receptorology and enzymology is desirable and follows in the next chapters.

ADDITIONAL READING

"The Human Body", by P. Lewis and D. Rubenstein, Hamlyn, Feltham (U.K.), 1979.
"Neurotransmitters and Drugs", by Z. L. Kruk and C. J. Pycock, Croom Helm, London, 1979.
"Biochemistry", by L. Stryer, Freeman, San Francisco, 1975.
"Cutting's Handbook of Pharmacology: The Actions and Uses of Drugs", 6th Edition, by T. Z. Czaky, Appleton-Century-Crofts, New York, 1979.
"The Pharmacological Basis of Therapeutics", 6th Edition, by L. S. Goodman and A. Gilman, Macmillan, New York, 1980.
"The Basis of Medicinal Chemistry: Burger's Medicinal Chemistry", 4th Edition, Vols. 1–3, (M. E. Wolff, ed.), Wiley (Interscience), New York, 1980.
"Drug receptor interactions", by E. W. Gill, in "Progress in Medicinal Chemistry" (G. P. Ellis and G. B. West, eds.), Vol. 4, p. 39, Butterworths, London, 1965.
"Basis of biological specificity" by A. R. Fersht, *Trends in Biochemical Sciences* **9,** 145 (1984).

CHAPTER 2

More about Receptors: Theories of Small Molecule–Receptor Interactions

B. WALKER

Her Majesty's Inspectorate
Department of Education and Science
London, England

I. THE NATURE OF RECEPTORS

Evidence for the existence of pharmacological receptors is derived from several observations: (i) many drugs cause marked effects following administration of very small doses; (ii) certain cellular responses are elicited only by a relatively few chemical substances which have similar electronic and structural properties, such that geometric and optical isomers may differ markedly in potency; (iii) a particular biological effect may be influenced by agonist/antagonist pairs of drugs with structural similarities; and (iv) the response of cells is always the same when activated by structurally similar agonists, and this response is determined by the properties of the cells.

All of these findings are consistent with the idea of discrete receptors which occupy a relatively small part of the cell. Furthermore, there is evidence, in the case of certain membrane-bound receptors, that these receptors face outwards: for example, acetylcholine elicits a response when applied to the outside of smooth muscle cells but not when it is injected intracellularly. Receptors are proteins or glycoproteins: these macromolecules have the conformational and configurational versatility to provide the basis of different receptor types. Receptors can be destroyed by proteolytic enzymes, thus confirming their protein nature. As mentioned in Chap. 1, reversible binding of drugs to receptors involves van der Waals forces, hydrogen, hydrophobic and ionic bonds rather than covalent bonds.

II. THEORIES OF DRUG–RECEPTOR INTERACTIONS

In reviewing the theories which have attempted to account for drug–receptor interactions, many authors have discouraged their readers by the presentation of numerous and complex mathematical terms. Those interested in such approaches should refer to the reviews included in the Additional Reading section at the end of the chapter. Whenever possible in this review verbal descriptions and simple rate equations will be used.

A. J. Clark (1926) was among the first to attempt to put drug–receptor interactions on a quantitative basis. He noticed that drug dose–response curves were similar in shape to oxygen–haemoglobin dissociation curves and those obtained from other biological phenomena. He proposed that the interaction between drugs and receptors was comparable to Langmuir's adsorption isotherm for the catalysis of gases on polished metal surfaces and believed that progress could be made by applying the law of mass action to drug–receptor interactions [Eq. (1)].

$$\text{Drug + Receptor} \underset{k_2}{\overset{k_1}{\rightleftharpoons}} \text{Drug–receptor complex} \tag{1}$$

He assumed that one molecule of drug interacted with only one receptor and that the amount of drug bound to receptors was negligible in relation to the rest of the drug in the receptor environment. Clark recognised that drugs must have the capacity to excite the receptors to which they bound and he proposed that a pharmacological response depended upon the number of receptors which were occupied, a maximum response only being obtained when all of the receptors were occupied. Thus if p is the proportion of receptors occupied by the drug (molar concentration x), then

$$\text{response} \propto p = \frac{Kx}{1 + Kx} \qquad \text{where } K = \frac{k_1}{k_2} = \text{affinity constant}$$

Hence in this theory the potency of any drug, agonist or antagonist, is determined solely by its affinity for its receptors.

The "occupancy theory" does not account for drugs which differ in potency and yet which occupy the same receptor, as demonstrated by the fact that they are inhibited by the same antagonist (Fig. 1).

Clark estimated that acetylcholine could elicit a response when only 1/10,000 of the cell surface was occupied by drug. More recent estimations have suggested that as much as 10% of the membranes of some cells may consist of cholinergic receptors. This apparent discrepancy may be accounted for by the difference in size of acetylcholine molecules and the acetylcholine receptor molecules. The complementary idea of "spare" receptors suggests that there may be receptors

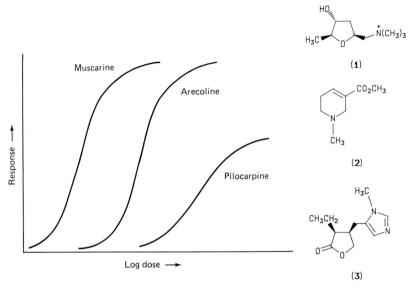

Fig. 1 Log dose–response curves of the agonists of the acetylcholine (ACh) receptors muscarine (**1**), arecoline (**2**), and pilocarpine (**3**).

which have the potential to contribute to a response although a maximum response can be achieved when less than 100% of the receptors are occupied.

Experiments with agonist/antagonist pairs of drugs have shown that the dose–response curve for an agonist can be progressively displaced to the right in a parallel manner by increasing concentrations of competitive antagonists (Fig. 2). This is consistent with the idea of spare receptors.*

"Intrinsic activity" was a concept introduced by Ariëns (1954) to attempt to explain the observation that not all members of an homologous series were active although all appeared to bind to the same population of receptors. Ariëns concluded that drugs possessed properties of "affinity" and "intrinsic activity" so that two different drugs could produce the same effect by one having a low affinity and a high intrinsic activity while the other had a high affinity and a relatively low intrinsic activity. Antagonists would have a relatively high affinity but zero intrinsic activity. Ariëns, like Clark, assumed that all the receptors needed to be occupied if a maximum response was to be obtained.

Stephenson (1956) expanded on the ideas of Clark and Ariëns, and took into account the idea that a maximum effect could be produced without the occupa-

---

*The potency of an antagonist is usually measured as a pA_2 value: this value is the reciprocal log of the molar concentration of antagonist required to return the dose–response curve to its original point after doubling the dose of the agonist.

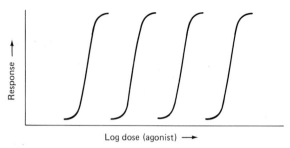

Fig. 2   Dose–response curves for an agonist drug in the presence of increasing concentrations of antagonist.

tion of the maximum number of receptors available and introduced the term "efficacy". This he defined as the capacity of a drug to initiate a response once it occupies receptor sites.

Stephenson assumed that the biological response to any kind of agonist to be a specific but unknown function of the stimulus (S) applied to the tissue; the stimulus is proportional to the proportion of receptors occupied (p) and to the efficacy (e) of the drug. Assuming steady state conditions in Eq. (1),

$$\text{Response} = f(S)$$

and

$$S = ep = \frac{eKx}{1 + Kx}$$

Stephenson's theory differs from Clark's in two important respects. First the biological response to an agonist is not assumed to be directly proportional to the proportion of receptors occupied by it, and, secondly, a maximum biological response is not taken to correspond to complete receptor occupancy.

In other words, different drugs may have varying capacities to initiate a response and consequently occupy different proportions of the receptors when producing equal responses. For an agonist of high efficacy a maximum effect would be produced with only a small proportion of receptors occupied. Partial agonists are not able to produce a maximal effect even when occupying all the available receptors. Since a partial agonist occupies receptors, it will exclude them, by competition, from occupation by more active agonists and thus exhibit some antagonistic activity. An antagonist has an affinity for its receptor but zero efficacy.

In the occupation theory of drug action outlined above, both agonists and antagonists are assumed to be effective for as long as their drug–receptor complexes exist.

Certain pharmacological phenomena are not readily explained by the occupancy theory or modifications of it: for example, some agonists can elicit a maximum response from, and then block, the receptors to which they are applied. To explain these phenomena, Paton (1961) proposed his rate theory of drug action which emphasised the importance of the *rate* with which receptors become occupied: the faster the rate of association (*A*) the greater the response produced. Expressed simply and using Eq. (1):

$$\text{Response} \propto A = k_2\, p = \frac{k_2 K x}{1 + K x}$$

Remember that *K* is a measure of the affinity of a drug for its receptor. Remember also that $K = k_1/k_2$: if k_2 is high then k_1 can also be high, and this is the condition which must be observed for a potent agonist.

Thus potent agonists are those which are able to maintain high rates of association with their receptors, a condition which demands the existence at any one time of a substantial proportion of unoccupied receptors. In rate theory, prolonged receptor occupation is incompatible with high potency for an agonist.

If k_2 is low or zero, k_1 will fall to a low level at equilibrium and an antagonistic action will ensue. The initial stimulant action and subsequent blockade by some agonists is also predictable by this theory, and so is the long duration and offset time of antagonist action.

Figure 3 illustrates that agonist drugs have a rapid onset and offset of action

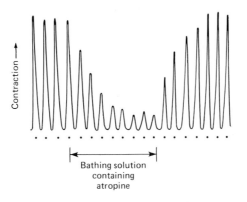

Agonist: acetylcholine $\quad CH_3COOCH_2CH_2\overset{+}{N}(CH_3)_3$

Antagonist: atropine

Fig. 3   An experiment with a piece of tissue [isolated ileum (smooth muscle) from the guinea-pig] to show the slow onset and offset rates of an antagonist drug. The same dose of acetylcholine has been administered every 2 min throughout the experiment, and the muscle contractions were inhibited for a period of time by changing the bathing solutions to one containing atropine.

while antagonist drugs have a relatively slow onset and offset at the receptor surface.

In considering the various attempts which have been made this century to find a unifying theory to explain all aspects of drug–receptor interactions, it may be that the final solution will have to accommodate several theories and that the nature of the association between drugs and receptors may be fundamentally different in different tissues.

III.   RECEPTOR CO-OPERATIVITY AND SENSITIVITY

From what has been presented so far, the impression may have been conveyed that a pharmacological receptor is a slightly flexible but permanent structure on a cell membrane. This is far from the truth, for a receptor is better considered as an inconstant, transient structure which can change in sensitivity, sometimes moving about in a fluid membrane, interacting and co-operating with its fellows in a positive or negative manner. These features may not be characteristic of all receptors all the time, but more consideration will be given to them as they contribute much to understanding the mechanisms of action of drugs and chemical transmitters on receptors.

Cutting through a nerve axon results in degeneration of that fibre with the result that the output of neurotransmitter becomes depleted. Subsequently, the post-synaptic membrane becomes supersensitive through the production of more receptors. This process provides an understanding of the way in which both drug tolerance and drug dependence can develop through receptor involvement. Consider a centrally acting drug (i.e., a compound which acts on the CNS) which produces its effect by the reduction of transmitter output in a particular nerve pathway. The passage of time allows post-synaptic membrane sensitivity to increase such that the original amount of activity in that pathway becomes restored although the amount of neurotransmitter remains reduced. To achieve the desired effect the dose of drug needs to be increased to further reduce neurotransmitter output: that is, tolerance has developed.* On withdrawal of the drug the neurotransmitter level is immediately restored while the post-synaptic membrane is still supersensitive, with the result that hyperactivity occurs in that pathway; that is, dependence has developed. (Withdrawal symptoms of centrally acting drugs are commonly the opposite effects of those induced by administration of the same drug: e.g., withdrawal of sedative drugs results in excitation and withdrawal of stimulating drugs results in depression.)

---

*Tolerance may develop to some drugs as a result of induction of those liver enzymes which bring about the more rapid metabolism of drugs to inactive molecules.

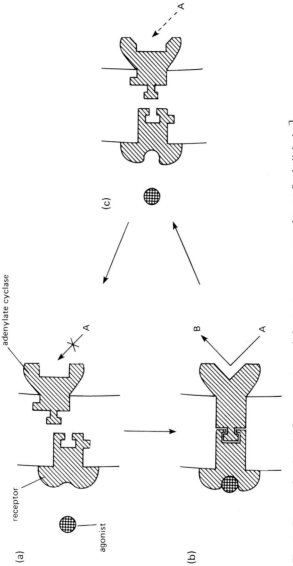

Fig. 4 Receptor function. (a) Receptor not occupied, receptor–enzyme complex not firmly linked. (b) Receptor occupied, receptor–enzyme complex forms, enzyme activated. (c) Receptor not occupied, enzyme dissociates and returns to inactive state.

During the past 20 years it has become increasingly clear that cell membranes may be considered as dynamic fluid structures with proteins free to diffuse laterally unless specifically anchored. In rat adipose cells there are at least eight different receptors coupled to adenylate cyclase. The molecular weight of each receptor makes arrangement of the receptors at the surface as a single complex, while in contact with the enzyme, difficult. Jacobs and Cuatrecasas (1976) and others have developed the idea that the association of any ligand with its receptor induces a conformational change which favours the further association of that receptor with the underlying cyclic nucleotide system. The temporary nature of this association allows other receptors subsequently to become attached to the same enzyme. Figure 4 of Chap. 1 should then be modified to Fig. 4 to provide a more accurate picture.

One last point needs to be made before the structure and function of enzymes are considered. While drugs induce conformational changes in their receptors, receptors in turn may induce conformational changes in drugs. During the docking procedure the drug may have to adopt a non-preferred conformation to fit exactly into the receptor. This means that while the conformation of a drug in a biological solution is of some interest, studies of drugs carried out with the aim of developing more useful analogues need to be extended, ideally, to the conformation of drugs associated with receptors in their natural environment of the cell membrane.

ADDITIONAL READING

"Textbook of Pharmacology", 2nd Edition, by W. C. Bowman and M. J. Rand, Blackwell, London, 1980.

"Lewis's Pharmacology", 5th Edition, by J. Crossland, Churchill-Livingston, London, 1980.

"Towards Understanding Receptors", edited by J. W. Lamble and G. A. Robinson, Elsevier, Amsterdam, 1981.

"More about Receptors", edited by J. W. Lamble and A. W. Cuthbert, Elsevier, Amsterdam, 1982.

"Important concepts of receptor theory", by R. R. Ruffolo, *J. Auton. Pharmacol.* **2,** 277 (1982).

CHAPTER 3

More about Enzymes: Structure and Catalytic Properties of Enzymes

M. G. DAVIS

Division of Biological and Environmental Sciences
The Hatfield Polytechnic
Hatfield, England

I. CONFIGURATION OF ENZYMES

Although some metabolic reactions can occur spontaneously, by far the majority require enzymes as catalysts. Each cell requires about 200 different enzymes to enable it to carry out all its functions, although the types of enzymes required will depend on the nature of the cell. Some enzymes are membrane bound, some are found only in particular sub-cellular organelles such as mitochondria and others are cytoplasmic. Over 1000 enzymes have been described, all of which are proteins (though many proteins, such as haemoglobin and insulin, are not enzymes). Although all enzymes are proteins, many also require additional non-protein components (known as co-factors) in order to be catalytically active: the role of co-factors will be discussed later.

Like all proteins, enzymes have characteristic primary, secondary and tertiary structures. The *primary structure* is based on the sequence of amino-acids linked by peptide bonds. Twenty-two amino-acids are available for use in the primary sequence and each polypeptide chain may contain several hundred amino-acid residues. An enzyme's *secondary and tertiary structure* give it its three-dimen-

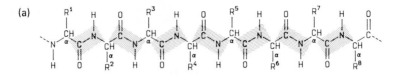

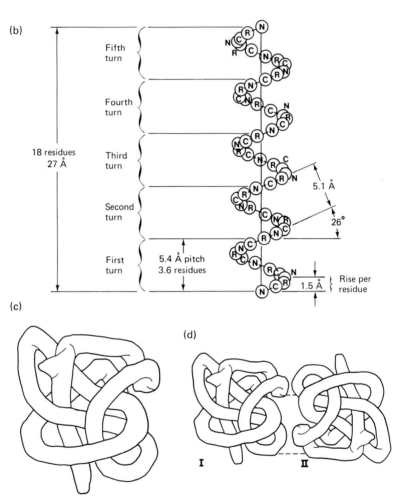

Fig. 1 (a) Primary structure. General formula of a polypeptide chain showing the linkage of adjacent amino-acid residues through peptide bonds. (b) Secondary structure. Representation of a polypeptide chain as an α-helical configuration. N, NH; C, CO; R, CHR. [From L. Pauling and R. B. Corey, *Proc. Int. Wool Textile Res. Conf., B,* 249 (1955), as redrawn in C. B. Anfinsen, *The Molecular Basis of Evolution,* Wiley, New York, 1955, p. 101.] (c) Tertiary structure. (d) Quaternary structure. A protein dimer unit illustrating the quaternary structure of a complex globular protein.

sional characteristics, as revealed by X-ray crystallography (Fig. 1). The secondary structure refers to the coiling and twisting of the polypeptide chain due to hydrogen bonding, and tertiary structure to the way in which the enzyme folds into its characteristic globular form and is retained in this configuration by a number of types of bonding including disulphide bonds formed between adjacent thiol groups and ionic bonds between adjacent free carboxylic acid and amino groups. Hydrogen-bonding and hydrophobic bonding are also crucial in determining the overall shape of an enzyme. The digestive enzymes such as pepsin and trypsin consist of single polypeptide chains and have molecular weights varying from 15,000 to 35,000.*

Most enzymes catalysing metabolic reactions inside cells have what is called a *quaternary structure,* which means that they consist of more than one polypeptide sub-unit. Ultra-centrifugation has shown that anything from two to 60 subunits can occur in a single enzyme, giving rise to molecular weights ranging from 35,000 to several hundred thousand. Most enzymes have from two to eight subunits. The enzyme may consist of aggregates of identical sub-units, or of more than one type of sub-unit. For example, the enzyme lactate dehydrogenase, important for carbohydrate metabolism in muscle, consists of four sub-units of which there are two types. Gel electrophoresis has shown that there are five different forms of this enzyme, depending on the combination of sub-units. Enzymes like this which can occur in more than one molecular form are called *isoenzymes.* These have an important role in the regulation of metabolism, and are also valuable clinically in diagnostic enzymology, as elevated plasma levels of a particular isoenzyme may indicate that damage has occurred in an organ such as liver or heart.

Some metabolic systems involve even more complex levels of organisation known as *multienzyme complexes* in which several different enzymes associate together physically to catalyse a series of sequential reactions. An example of this occurs in fatty acid synthesis in which seven different enzymes aggregate together to give a highly ordered and efficient system.

Because of their protein structure, enzymes are highly sensitive to their physical environment. Organic solvents, high salt concentrations, oxidation or reduction and extremes of pH or temperature will readily cause *denaturation,* precipitation due to breakdown of the tertiary and secondary structure. Loss of enzyme activity without denaturation can also occur due to relatively small changes in temperature and pH. Most enzymes have their optimal activity at physiological pH and temperature, that is, pH 7 and 37°C.

---

*These enzymes, incidentally, have an inactive precursor form called *zymogens* or pro-enzymes, which have to be converted to the active form by hydrolytic removal of a protective section of the peptide chain.

II.   ENZYME SPECIFICITY, CLASSIFICATION, AND NOMENCLATURE

One of the properties of enzymes that most distinguishes them from inorganic catalysts is their high degree of specificity. This is due to the chemical and physical characteristics of an enzyme's protein structure. Enzymes are normally specific for one particular type of reaction and one particular type of substrate only. For example, a hydrolytic enzyme such as a peptidase or a lipase will not catalyse oxidation–reduction or group transfer reactions. Likewise the enzyme alcohol dehydrogenase, which catalyses the oxidation of ethanol to acetaldehyde, will also convert a variety of other alcohols to their corresponding aldehydes, with differing affinities for the substrates, but will have no effect on non-alcoholic substrates. Most enzymes will accept a range of chemically related compounds as their substrates; relatively few enzymes show absolute specificity for a single substrate.

TABLE I

Enzyme Classification

Enzyme category	Examples	Types of reaction catalysed
Oxidoreductases		Oxidation or reduction of substrate
	Dehydrogenases	Transfer of H from substrate to co-factor
	Reductases	Addition of H to substrate
	Oxidases	Transfer of H from substrate to oxygen
Transferases		Transfer of group from one molecule to another
	Transaminases	Transfer of amino groups
	Transacetylases	Transfer of acetyl groups
	Phosphorylases	Transfer of phosphate groups
Hydrolases		Hydrolysis of substrate (irreversible)
	Disaccharidases	Hydrolysis of glycosidic bonds
	Esterases	Hydrolysis of ester bonds
	Peptidases	Hydrolysis of peptide bonds
Lyases		Elimination and addition reactions
	Hydratases	Addition of water to double bonds (reversible)
	Decarboxylases	Removal of CO_2 from substrate (reversible)
	Aldolases	Aldol condensations (reversible)
Isomerases		Molecular rearrangement
	Racemases	D- and L-Isomer interconversion
	cis-trans Isomerases	Geometrical isomerisation
	Mutases	Intra-molecular group transfer
Ligases		Energy-dependent bond formation (generally irreversible)
	Synthetases	Condensation of two molecules
	Carboxylases	Addition of CO_2 to substrate

Enzymes also display stereochemical specificity, and may be specific for particular optical or geometric isomers of a substrate. For example, D-amino-acid oxidase will oxidise a variety of D-amino-acids but has little or no activity with L-amino-acids, and fumarase catalyses the hydration of the trans unsaturated dicarboxylic acid fumaric acid but not the cis isomer of maleic acid.

Enzymes are generally classified as belonging to one of the six categories shown in Table I.

Enzymes have complex systemic names based on further sub-divisions of the categories in Table I. These are used for precise identification in technical literature, but trivial names are normally used in laboratories. These usually include the name of the substrate and type of reaction (e.g., alcohol dehydrogenase). Other common trivial names simply add the suffix -ase to the name of the substrate (e.g., ribonuclease), while many of the digestive enzymes are known by very old names (e.g., amylase, lipase, pepsin and trypsin).

III. CHARACTERISTICS OF ENZYME CATALYSIS

Although enzymes show much greater specificity and sensitivity to temperature and pH than inorganic catalysts, they have the same function as all catalysts, accelerating the rate of reaction by lowering the activation energy required for a reaction to proceed. Enzymes also obey the normal rules of catalysis: (1) enzymes will not catalyse thermodynamically unfavourable reactions; (2) they will not change the direction of a reaction; (3) they will not change the equilibrium of a reaction; (4) they remain unchanged at the end of the reaction (though some enzymes undergo temporary covalent changes such as phosphorylation during the course of a reaction). Enzymes normally catalyse reactions much more efficiently than inorganic catalysts. For example, both platinum and the enzyme peroxidase (also known by its old name catalase) catalyse the decomposition of hydrogen peroxide into water and oxygen. The effects of the different catalysts on the activation energy (in kilojoules per mole) are as follows:

No catalyst	75
Platinum	50
Peroxidase	8

One mole of peroxidase can catalyse the decomposition of over one million moles of H_2O_2 per minute.

Enzymes are able to lower the activation energy for a reaction though the formation of an intermediate *enzyme–substrate complex,* which in turn can break down to enzyme and product as follows:

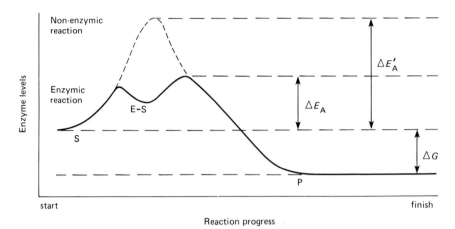

Fig. 2   The effect of enzyme catalysis on activation energy. ΔE_A is the activation energy for the enzyme-catalysed reaction and $\Delta E'_A$ for the non-enzymic reaction.

$$E + S \rightleftharpoons E\text{—}S \rightarrow E + P$$

S may consist of more than one substrate and P of more than one product. The effect of the formation of this complex is shown in Fig. 2.

The formation of this enzyme–substrate complex occurs at a small region on the surface of the enzyme called the *active site* or *centre,* usually present as a crevice or pit. Only a few amino-acids (5–10) are directly involved in the formation of this complex and subsequent catalysis at the active site. These amino-acid residues are not normally consecutive, as different parts of the polypeptide chain come together at the active site due to the characteristic folding of the protein. The amino-acids not directly involved at the active site are still important, however, as they are essential for maintaining the configuration of the protein required for the active site to function. This explains why some modifications to an enzyme's structure are more crucial than others. A modification or mutation leading to a change in amino-acid sequence at the active centre will lead to complete loss of enzyme activity, while a change in sequence elsewhere may have far less effect.

The amino-acids most frequently found at the active site are shown in Table II; these amino-acids possess groups on the side chain that are known to interact with substrate.

As well as hydrogen-bonding and electrostatic interactions being involved between the substrate and complex, hydrophobic interactions are also important.

It has been shown that some of the amino-acids at the active centre are only involved in binding the substrate to the enzyme. This part of the active site is called the *binding site.* Other amino-acids at the active site are exclusively

TABLE II

Amino-Acids Frequently Involved in the Active Centre

Amino-acid	Side group	Interaction with substrate
Serine	—OH	Hydrogen-bonding
Cysteine	—SH	Hydrogen-bonding
Histidine	—Imidazole	Electrostatic
Lysine	$-NH_3^+$	Electrostatic
Arginine	$-NH_3^+$	Electrostatic
Aspartic acid	$-COO^-$	Electrostatic
Glutamic acid	$-COO^-$	Electrostatic

involved in catalysis, making up the *catalytic site*. The active site thus consists of binding and catalytic sites. Both binding and catalysis are essential for conversion of substrate(s) to product(s). The active site of an enzyme is shown diagramatically in Fig. 3.

The presence of the binding and catalytic sites at the active site account for the specificity of enzyme reactions discussed earlier. Only the correct substrate (and closely related analogues) can bind to the enzyme, and only the appropriate type of reaction can be catalysed by a particular enzyme.

The old analogy of a rigid lock and key mechanism introduced in the nineteenth century by Emil Fischer has been largely superseded since the 1960s by Koshland's induced fit hypothesis, in which the substrate is believed to induce the required orientation of groups in the active site required for binding and catalysis.

Formation of the enzyme–substrate complex leads to a lowering of activation energy and subsequent catalysis due to the interaction between the substrate and the catalytic site. The binding between the substrate and amino-acid groups at the active centre causes changes in bond energies and electron densities within the

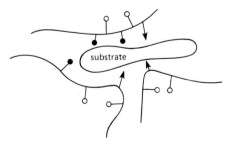

Fig. 3   Active site of an enzyme: —●, amino-acids involved in binding site; arrow, amino-acids involved in catalytic site; —○, amino-acids not directly involved in active site.

substrate, possibly accompanied by physical distortion and strain, resulting in a thermodynamically unstable conformation from which the reaction can readily proceed. When there is more than one substrate for a reaction, the enzyme catalyses the reaction by bringing the substrates together at the binding site in the juxtaposition required for the reaction to proceed. Provided the affinity of the product for the binding site is lower than that of the substrate, the product will dissociate from the active site, leaving it free for further reactions. As will be seen later, certain inhibitors have their effect by binding to the active site without further reaction and thus remain there, blocking the site.

Many enzymes require additional non-protein substances called co-factors for catalysis to occur. These substances can be either metal ion *activators* or relatively small organic compounds called *co-enzymes*. These co-factors are normally attached to the enzyme by electrostatic bonds, but some co-enzymes are linked covalently.

Metal ion activators include Mg^{2+}, Ca^{2+}, Zn^{2+}, Fe^{2+}, Fe^{3+}, Cu^{2+}, Co^{2+}, Mo^+, K^+ and Na^+, and account for the trace metal elements required in the diet. Their requirement for enzyme activity also explains the inhibitory effect of chelating agents.

Co-enzymes are derived from water-soluble vitamins and are involved in a variety of reactions, as shown in Table III. They operate as second substrates, undergoing chemical modifications during the course of a reaction and reverting back to the original form by a further reaction. Diseases (such as scurvy) caused by the deficiency of a water-soluble vitamin are due to the resultant loss of enzyme activity.

TABLE III
Some Commonly Occurring Co-Enzymes

Co-enzyme	Function	Vitamin processor	Defining disease
Nicotinamide adenine dinucleotide (NAD)	Hydrogen-transfer	Nicotinamide (niacin)	Pellagra
Thiamine pyrophosphate	Decarboxylation	Thiamine (B_1)	Beriberi
Flavine mononucleotide	Hydrogen-transfer	Riboflavin (B_2)	Skin lesions
Flavine adenine dinucleotide (FAD)	Hydrogen-transfer	Riboflavin (B_2)	Skin lesions
Pyridoxal phosphate	Amino-transfer	Pyridoxine (B_6)	Neurological disturbances
Ascorbic acid	Hydroxylation	Vitamin C	Scurvy
Cobalamine	Methylation	Vitamin B_{12}	Pernicious anaemia

IV. ENZYME REACTION RATES

Enzyme activity is measured in units which indicate the rate of reaction cata-lysed by that enzyme expressed as micromoles of substrate transformed (or product formed) per minute. An enzyme unit is the amount of enzyme which will catalyse the transformation of one micromole of substrate per minute under specified conditions of pH and temperature. The specific activity of an enzyme is expressed as the number of units per milligram of protein.

The rate of a biochemical reaction at a given temperature and pH depends on the enzyme concentration and the substrate concentration. Provided the substrate concentration remains in excess, the initial rate is directly proportional to enzyme concentration, as shown in Fig. 4.

When the enzyme concentration is kept constant and the substrate concentra-tion varies, the effect of the substrate concentration on the rate of reaction is as shown in Fig. 5. Initially the reaction follows first-order kinetics with the rate proportional to substrate concentration, and eventually zero-order kinetics are followed with the velocity reaching a limiting value V_{max}. V_{max} is the reaction rate when the enzyme is fully saturated by substrate, indicating that all the binding sites are being constantly reoccupied. V_{max} is constant for a given amount of enzyme. The substrate concentration corresponding to half maximum velocity is known as K_m, the Michaelis constant, which is inversely proportional to the affinity of the enzyme for the substrate. K_m is constant for a particular enzyme and is independent of the amount of enzyme. A useful rule of thumb is that the substrate concentration has to be about $100 \times K_m$ to achieve maximum velocity. The relationship between reaction rate and substrate concentration is described by the Michaelis–Menten equation:

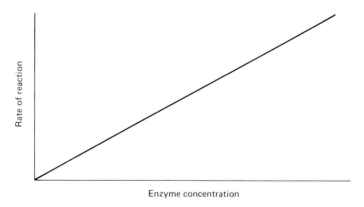

Enzyme concentration

Fig. 4   The effect of enzyme concentration on the rate of reaction.

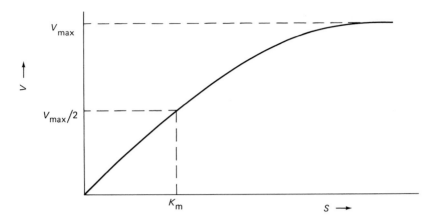

Fig. 5   The effect of substrate concentration (*S*) on the rate of reaction (*V*).

$$V = \frac{V_{max}S}{K_m + S}$$

This can also be expressed in the form

$$\frac{1}{V} = \frac{K_m}{V_{max}}\frac{1}{S} + \frac{1}{V_{max}}$$

A graph showing the reciprocal of the rate against the reciprocal of the substrate concentration, called the Lineweaver–Burk plot, will therefore give a straight line, as shown in Fig. 6. As the intercepts correspond to $1/V_{max}$ and $-1/K_m$, and the slope is K_m/V_{max}, this plot provides a useful way of determining

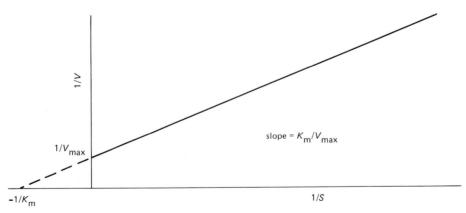

Fig. 6   A Lineweaver–Burk plot.

the kinetic constants V_{max} and K_m from experimental data. As will be shown shortly, it is also a useful way of showing what type of inhibition may be occurring.

V.   ENZYME SUBSTRATES AS DRUGS

Many of the basic building blocks (e.g., amino-acids, sugars) for enzyme-controlled biosynthesis of complex natural products are provided in the diet. In contrast, there are few cases where an enzyme substrate is given to counter a disease, but one excellent example is in the treatment of Parkinson's disease.

Parkinson's disease is a disorder characterised by rigidity of the limbs, torso, and face, and tremor, abnormal body posture, and an inability to initiate voluntary motor activity (akinesia). It occurs mainly in elderly people and is a chronic and progressive degenerative disorder.

The disease is associated with decreased dopaminergic function in the brain,

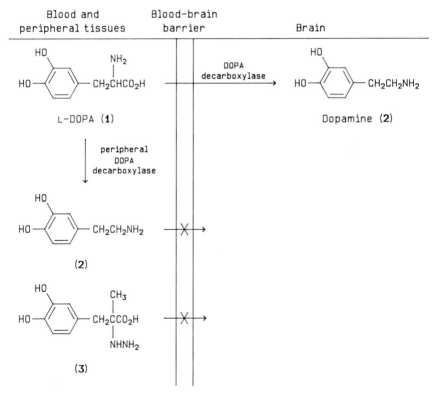

Fig. 7   Structural relationship of DOPA, dopamine and carbidopa.

and many of the symptoms of the disease can be alleviated by oral administration of L-DOPA (L-dihydroxyphenylalanine) (**1**). L-DOPA is given orally, absorbed from the gastro-intestinal tract, and carried to the brain by the bloodstream. In the brain the compound is a substrate for the enzyme DOPA decarboxylase and dopamine (**2**) is produced, thus raising the activity of the dopaminergic neurones in the brain. Dopamine cannot be given itself because it does not have the lipophilic properties necessary to cross the blood–brain barrier (Fig. 7).

The enzyme DOPA decarboxylase is also present in the liver and other tissues in the periphery. The action of periphral DOPA decarboxylase decreases the amount of L-DOPA reaching the brain. To obtain a sufficient amount of compound at the necessary sites, large doses must be given with a consequent increase in side effects (nausea and vomiting). The administered dose of L-DOPA can be reduced by inhibiting the peripheral DOPA decarboxylase enzyme using a compound such as carbidopa (**3**) which does not cross the blood–brain barrier.

VI.   ENZYME INHIBITION AND ENZYME INHIBITORS AS DRUGS

As was seen earlier, a variety of physical and chemical conditions such as extremes of temperature and pH and the presence of organic solvents can lead to a loss of enzyme activity. This, however, is due to gross damage to the protein's secondary and tertiary structure, resulting in denaturation rather than a specific effect on the enzyme's active site. In contrast, enzyme inhibitors are substances which bind to the enzyme with resulting loss of activity, without damaging the enzyme's protein structure. Inhibitors exert their effect by decreasing the affinity of the enzyme for the substrate, or by decreasing the amount of active enzyme available for catalysis, or by a combination of these effects. Different categories of inhibitor are described below.

A.   Irreversible Inhibitors

These are compounds which bind covalently to specific groups on the protein's surface, preventing binding and catalysis of the reaction. These compounds will inhibit a wide range of enzymes. Examples include iodoacetamide (**4**) and *p*-chloromercuribenzoate (**5**) (which bind to the sulphydryl group of cysteine residues), diisopropylfluorophosphate (**6**) (which binds to the hydroxyl groups of serine residues), and 1-fluoro-2,4-dinitrobenzene (**7**) (which binds to the amino groups in lysine residues and to the phenolic groups in tyrosine residues). Compounds such as these are only used for *in vitro* research studies.

ICH_2CONH_2 $ClHg$ —⟨benzene⟩— CO_2H F—$\overset{\displaystyle O}{\overset{\|}{P}}$—$OCH(CH_3)_2$

$OCH(CH_3)_2$

(4)   (5)   (6)

O_2N
F—⟨benzene⟩—NO_2

(7)

B. COMPETITIVE INHIBITORS

These compounds structurally resemble the substrate and can thus compete with the substrate for the enzyme's binding site. Such inhibitors are highly specific for a particular enzyme. Binding of the inhibitor is reversible, so the inhibitor can be displaced from the binding site by excess substrate. The affinity of the enzyme for the substrate is thus lowered in the presence of a competitive inhibitor (i.e., K_m is increased) but as catalysis is not directly affected, V_{max} can still be attained, even though a higher concentration of substrate will be required for this. The competitive inhibitor may be a naturally occurring alternative substrate for the enzyme which is also metabolised by it, though with a different degree of affinity, or it may be a chemical analogue of the substrate which binds to the enzyme without being further metabolised. A number of toxins and drugs operate in the latter manner. One of the earliest examples to be recognised was sulphanilamide (8), which inhibits a bacterial enzyme dihydropteroate synthetase (Scheme 1) required for folic acid synthesis, through its chemical similarity to *p*-aminobenzoic acid (9), a component of folic acid.

Since the existence of many bacteria depends on the production of folates by this process (whereas in humans folic acid is used and supplied in the diet as a preformal vitamin), sulphanilamide (and related sulphur drugs) will destroy the infecting bacteria but not the human host.

A different situation arises when it is required to inhibit an enzyme which is

Sulphamethoxypyridazine

$R =$ —⟨pyridazine⟩— OCH_3
$N=N$

H_2N—⟨benzene⟩—SO_2NHR

Sulphamethoxazole

(8)

$R =$ —⟨isoxazole⟩
N—O
CH_3

common to bacteria and man. Consider transformation 2 in Scheme 1. This step is essential for the well-being of both bacteria and man; in order to have an anti-bacterial agent that is non-toxic to the host, advantage must be taken of the fact that the structures of bacterial dihydrofolate reductase and mammalian dihydrofolate reductase are different. Selective inhibitors of the bacterial enzyme have been found: for example the anti-bacterial drug trimethoprim (**10**) is bound to dihydrofolate reductase from the bacterium *Escherichia coli* about 10^4 times more strongly than the same enzyme derived from rat liver.

Methotrexate (**11**) is another dihydrofolate inhibitor that is in clinical use, in this case for the treatment of the widespread and sometimes crippling disease psoriasis. The effect of reducing purine synthesis and cell division by blocking tetrahydrofolate production in psoriatic cells is beneficial: however, the drug must be used with caution since other, structurally similar and in many cases indistinguishable, dihydrofolate reductase enzymes in other tissues are affected, leading to the severe toxicity on long-term treatment.

Another important enzyme inhibitor is allopurinol (**12**), which is used in the treatment of gout. This condition is due to a build-up in concentration of uric acid in joints. The enzyme controlling the production of urate from xanthine is xanthine oxidase (Scheme 2); on inhibition of this enzyme with allopurinol the cascades from guanine and hypoxanthine are stopped at xanthine and this compound is rapidly excreted. Such enzymes, having a very limited function in the body, may be safely and usefully inhibited by drugs.

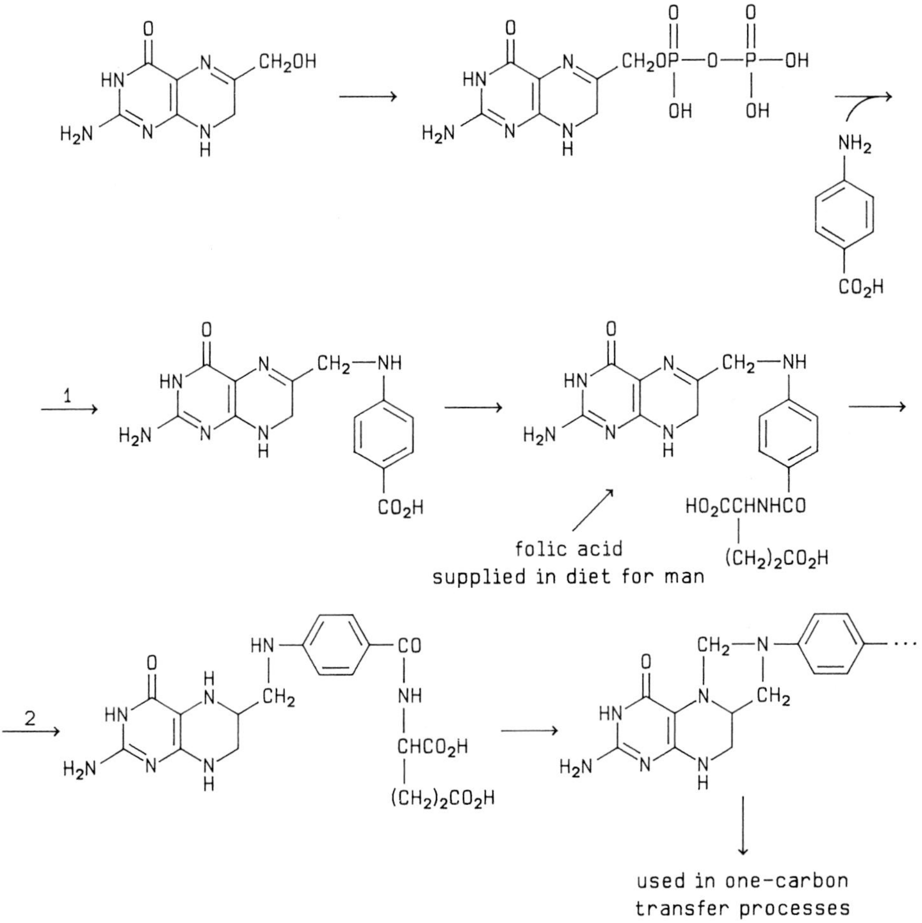

Scheme 1   Biosynthesis of the folates. Transformation 1 is catalysed by dihydropteroate synthetase. This enzyme is inhibited by sulphanilamide (**8**). Transformation 2 is catalysed by dihydrofolate reductase. The bacterial enzyme is inhibited by trimethoprim (**10**).

The above examples of drugs acting as enzyme inhibitors, and other examples of useful enzyme inhibitors described later in the book, are summarised in Table IV.

C. NON-COMPETITIVE INHIBITORS

These substances, which are generally structurally unrelated to the substrate, bind reversibly to groups distant from the binding site of the enzyme, and are thus less specific than competitive inhibitors. The rate of reaction is decreased

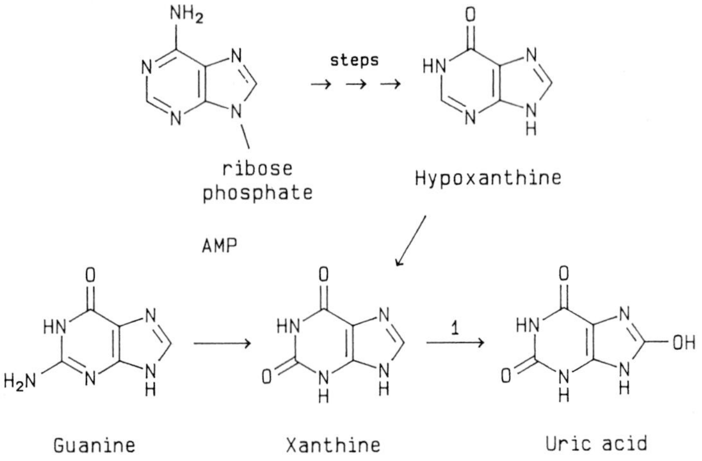

NH₂ ... (chemical structures)

steps
→ → →

ribose
phosphate

Hypoxanthine

AMP

Guanine → Xanthine —1→ Uric acid

Scheme 2   Biosynthesis of uric acid. Transformation 1 is catalysed by xanthine oxidase. This enzyme is inhibited by allopurinol (**12**).

TABLE IV
Drugs Acting as Enzyme Competitive Inhibitors

Drug	Enzyme inhibited	Disorder treatment
Sulphanilamides	Dihydropteroate synthetase	Bacterial infections
Trimethoprim	Bacterial dihydrofolate reductase	Bacterial infections
Penicillins and cephalosporins	Bacterial peptidoglycan transacylases	Bacterial infections
Ketoconazole	Steroid demethylase	Fungal infections
Allopurinol	Xanthine oxidase	Hyperuricaemia (primary metabolic gout)
Methotrexate	Dihydrofolate reductase	Psoriasis

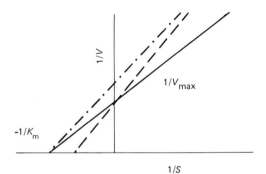

Fig. 8   Effects of competitive and non-competitive inhibition in enzyme kinetics: ———, no inhibitor present; — — —, competitive inhibitor present; — · —, non-competitive inhibitor present.

TABLE V
Poisons Acting as Non-competitive Enzyme Inhibitors

Compound	Mode of action	Biological effect
Organophosphate nerve gases and pesticides	Binds to —OH groups in acetyl- cholinesterase	Paralysis
Mercuric salts and arsenic salts	Bind to —SH groups in many enzymes	Widespread cellular damage
Cyanide	Binds to cytochrome oxidase	Respiratory failure
Digitoxin	Binds to Na,K-ATPase	Inhibits sodium ion migration

because the catalytic site is affected by the presence of the inhibitor. V_{max} is thus reduced, but because the binding site is not affected, the affinity of the enzyme for the substrate and therefore K_m remains unchanged. The effect of non-competitive inhibition is the same as that of less enzyme being present. Competitive and non-competitive inhibition can be distinguished from each other by the Lineweaver–Burk plot discussed earlier, as shown in Fig. 8.

A number of poisons are harmful to cells because they are potent non-competitive inhibitors. Some examples are shown in Table V.

VII. ENZYME REGULATION

Metabolic systems require regulation to ensure that adequate production output occurs (whether this be energy production from nutrients or biosynthesis of complex molecules) while avoiding the wasteful and potentially harmful consequences of over-production. In general this fine control is achieved by a co-ordination of the regulation of enzyme synthesis and the regulation of enzyme activity. Enzyme activity is mainly controlled by the process of *allosteric regulation,* which can produce activation or, more commonly, inhibition of enzyme activity. The regulator or *effector* molecule is normally structurally unrelated to the substrate, but binds specifically and reversibly to the enzyme. However, this does not occur at the substrate binding site, but at a quite separate regulatory site (the name allosteric is derived from the Greek *allos steros,* meaning other space). Binding of the effector induces a conformational change which either increases or decreases the affinity of the enzyme for the substrate, depending on the nature of the effector.

Only certain enzymes, called regulatory or allosteric enzymes, are sensitive to this form of control, and all such regulatory enzymes have been shown to have quaternary structure, that is, two or more sub-units. In many cases the regulatory site is on a different sub-unit to the active site, though in some enzymes both sites are on the same sub-unit. Some enzymes are regulated by more than one al-

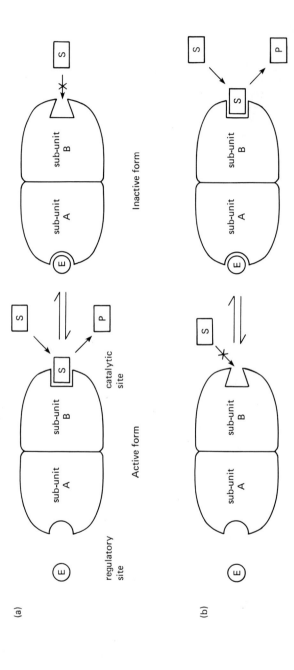

Fig. 9 Allosteric regulation of enzyme activity showing (a) inhibition and (b) activation. The effector is E, the substrate S and the product P.

losteric effector; in such cases there are separate regulatory sites for each effector. Allosteric regulation is illustrated in Fig. 9.

In biosynthetic pathways a system of feedback inhibition frequently occurs whereby the end product of the pathway allosterically inhibits the first enzyme specific to that pathway. In branched-chain pathways, as occur in amino-acid biosynthesis, the different products can separately inhibit the primary enzyme in the pathway and also the enzymes immediately after branching, as shown in Fig. 10.

This system of regulating biosynthesis ensures that the pathways operate normally when the products are required, but can be partially or completely shut down when adequate supplies of product have been formed. Some examples of allosteric regulation are shown in Table VI.

As well as the change in activity achieved through allosteric regulation, some enzymes undergo changes in activity due to covalent modification, normally phosphorylation. Well studied examples of this form of regulation occur in the synthesis of the polysaccharide glycogen. Glycogen synthetase exists in an inactive phosphorylated form and an active dephosphorylated form. Through mechanisms not yet fully elucidated the protein–hormone insulin stimulates the dephosphorylation of the inactive form of the enzyme, thus increasing its activity in synthesising glycogen. (Insulin also stimulates the uptake of the precursor glucose into the cells, further enhancing glycogen synthesis.) Glycogen breakdown (producing blood glucose in the liver and energy in muscle) requires the enzyme phosphorylase, which exists as a relatively inactive dimer or as a highly active phosphorylated dimer. Conversion to the active form requires intracellular

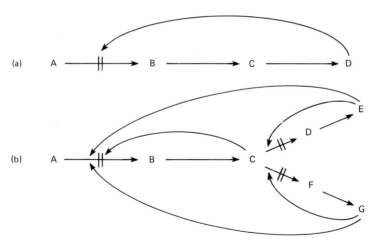

Fig. 10 Allosteric regulation of biosynthetic pathways by end product feedback inhibition illustrating (a) an unbranched pathway and (b) a branched pathway.

TABLE VI
Some Examples of Allosteric Regulation

Regulatory enzyme	Effector	Effect	Biochemical pathway
Phosphofructokinase	AMP	Activation	Glycolysis
	ATP	Inhibition	
Pyruvate carboxylase	Acetyl-CoA[a]	Activation	Gluconeogenesis
Mevalonate synthetase	Cholesterol	Inhibition	Steroid synthesis
Aspartokinase	Threonine, isoleucine, methionine, lysine	Inhibition	Amino-acid synthesis

[a] CoA, co-enzyme A.

cyclic AMP, which is produced from ATP by the membrane enzyme adenylate cyclase in response to the extracellular hormones adrenaline (Chap. 1) or glucagon binding to specific receptors on the membrane. Cyclic AMP also leads to phosphorylation and hence inactivation of glycogen synthetase. The opposite effects of the hormones adrenaline and glucagon from that of insulin can thus be explained by their indirect effects on enzyme activity.

Cyclic AMP is referred to as a secondary messenger as it is produced inside cells in response to plasma hormones binding to specific receptors on the outer surface of cell membranes. Many hormones other than adrenaline and glucagon operate in this way, including noradrenaline.

As well as this indirect effect on enzyme activity, many hormones help to control metabolism by their effect on enzyme synthesis. An increase in synthesis and subsequently the amount of enzyme is called *induction,* and a decrease in synthesis is called *repression.* In bacterial cells these processes frequently occur as a direct response to levels of nutrients present, and do not involve hormones. For example, when bacteria are grown in media rich in carbohydrates, the enzymes involved in carbohydrate absorption and breakdown are induced in order to optimise their utilization whereas when bacteria are grown in media rich in amino-acids, enzymes required for their synthesis are repressed in order to avoid wasteful over-production.

In animals, however, induction and repression of enzyme activity occur in response to hormones and some drugs. Most hormones cannot readily cross the cell membrane and will therefore achieve this effect by secondary messengers, but the steroid hormones and possibly the thyroid hormones do cross the membrane and exert a direct influence on protein synthesis.

The steroid hormones affect *transcription,* the transfer of genetic information required for protein synthesis from DNA to messenger RNA. Other hormones affect *translation,* the production of proteins at the ribosomes. In both cases metabolism is being controlled through the regulation of enzyme synthesis. The mechanisms by which such hormones operate are not well understood at a molecular level, and the nature of these interactions will only be determined by further research in this area.

ADDITIONAL READING

"The potential of microbial enzymes as diagnostic reagents", T. Atkinson, *Philos. Trans. R. Soc. London, Ser. B* **300**, 399 (1983).

"Enzyme kinetic constants: the double reciprocal plot", D. Burk, *Trends Biochem. Sci. (Pers. Ed.)* **9**, 202 (1984).

"Control of Enzyme Activity", 2nd Edition, by P. Cohen, Chapman & Hall, London, 1983.

"Enzyme Structure and Mechanism", A. Ferscht, Freeman, Oxford, 1977.

"Control of enzyme activity and metabolic pathways", D. E. Koshland, *Trends Biochem. Sci. (Pers. Ed.)* **9**, 155 (1984).

"Structure and catalysis of enzymes", W. N. Lipscomb, *Annu. Rev. Biochem.* **52**, 17 (1983).

"Understanding Enzymes", by T. Palmer, Ellis Horwood, Chichester, 1981.

"Enzymes as reagents in clinical chemistry", C. P. Price, *Philos. Trans. R. Soc. London, Ser. B* **300**, 411 (1983).

"Biochemistry", 2nd edition, by L. Stryer, Freeman, Oxford, 1981.

"Enzyme mechanisms", C. T. Walsh, *Trends Biochem. Sci. (Pers. Ed.)* **9**, 159 (1984).

"The Structure and Function of Enzymes", 2nd Edition, by C. H. Wynn, Arnold, London, 1979.

Salbutamol: A Selective β_2-Stimulant Bronchodilator

L. H. C. LUNTS
Glaxo Group Research Ltd.
Ware, England

I. INTRODUCTION AND BIOLOGICAL BACKGROUND

Bronchial asthma is a widespread disease from which about 5% of Western society will suffer at some time in their lives (*1*). It affects about one in 25 children and kills at least 1500 people a year in the United Kingdom (*2*). The aetiology of the disease is often of allergic origin but its causes are complicated and not completely understood.

Bronchial asthma is characterised by breathlessness and wheezing; in the early stages of the disease this is due to constriction of respiratory smooth muscle (bronchoconstriction) which is easily reversed by administration of a bronchodilator. In more severe cases, physical obstruction of the airways also occurs due to inflammation of the bronchial mucosal cells and by the formation of a viscous bronchial secretion. This condition is not reversible by bronchodilators, and glucocorticoid steroids (Chap. 9) are the only drugs that will reverse the inflammatory process and re-establish the response to bronchodilators.

49

Many natural mediators have been implicated in causing bronchoconstriction. Some are stored inside specialised cells, called mast cells, which, in allergic individuals, rupture in response to a signal at the cell surface and initiate an asthmatic attack.

Blocking the actions of the released mediators is a potential method for treatment but this requires knowledge of which mediators are the most significant and the availability of suitable antagonists. Although histamine is one of the substances released from the mast cell and causes bronchoconstriction, antihistamines (H_1-antagonists and H_2-antagonists) are of little value in the treatment of asthma.

Nature's own method of bronchodilation utilises the hormone adrenaline (2) which is released from the adrenal gland and mediates its actions through stimulation of the enzyme adenylate cyclase. This enzyme converts adenosine $3',5'$-triphosphate to cyclic adenosine monophosphate (cAMP) which is responsible for the relaxation of smooth muscle.

However, while adrenaline (2) is effective in relaxing bronchial muscle, it also causes unwanted stimulation of the heart and elevation of blood pressure.

HO

HO — CH(OH)CH$_2$NHR

(1) R = H   Noradrenaline
(2) R = Me   Adrenaline
(3) R = *i*-Pr   Isoprenaline
(4) R = *t*-Bu

It was clearly desirable, therefore, to find a compound that would reverse the constriction of the airways without causing cardiac or other side effects. It should also be effective given by mouth or inhaled and have a long duration of action.

An important step forward was the classification of adrenoceptors into α and β sub-types by Ahlquist (3). This was based on their sensitivities to noradrenaline and adrenaline and some close analogues of these natural stimulants. α-Adrenoceptors were defined as those very sensitive to adrenaline and insensitive to isoprenaline and β-receptors as those most sensitive to isoprenaline and least sensitive to noradrenaline (1) (Table I).

Isoprenaline (3) largely replaced adrenaline as a bronchodilator because of its greater selectivity of action on β-receptors but it still had substantial disadvantages. It has marked cardiovascular side-effects causing an increase in both the force and rate of contraction of the heart and could only be used by the inhaled route.

Lands and his colleagues (4) were responsible for defining that further selectivity for bronchial smooth muscle was possible using techniques similar to those

TABLE I
Some Properties of α- and β-Adrenoceptor Stimulants

Tissue	α-Effect	β-Effect
Bronchus	NSE[a]	Relaxation
Uterus	NSE	Relaxation
Blood vessel	Constriction	Dilatation
Skeletal muscle	NSE	Decrease in duration of muscle twitch
Heart muscle	NSE	Increase in force and rate
Alimentary tract	Constriction of sphincters	Relaxation

[a] NSE, No significant effects.

employed by Ahlquist. They found that catecholamines with a relatively large *N*-alkyl substituent (**4**) in the side-chain were more active at some β-receptors than others. On the basis of the observed order of activity, they sub-classified β-receptors into β_1 and β_2 types. Lands's work indicated that a selective β_2-stimulant given by inhalation or by mouth would be an excellent bronchodilator free from cardiovascular side-effects (Table II).

Isoetharine (**5**), which was distinctly more active on respiratory smooth muscle than on the heart, proved to be a useful selectively acting bronchodilator in

$$HO-\!\!\!\bigcirc\!\!\!-CH(OH)CH(Et)NH\text{-}i\text{-}Pr$$

(with an additional HO group at the top of the ring)

(**5**)
Isoetharine

man, but it and the *t*-butyl substituted compound (**4**) were short-acting compounds, which limited their therapeutic value.

TABLE II
Lands Classification and Distribution
of β-Adrenoceptor Sub-types

Organ	Main receptor type or sub-type
Heart	β_1
Lung (bronchial smooth muscle)	β_2
Blood vessels (vascular smooth muscle)	α, β_2
Uterus	β_2
Skeletal muscle	β_2

II.   BIOLOGICAL TEST PROCEDURES

In our laboratories, primary screening for bronchodilator activity is carried out using the guinea-pig isolated tracheal smooth muscle preparation or in anaesthetised guinea-pigs. In these tests, the abilities of new compounds to inhibit contractions of smooth muscle elicited by a variety of chemical stimuli is determined.

That the mechanism of the bronchodilatation is via β receptors is shown by blocking its effect with a β-blocking agent. To ensure that the compound has little or no activity on the heart (β_1 receptor) its ability to cause an increase in the rate of contraction of the guinea-pig isolated right atrium preparation is determined. The ratio of $\beta_2 : \beta_1$ activities gives a measure of selectivity.

To quantify the results, the *in vitro* test potency is expressed either as the EC_{50} value [the concentration of drug required to cause a 50% decrease in tracheal contractions (β_2) or a 50% increase in the heart rate (β_1)]. An alternative way of expressing potency is to calculate the equipotent dose ratio relative to isoprenaline.

Further bronchodilator tests may be carried out in anesthetised cats and these can simultaneously determine other parameters such as the effect on blood pressure and heart rate. In man the efficacy of bronchodilators is measured by other abilities to (a) increase the volume of air that can be expired in one second (FEV_1, forced expiratory volume in 1 second) or (b) the increase in the peak expiratory flow rate (PEFR).

III.   STRUCTURE–ACTIVITY RELATIONSHIPS AND METABOLISM OF CATECHOLAMINES

Adrenaline (**2**) and noradrenaline (**1**) are the natural hormones of the sympathetic nervous system. They are substituted phenylethanolamines with a catechol (1,2-benzenediol) nucleus so are referred to as catecholamines. On the above classification noradrenaline (**1**) acts mainly as an α-adrenergic stimulant whereas adrenaline (**2**) acts both as an α- and a β-stimulant. An increase in the bulk of the substituent on the nitrogen atom, from hydrogen (noradrenaline) to isopropyl (isoprenaline), results in a loss of potency of the compound as an α-stimulant and an increase in its potency as a β-stimulant. Isoprenaline (**3**) is a powerful β-stimulant devoid of α-agonist properties. This makes it a more satisfactory bronchodilator than adrenaline since it causes no vasoconstrictor (α) side effects.

As mentioned earlier, the two catecholamines **4** and **5** have a higher selectivity than isoprenaline (**3**) for β_2 than for β_1 sites and so produce less unwanted cardiac stimulant actions.

TABLE III
Bronchodilator Activity
of Some Substituted Catecholamines

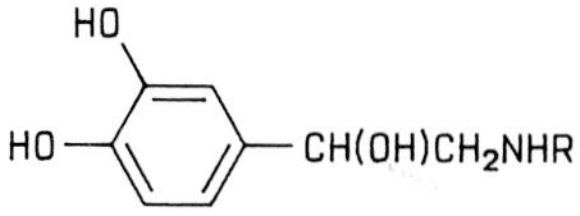

HO—, HO—⟨benzene ring⟩—CH(OH)CH₂NHR

R	Activity (isoprenaline = 1)
i-Pr	1
t-Bu	1.5–2[a]
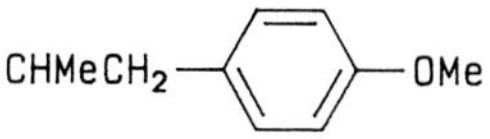 CHMeCH₂—⟨benzene ring⟩—OMe	2[b]
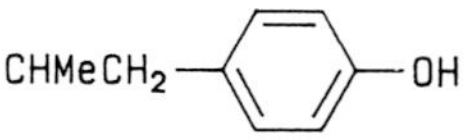 CHMeCH₂—⟨benzene ring⟩—OH	8[c]

[a] Various sources (4,6).
[b] Perfused guinea-pig lung: constriction induced by histamine (5).
[c] Anaesthetised guinea-pig: constriction induced by acetylcholine (6).

The isopropyl or t-butyl substituent of β-stimulant catecholamine and similar amines can also be replaced by certain aralkyl groups and potency is maintained or increased. Some examples are shown in Table III.

Phenylethanolamines have an asymmetric centre at the carbon atom that bears the hydroxyl group. The natural hormones have the (R) configuration, and biological activity in all phenylethanolamines resides in these enantiomers.

The shortcomings of the catecholamines (**3–5**) are that they have a short duration of action and are inactive when given by mouth. Catecholamines are readily taken up into tissues and inactivated by enzymes such as catechol O-methyltransferase (COMT). This results in methylation of the *meta*-hydroxy group to give an inactive ether:

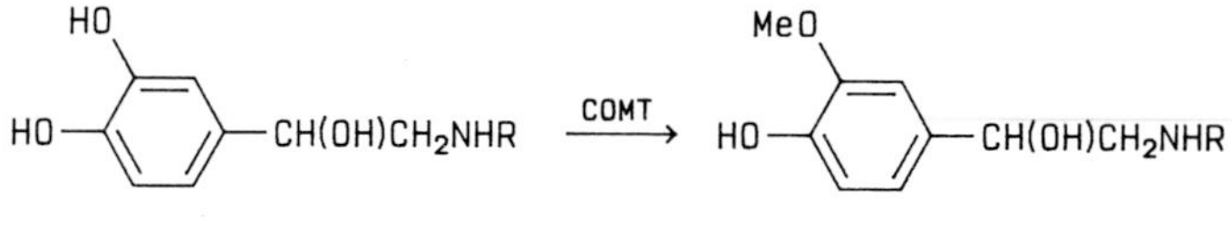

HO—, HO—⟨benzene ring⟩—CH(OH)CH₂NHR $\xrightarrow{\text{COMT}}$ MeO—, HO—⟨benzene ring⟩—CH(OH)CH₂NHR

IV. CHEMICAL APPROACH TO FIND AN ALTERNATIVE β-STIMULANT

In order to obtain an improved bronchodilator we needed a compound (a) that was stable to metabolic inactivation and (b) that was more selective for β-adrenoceptors in the lung than for those in the heart.

Our approach was to endeavour to replace the *meta*-hydroxy group of catecholamines with another group which in conjunction with the *para*-hydroxy group would possess the characteristics that were necessary for biological activity.

An analysis of the properties of this *meta*-hydroxy group identifies the following parameters that may be significant:

1. Size
2. Electronic effects on the aromatic system (resonance and inductive)
3. Capacity to form hydrogen bonds
4. Acidity
5. Ability to chelate with metals, particularly assisted by the *para*-hydroxy group
6. Capacity to form a redox system, again assisted by the *para*-hydroxy group.

Hydrogen-bonding and chelation powers were considered to be important properties because they had been invoked as the major binding features of the catecholamines at the receptor level. These properties together with acidity would be provided by a carboxylic acid group.

The synthesis of this salicylic acid derivative (**11**) is outlined in Scheme 1 (7). The ketoacid (**7**) was prepared by a Fries rearrangement of aspirin (**6**) and its methyl ester (**8**) was converted *via* a bromoketone (**9**) into the aminoketone (**10**) which was demethylated with hydrobromic acid. Catalytic hydrogenation then removed the protecting benzyl group and reduced the ketone to give the salicylic acid analogue (**11**) of isoprenaline. Reduction before hydrolysis afforded the methyl ester (**12**).

If the bromoketone (**9**) was condensed with isopropylamine a very poor yield of a secondary aminoketone was obtained.

The ester (**12**) reacted with ammonia to give a salicylamide derivative (**13**) (8). These three compounds **11, 12** and **13** proved not to be β-stimulants, but the ester (**12**) and particularly the amide (**13**) were β-adrenergic *antagonists*. In fact, the closely related *t*-butylamine (**14**) was about one-tenth as active as the standard β-blocker propranolol (**15**) (see Chap. 5). This result afforded some encouragement since it showed that the compounds had an affinity for the receptor, but had not the capacity to elicit a biological response.

A similar approach to finding an improved bronchodilator was carried out

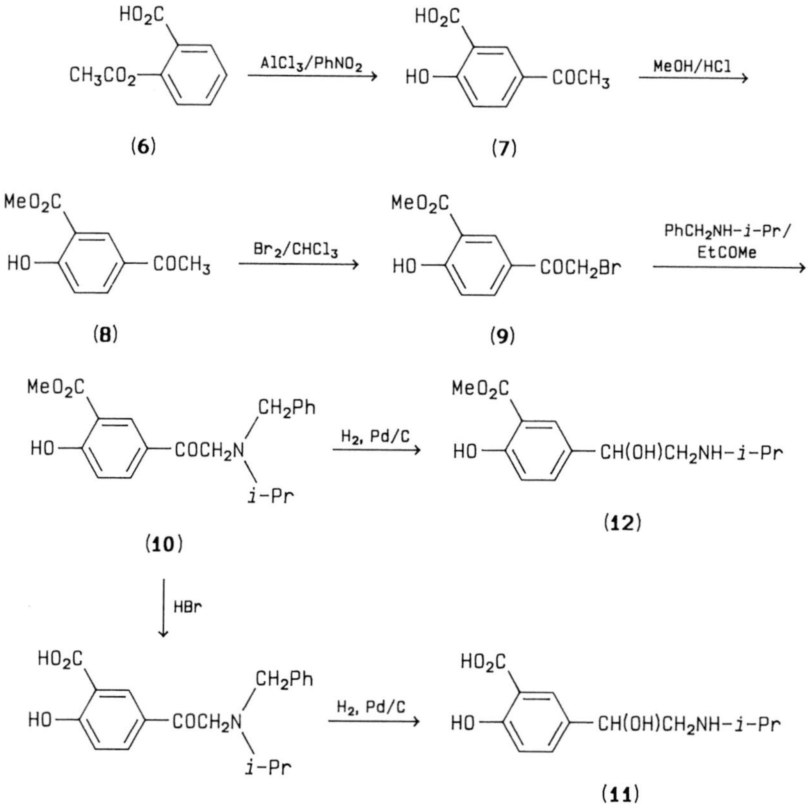

Scheme 1

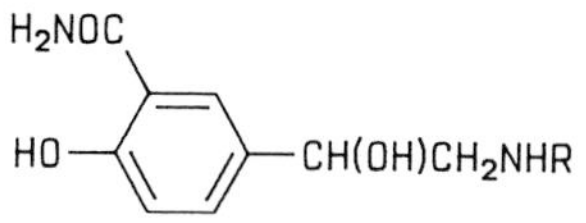

(13) R = *i*-Pr
(14) R = *t*-Bu

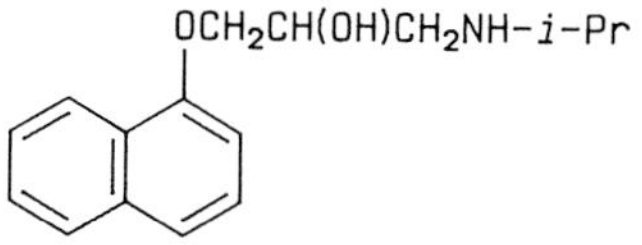

(15)
Propranolol

concomitantly by workers at Mead Johnson. They considered that the important property of the meta substituent was its acidity and that it would be mimicked by the methanesulphonamide group (pK_a 8.35) since it was of a comparable acidity to a phenol (pK_a 9.56); the bulky MeSO$_2$ moiety could be oriented in such a way that it would not interfere with binding to a receptor (9). Their compound soterenol (16) was a long-acting, selective β-stimulant, but it does not appear to have found clinical application. The isomer (17) was inactive (10).

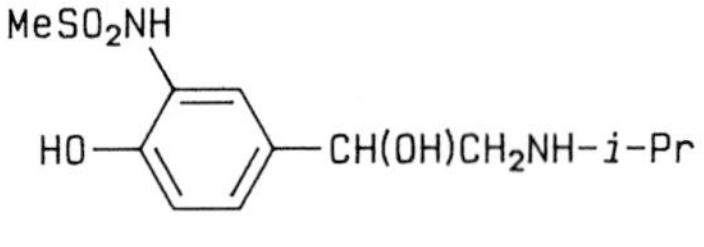

(16)
Soterenol

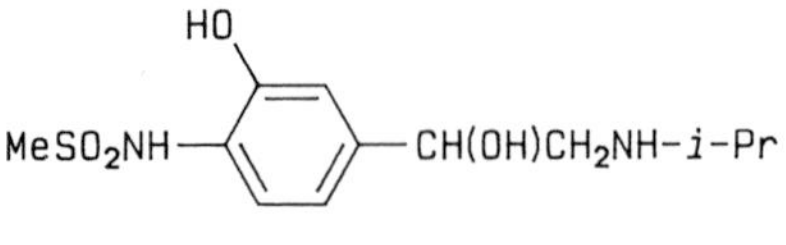

(17)

Another suitable candidate was a saligenin (2-hydroxybenzenemethanol) derivative since it retained a hydrogen-bonding and a chelating ability. Consequently the keto-esters (18) were reduced by lithium aluminium hydride and debenzylated (Scheme 2).

The products were indeed potent β-stimulants. The isopropyl compound (19) had almost half of the activity of isoprenaline as a bronchodilator in the guinea-pig (β_2) but with only one-thousandth of its activity on guinea-pig cardiac muscle (β_1). The *t*-butyl homologue (20) was even more selective [as was to be expected by comparison with the catecholamine analogue (4)]. It was equipotent with isoprenaline on bronchial muscle but two thousand times less potent on the heart.

This compound, salbutamol, was developed as a bronchodilator drug.

ENANTIOMERS OF SALBUTAMOL

A very convenient method to prepare the enantiomers of salbutamol was by resolution of an intermediate protected ester (*11*) (Scheme 3). Only one of the diastereoisomers of the di-*p*-toluoyltartrate salt (21) was insoluble in ethyl acetate. This was recrystallised twice and converted into the free base which after reduction with lithium aluminum hydride and catalytic debenzylation gave enantiomerically pure salbutamol. By using (−)-di-*p*-toluoyltartaric acid, (R)-(−)-

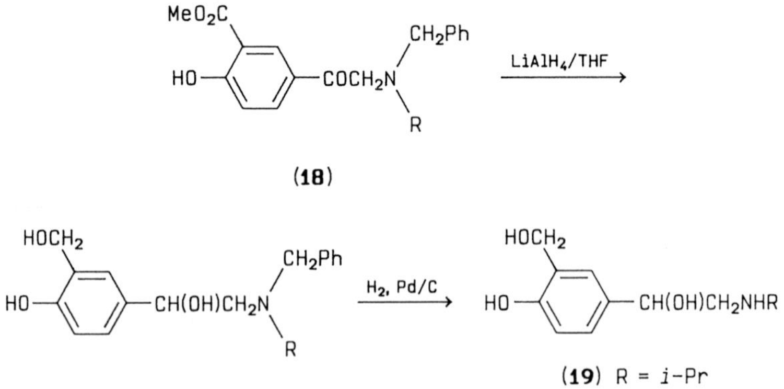

(18)

(19) R = *i*-Pr
(20) R = *t*-Bu

Scheme 2

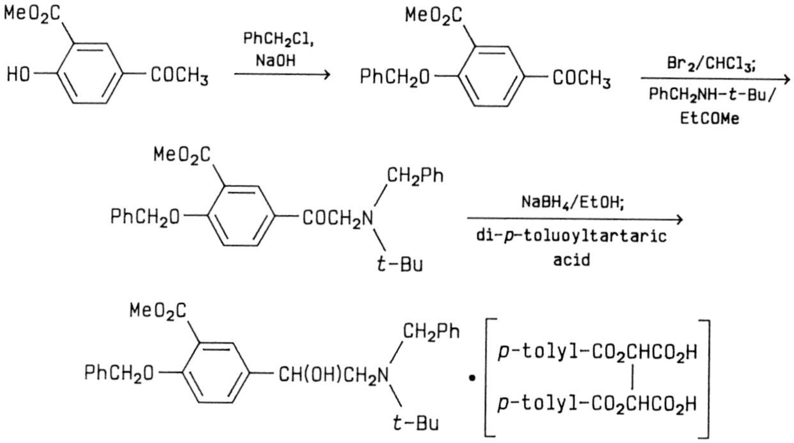

(21)

Scheme 3

salbutamol was obtained; the other enantiomer was formed similarly after resolving the original ester as its (+)-di-*p*-toluoyltartrate.

The absolute configuration of (*R*)-(−)-salbutamol (**20a**) was determined by comparison of its CD spectrum with that of (*R*)-(−)-octopamine (**22**). They both showed a negative Cotton effect at 276–280 nm.

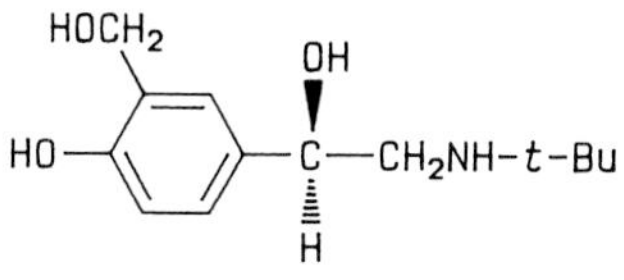

(20a) 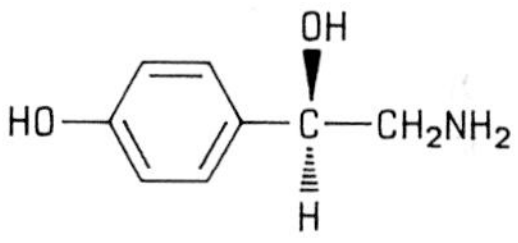   (22)

When tested on the guinea-pig trachea this enantiomer was 68 times as active as the (*S*)-(+)-isomer as a β_2-stimulant, as was to be expected by analogy with other phenylethanolamines which have been referred to already (*12*).

V. STRUCTURE–ACTIVITY RELATIONSHIPS BETWEEN SALBUTAMOL AND CONGENERS

A. OTHER SALIGENIN DERIVATIVES

Salbutamol analogues with substituents on nitrogen similar to those on active catecholamines described in Section III had high potency and also β_2-selectivity (Table IV). One of these, the 4-methoxy-α-methylphenethyl derivative (salm-

TABLE IV
Bronchodilator and Cardiac Stimulating Activity
of Some Substituted Saligenin Ethanolamines[a]

	Activity (isoprenaline = 1)	
R	Bronchodilator[b]	Cardiac stimulant[c]
i-Pr	0.4	0.001
t-Bu Salbutamol (**20**)	1	0.005
CHMeCH₂—⟨OMe⟩ Salmefamol (**27**)	1.5	0.00075
CHMeCH₂—⟨OH⟩	3	0.0005

[a] Adapted from Ref. 1.
[b] Anaesthetised guinea-pig (Konzett–Rössler preparation).
[c] Guinea-pig isolated atria.

efamol) (**27**), was one and a half times as active as salbutamol. It is a clinically effective bronchodilator with a duration of action of up to 6 hours.

Chemically these analogues were usually prepared by methods using reductive alkylation of the primary amine with an aldehyde or a ketone. There are several ways of accomplishing this reaction as illustrated in Scheme 4 for the preparation of salmefamol (**27**).

The intermediate esters could be prepared from a primary phenylethanolamine (**25**) which itself was derived by hydrogenolysis of a dibenzylamino precursor (**24**). It was more convenient to use the latter compound directly, when concomitant debenzylation and reductive alkylation can occur, so that the reaction may proceed via a tertiary benzylamine (**28**). The reaction sequence could be further shortened by starting from the dibenzylamino ketone (**23**).

Esters were then reduced by lithium aluminium hydride as before. Of course the reductive alkylations can be undertaken with saligenin precursors instead of esters.

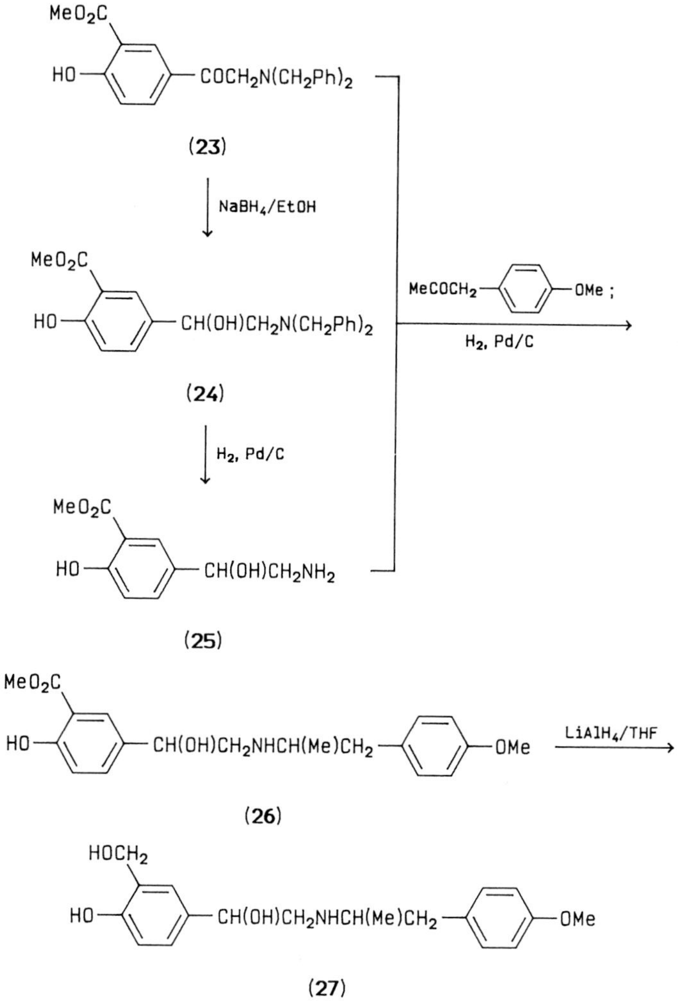

(23)

NaBH₄/EtOH

(24)

MeCOCH₂——OMe ;

H₂, Pd/C

H₂, Pd/C

(25)

(26)

LiAlH₄/THF

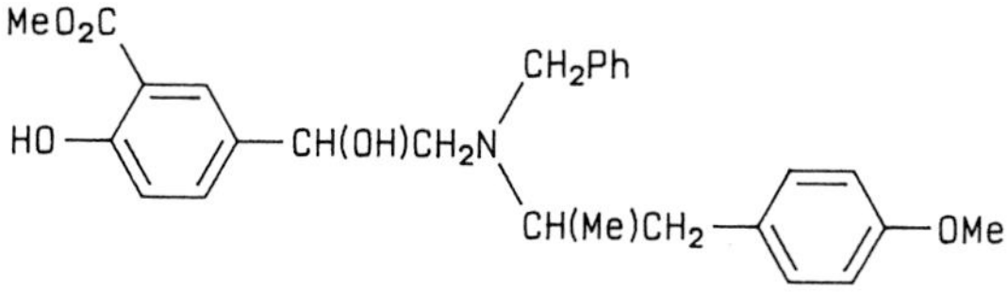

(27)

Scheme 4

(28)

The more active of these aralkyl phenethanolamines were prepared from methyl ketones and thus contain another asymmetric carbon atom (which bears the methyl group). In these instances the products exist as a mixture of four diastereoisomers. Each isomer of salmefamol (**27**) has been tested, and β-stimulant activity resides mainly in the (*R,R*)-enantiomer.*

B.   Variants of the Saligenin Moiety of Salbutamol

When the activity of salbutamol had been established it was necessary to prepare other analogues and derivatives to gain an insight into the influence of structure on activity.

Modification of the Hydroxymethyl Group

As the catecholamines and their saligenin analogues had similar β_2-stimulant activity it was likely that they interacted in a similar fashion at the β_2-adrenoceptor. In contrast only the catecholamines had potency at β_1-adrenoceptors. To investigate the sensitivity of these interactions and effects on β_1:β_2 selectivity we introduced steric hindrance at the benzylic carbon atoms and extended the methylene group to move the alcohol group further from the ring. We also put a second hydroxy group into the meta side-chain.

An aldehyde (**29**) was obtainable by oxidation of salbutamol with manganese dioxide and this or a protected derivative was a convenient source of a secondary alcohol (**30**), the hydroxypropyl compound (**31**) and a 1,3-diol (**32**) (Schemes 5, 6, 7 and 8).

Grignard reactions on ester derivatives afforded tertiary alcohols (**33**) and (**34**) (Schemes 9 and 10).

The hydroxyethyl homologue (**35**) of salbutamol was built up from phenol, protected as a tetrahydropyranyl ether (Scheme 11).

The most interesting compound from this selection was the hydroxyethyl derivative (**35**) which was very potent and selective as a β_2-adrenergic stimulant. We found the hydroxypropyl homologue (**31**) to be much less active as were the other compounds described in these schemes (*13*).

Therefore it seems that the methylene of the hydroxymethyl group of salbutamol cannot be substituted without causing significant loss of potency. Even polyfunctional groups such as diols cannot replace the hydroxymethyl substituent. Only homologation to a two-carbon chain afforded a very active stimulant.

---

*The first assignment of configuration refers to the carbon atom which bears the hydroxy group; the second is that of the carbon atom with the methyl group.

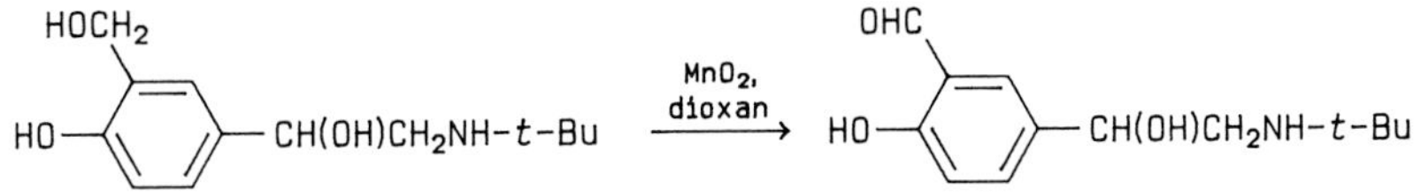

HOCH$_2$

HO— ⬡ —CH(OH)CH$_2$NH–t–Bu $\xrightarrow[\text{dioxan}]{\text{MnO}_2,}$ OHC

HO— ⬡ —CH(OH)CH$_2$NH–t–Bu

(29)

Scheme 5

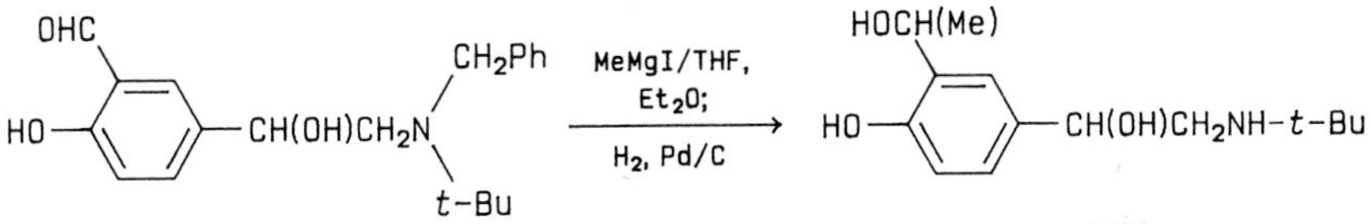

OHC

HO— ⬡ —CH(OH)CH$_2$N(CH$_2$Ph)(t–Bu) $\xrightarrow[\text{H}_2,\ \text{Pd/C}]{\substack{\text{MeMgI/THF,} \\ \text{Et}_2\text{O};}}$ HOCH(Me)

HO— ⬡ —CH(OH)CH$_2$NH–t–Bu

(30)

Scheme 6

OHC

PhCH$_2$O— ⬡ —CH(OH)CH$_2$N(CH$_2$Ph)(t–Bu) $\xrightarrow[\text{HCl}]{(\text{EtO})_2\overset{+}{\text{P}}\text{CH}_2\text{CO}_2\text{Et, NaH};\ \text{O}^-}$

EtO$_2$CCH=CH

PhCH$_2$O— ⬡ —CH(OH)CH$_2$N(CH$_2$Ph)(t–Bu) $\xrightarrow[\text{H}_2,\ \text{Pd/C}]{\text{LiAlH}_4/\text{THF};}$

HO(CH$_2$)$_3$

HO— ⬡ —CH(OH)CH$_2$NH–t–Bu

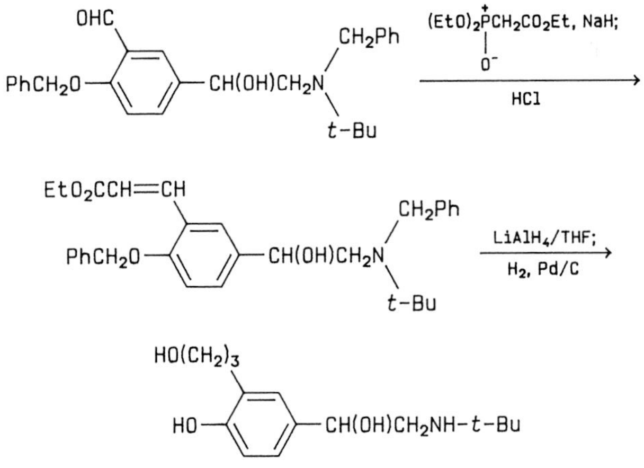

(31)

Scheme 7

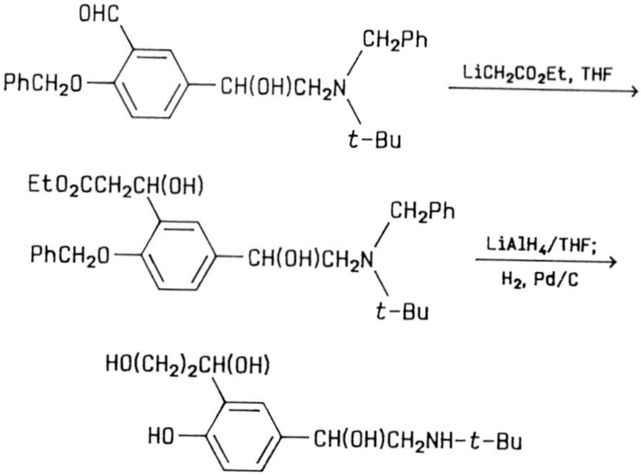

(32)

Scheme 8

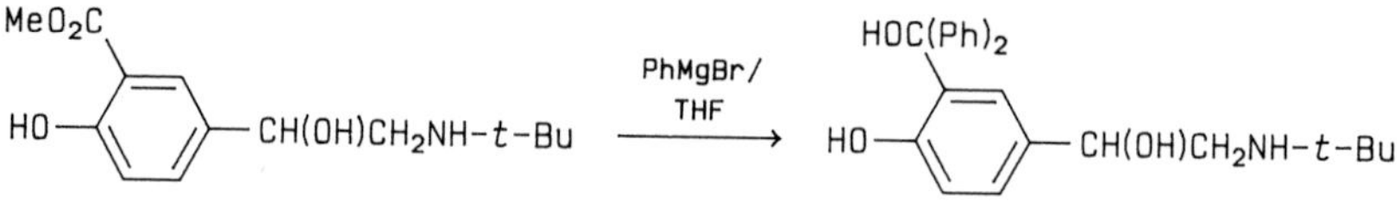

(33)

Scheme 9

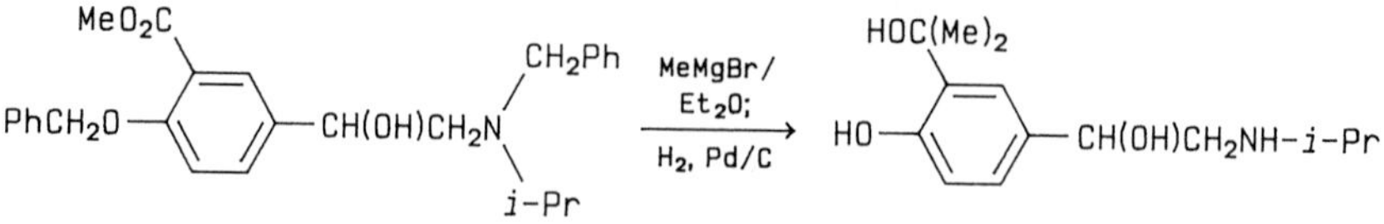

(34)

Scheme 10

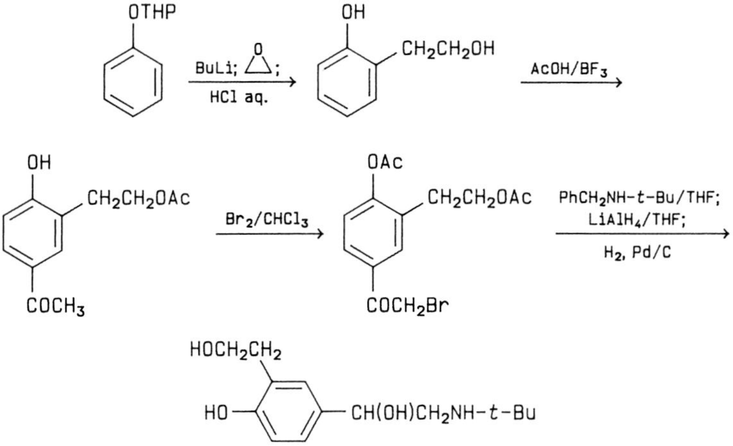

(35)

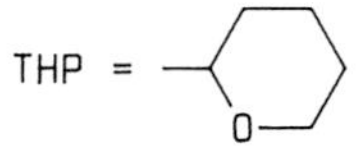

THP =

Scheme 11

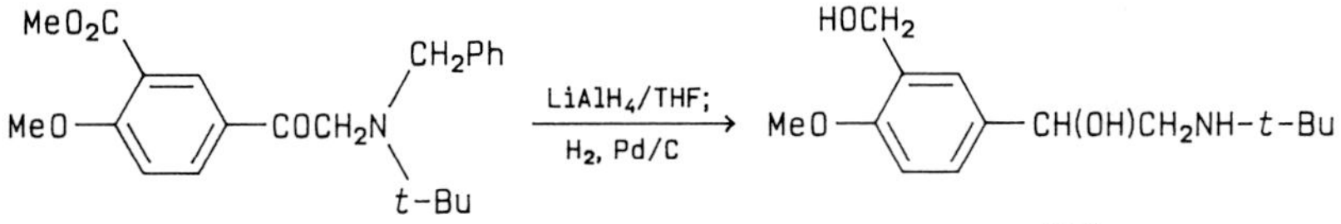

(36)

Scheme 12

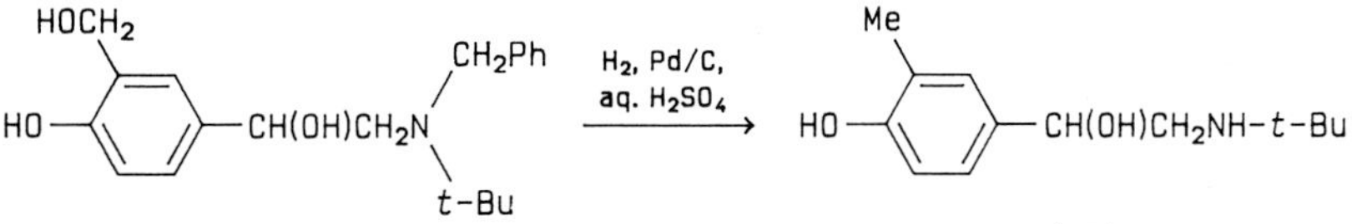

(37)

Scheme 13

Neither the phenolic ether (**36**) nor the methyl phenol (**37**) had any β-stimulant activity (*7*). Their syntheses are shown in Schemes 12 and 13.

C. SALICYLAMINE DERIVATIVES

Reduction of derivatives of the amide mentioned in Section IV gave salicylamine derivatives (Scheme 14). This replacement of one of the hydroxy

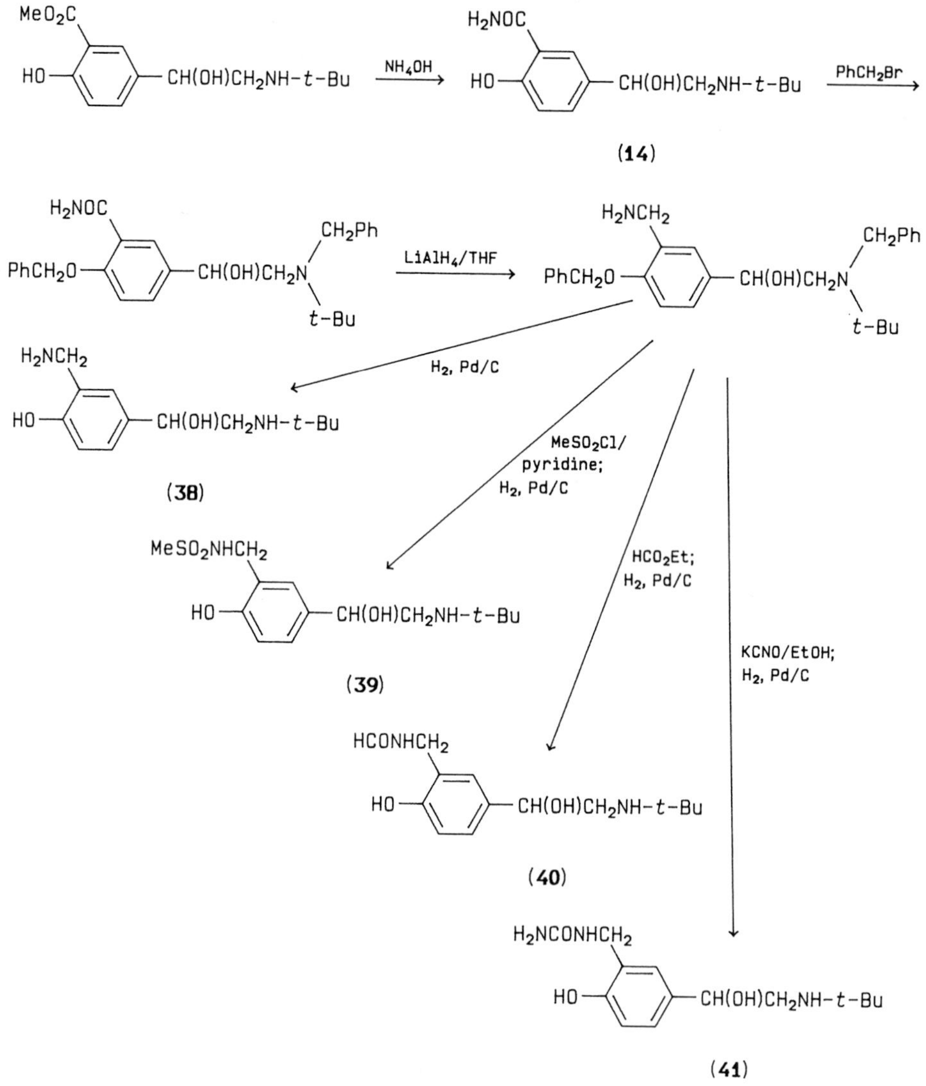

Scheme 14

TABLE V

Bronchodilator and Cardiac Stimulating Activity
of Some Salicylamine Derivatives[a]

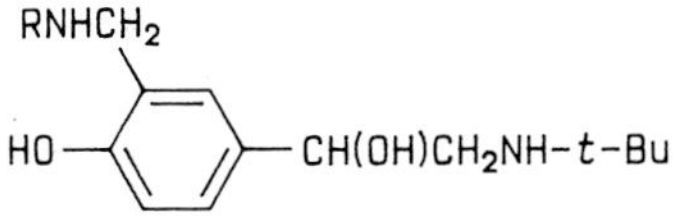

RNHCH$_2$

HO—⟨ ⟩—CH(OH)CH$_2$NH-*t*-Bu

	Activity (isoprenaline = 1)	
R	Bronchodilator[b]	Cardiac stimulant[c]
H	0	NT[d]
MeSO$_2$	0.2	0.001
HCO	0.05	0
NH$_2$CO	0.1	<0.0001

[a] Adapted from Ref. *13*.
[b] Anaesthetised guinea-pig (Dixon–Brodie preparation).
Salbutamol = 0.1.
[c] Guinea-pig isolated atria (rate).
[d] NT, not tested.

groups of salbutamol by an amino group afforded an inactive compound (**38**), but when it was converted into a variety of amides it yielded some very active and selective β_2-stimulants (Table V). A methanesulphonamide (**39**), formamide (**40**) and urea (**41**) stand out with potencies of the order of salbutamol.

Their mobile hydrogen atoms were situated relative to the phenolic group in a manner similar to that of the alcoholic group of salbutamol.

D.   CONCLUSIONS REGARDING STRUCTURE–ACTIVITY RELATIONSHIPS

The common features in the aromatic ring of the β-stimulants that we have obtained by chemical derivation from salicylic acid are

1. A phenolic hydroxyl group in the 4-position relative to the ethanolamine side-chain
2. A substituent in the 3-position which is capable of taking part in hydrogen bonding and which does not have an electron-withdrawing effect on the phenyl ring
3. A steric arrangement such that the functional moiety on the 3-substituent is not restricted by nearby bulky groups, and is not removed from the aromatic ring by more than two carbon atoms

Properties possessed by catechols but which do not seem to be relevant to β_2-stimulant activity are

1. Chelation *per se* since the aldehyde (29) and its oxime are not very active
2. Redox capacity
3. Acidity of the 3-substituent, since the hydroxymethyl group is not acidic, the methanesulphonamidomethyl substituent of 39 is acidic and the methanesulphonanilide group in soterenol (16) is more acidic than phenol* (*10*)

VI. SUMMARY AND FINAL COMMENTS

This chapter has outlined the problems presented by the requirement for a bronchodilator therapy for asthma and how several selective β-stimulant bronchodilators were devised and synthesised.

The principle was to modify an active drug (isoprenaline) by replacement of the functional group that was responsible for its deficiencies to give an analogue that would retain the key physicochemical properties of the original. Simple chemical manipulation of an abundant starting material, aspirin, generated the anti-asthmatic drug salbutamol. Effects of changes in structure on biological activity were applied to the preparation of further potent and selective β_2-adrenoceptor stimulants.

The success of this project has had profound beneficial effects for asthmatics who are now able to obtain rapid and sustained relief from their distressing symptoms without significant side effects.

Salbutamol† is efficacious in man in relieving attacks of asthma, active by inhalation and orally with minimal side effects and having a duration of about 4 hours. It is not metabolised by COMT. In man it is converted into a phenolic sulphate.

Salbutamol was introduced as a bronchodilator in the United Kingdom in 1969 where it quickly became the most widely prescribed treatment for asthma and is in fact the top-selling drug in the United Kingdom. It is marketed throughout the world and is the market leader in 26 countries.

Bronchodilator and other properties of salbutamol have been reviewed extensively (*13*).

VII. THE FUTURE

Salbutamol has proved to be a highly successful drug, so what properties can be expected from an improved bronchodilator? One possibility is an increase in

---

*The irrelevance of comparative acidities of the 3- and 4-substituents is confirmed by the inactivity of the 3-hydroxy-4-methanesulphonamide isomer (17).

†Albuterol in the United States.

its duration of action. Apart from convenience in administration it might relieve the acute bronchoconstriction that some asthmatics experience at about 4 a.m. (the so-called morning dip), so that medication at night would last until the following day. Another improvement would be to alter the profile of action to minimise effects on skeletal muscle to avoid the side effect of tremor associated with orally administered β_2-stimulants.

REFERENCES

1. P. H. Howarth and G. F. George, *Adverse Drug React. Acute Poisoning Rev.* **2**, 25 (1983).
2. L. J. Colmer and D. J. P. Gray, *Practitioner* **227**, 271 (1983).
3. R. P. Ahlquist, *Am. J. Physiol.* **153**, 586 (1948).
4. A. M. Lands, A. Arnold, J. P. McAuliff, F. P. Luduena, and T. G. Brown, *Nature (London)* **214**, 597 (1967).
5. J. H. Biel, E. G. Schwarz, E. P. Sprengler, H. A. Leiser, and H. L. Friedman, *J. Am. Chem. Soc.* **76**, 3149 (1954).
6. H. D. Moed, J. van Dijk, and H. Niewind, *Recl. Trav. Chim. Pays-Bas Belg.* **74**, 919 (1955).
7. D. T. Collin, D. Hartley, D. Jack, L. H. C. Lunts, J. C. Press, A. C. Ritchie, and P. Toon, *J. Med. Chem.* **13**, 674 (1970).
8. J. E. Clifton, I. Collins, P. Hallett, D. Hartley, L. H. C. Lunts, and P. D. Wicks, *J. Med. Chem.* **25**, 670 (1982).
9. A. A. Larsen and P. M. Lish, *Nature (London)* **203**, 1283 (1964).
10. A. A. Larsen, W. A. Gould, H. R. Roth, W. T. Comer, R. J. Uloth, K. W. Dungan, and P. M. Lish, *J. Med. Chem.* **10**, 462 (1967).
11. D. Hartley and D. Middlemiss, *J. Med. Chem.* **14**, 895 (1971).
12. R. T. Brittain, J. B. Farmer, and R. J. Marshall, *Br. J. Pharmacol.* **48**, 144 (1973).
13. R. T. Brittain, C. M. Dean, and D. Jack, *Pharmacol. Ther., Part B.* **2**, 423 (1976).

CHAPTER 5

Beta Blockers

B. G. MAIN and H. TUCKER

Chemistry Department
ICI Pharmaceuticals Division
Macclesfield, England

I. INTRODUCTION

In this chapter we trace the development of compounds which selectively block β_1-receptors: these compounds have found many uses in the clinic including the treatment of angina and high blood pressure. In addition we show the origin of compounds which selectively block β_2-receptors: these latter compounds will allow the physiological importance of these receptors to be delineated.

69

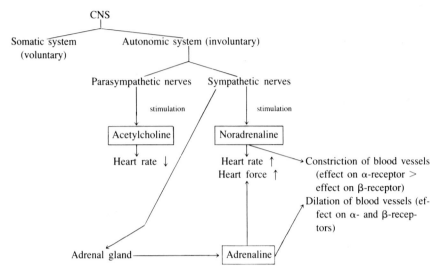

Fig. 1   Factors contributing to the control of heart rate and blood vessels.

II.   NERVOUS CONTROL OF THE HEART AND CIRCULATION

The nervous system which co-ordinates many of the body's functions is divided into two branches, the somatic system, which controls the activity of the skeletal (voluntary) muscles, and the autonomic system, which is concerned with the (involuntary) maintenance of a stable internal environment, and which is subdivided into the parasympathetic and sympathetic nervous systems (Fig. 1). In the heart, stimulation of the parasympathetic nerves (vagi) leads to a reduction in heart rate while stimulation of the sympathetic nerves increases the rate and force of contraction of the heart. The response of the heart to a given situation is governed by a fine balance between these two systems. Neural impulses along the parasympathetic or sympathetic nerves achieve their effect by the release from the nerve endings of the neurotransmitters acetylcholine (**1**) and noradrenaline (**2**), which bind to their respective receptors, eliciting biochemical reactions which ultimately express themselves in a physiological response. In addition, in response to stress the adrenal glands secrete into the blood stream a hormone, adrenaline (**3**), which is responsible for the "flight or fight" syndrome by which the body prepares to protect itself or run away when threatened. Adrenaline stimulates the heart, and dilates some blood vessels to supply the muscles with more blood; noradrenaline has the same cardiac actions but constricts the blood vessels (see Table III, Chap. 1).

In a search for bronchodilator agents Konzett (*1*), in 1940, synthesised iso-

(1) Acetylcholine

(2) Noradrenaline

(3) Adrenaline

(4) Isoprenaline

prenaline (4), the *N*-isopropyl analogue of noradrenaline, which has found widespread clinical use both as a bronchodilator and cardiac stimulant. Unlike noradrenaline and adrenaline, which are produced in the body, isoprenaline is a purely synthetic material.

In 1948 Ahlquist (2) studied the effects of a number of sympathomimetic amines (agonists) including adrenaline, noradrenaline and isoprenaline on various tissues innervated by the sympathetic nervous system and concluded that there were two types of adrenergic (sympathetic) receptors which he termed α and β. Stimulation of the α-receptor mainly causes a contractile response while β-receptor responses are largely relaxant. The major exception to this is the cardiac β-receptor, stimulation of which increases the rate and force of contraction of the heart. From this, it follows that noradrenaline exhibits mainly α-stimulant activity with some (important) β-agonism, adrenaline has equipotent stimulant activity on α- and β-receptors and isoprenaline is a pure β-agonist.

In 1967 Lands (3) studied the effects of 15 sympathomimetic amines on a series of tissues and showed by statistical analysis of the results that there were two different populations of β-receptor which he designated as β_1 and β_2. The cardiac β-receptors are β_1 while those in the bronchial smooth muscle and in blood vessels are β_2 (see Table I, Chap. 4). Evidence is now emerging that mixed populations of β_1 and β_2 receptors exist in many tissues, the overall response of the tissue depending on the proportions of receptor present (4).

III.   NATURE OF THE β-RECEPTOR

Despite intensive biochemical studies (reviewed in Ref. 5), the exact nature of the β-receptor is not known. It is a protein, and is located on the outer surface of the target cell membrane. It is currently accepted that binding of the agonist to the receptor results in an activation of the enzyme adenyl cyclase, located on the inside of the membrane, which converts ATP to cyclic AMP. This second messenger initiates a complex biochemical cascade which eventually leads to a physiological response.

IV.   β-BLOCKADE AND CARDIAC DISEASE

Ahlquist's hypothesis of α- and β-receptors was ignored for the first 10 years largely because no agent was known that would selectively block β-receptors in the same way that, for example, ergotamine blocks the α-receptors. In 1958, Mills of the Eli Lilly Company prepared the dichloro analogue of isoprenaline, commonly known as DCI (5).

(5) Dichloroisoprenaline (DCI)   (6) Pronethalol

DCI was shown to inhibit the relaxation of bronchial smooth muscle elicited by isoprenaline (6) and also the cardiac actions of isoprenaline (7), that is, it was the first β-adrenoreceptor blocking agent, now more commonly referred to as a β-blocker. In addition to its β-blocking actions DCI also had a stimulant action, that is, it was a partial agonist, and at that time no clinical application was perceived for such a compound.

The true clinical potential of β-adrenoreceptor blocking agents was first recognised by Black (8) at ICI when in 1959 he formulated a theory for a possible treatment for coronary artery disease and, in particular, angina. One of the body's responses to physical and mental stress is stimulation of the sympathetic nervous system causing (via β-receptors) an increase in the heart rate and force of contraction. These are energy-consuming processes and the heart muscle itself requires a greater supply of oxygen. If an adequate supply of blood cannot be maintained because of coronary arterial disease then the resulting oxygen deficiency in the cardiac muscle manifests itself in the intense pain of angina. Attempts to increase the oxygen supply to the heart by vasodilator drugs had not been successful so Black proposed that reduction of the heart's demand for oxygen by blocking the effects of sympathetic nerve stimulation should be an effective means of treating angina. In particular Black wanted a specific β-blocker without the stimulant properties of DCI. Within 18 months he had set up

screening tests for this type of activity and his colleague Stephenson had synthesised pronethalol (*6*), an agent which effectively blocked cardiac (and other)
β-receptors and which only had marginal partial agonist activity.

V. EARLY β-BLOCKERS

Pronethalol became the first clinically available β-blocker and was effective
not only in the treatment of angina but also controlled certain kinds of cardiac
arrhythmia and reduced elevated blood pressure. The discovery of these properties led to a systematic investigation around the pronethalol structure both within
ICI and at other pharmaceutical companies. The structure–activity relationships
of these arylethanolamines have been discussed elsewhere (*9*) and will not be
considered further. In the main, the ethanolamines are associated with varying
degrees of partial agonism, with the notable exception of sotalol [(*7*), Table I]
and have achieved their greatest success as β-stimulants (see Chap. 4). Sotalol
itself, however, is used clinically as a β-blocker.

Pronethalol was withdrawn from the clinic in 1963 due to concern over toxic
symptoms (thymic tumours) in animals, but during the development period of
pronethalol chemical work to optimise β-antagonist activity had continued. Be-
sides studying the effects of aryl ring and amine substitutions in the molecule, the
researchers modified the ethanolamine chain itself by, *inter alia,* the introduction
of linking groups between the aryl ring and ethanolamine chain. Of the many
linking groups tried, oxymethylene proved to be the best with the first analogue
prepared, the α-naphthyloxypropanolamine propranolol (*8*), being 10–20 times

(**8**) Propranolol   (**9**)

(**10**) R = Me
(**11**) R = H

TABLE I
Early β-Blockers in Clinical Use

Structure	Name (manufacturer)	Relative potency[a]	isa[b]	msa[c]
(structure) O–CH₂–CH(OH)–CH₂–NH–*i*-Pr on naphthalene	(8) Propranolol (ICI)	1	−	+
(structure) OH; O–…–NH–*i*-Pr; allyl on benzene	(12) Alprenolol (Hassle)	1	+	+
(structure) OH; O–…–NH–*i*-Pr; O–allyl on benzene	(13) Oxprenolol (Ciba-Geigy)	0.3	+	+
(structure) O–…–NH–*i*-Pr; OH on indole	(14) Pindolol (Sandoz)	30	+ +	+
(structure) O–…–NH–*t*-Bu; OH; HO, HO on tetrahydronaphthalene	(15) Nadolol (Squibb)	1	−	?
(structure) O–…–NH–*t*-Bu; OH; morpholino-thiadiazole	(16) Timolol (Merck)	4	−	?
(structure) OH; CH(OH)–CH₂–NH–*i*-Pr; MeSO₂NH on benzene	(7) Sotalol (Mead Johnson)	0.08	−	−

[a] Ratio of ED_{50} values in the test described by (*18*).
[b] isa, intrinsic sympathomimetic activity.
[c] msa, membrane stabilising activity.

more potent than pronethalol (*10*). Smith, one of the chemists involved, has related that he used α-naphthol as a model compound since at the time he could not find the bottle of β-naphthol. Ten days later the β-naphthyloxy derivative (**9**), which is the direct analogue of pronethalol, was synthesised and found to be only slightly more potent than pronethalol. It is interesting to note that some years before the discovery of DCI, BDH workers (*11*) published papers on the local anaesthetic properties of a series of aryloxypropanolamines, which included the *n*-propylamino analogue of propranolol and compounds **10** and **11** which were later found to be β-adrenergic agonists. "Where observation is concerned, chance favours only the prepared mind" (Louis Pasteur).

Many companies at this time began working in the aryloxypropanolamine area, and a number of successful drugs have emerged. A selection of these is listed in Table I. Propranolol has become the reference compound, and established the clinical concept of beta-blockade for the treatment of angina. In addition it pioneered the clinical use of β-blockers in many other disease states.

It is appropriate at this stage to summarise the pharmacology, clinical properties and toxicological problems common to all the drugs of this early type.

VI.   PHARMACOLOGY OF β-BLOCKERS

All β-blockers have two properties in common; namely, they are competitive antagonists, and they are specific for β-receptors. For any β-blocker the following parameters are used in defining its profile: potency, partial agonism and membrane stabilising activity (msa).

A.   POTENCY

Potency is usually expressed, *in vivo*, as an ED_{50}, or *in vitro*, as a pA_2. ED_{50} is the dose of antagonist required to reduce the response to an agonist by 50%, and pA_2 has been defined in Chap. 2. Because many different species and tissue types have been used throughout the world to evaluate β-blockers, wherever possible potencies relative to propranolol are used in this text.

B.   PARTIAL AGONISM

Partial agonism has generally been termed "intrinsic sympathomimetic activity" (isa), and is a measure of the ability of a compound to stimulate β-receptors directly. The majority of β-blockers have isa, and the usual value quoted is the absolute increase in heart rate observed when a compound is given at a fixed (high) dose of 2.5 mg/kg i.v. to rats whose natural catecholamine stores have been depleted by pre-treatment with syrosingopine (a reserpine derivative).

In this test propranolol causes no increase in heart rate, pronethalol causes a 70 beat per minute (bpm) rise, and isoprenaline causes the maximum rise of 200 bpm (from about 300 to 500). There is still much speculation about the clinical relevance of low (up to ~100 bpm) amounts of isa.

C. MEMBRANE ACTIVITY

In 1964 it was shown that pronethalol had local anaesthetic activity, more potent than procaine, and it was suggested that this might be the mode of action of β-blockers in angina and arrhythmias. Subsequent investigations showed, however, that this activity, which is believed to be caused by electrical stabilisation of cell membranes, was not present at normal clinical doses.

Hellenbrecht (12) showed that, for a series of related β-blockers, this membrane stabilising activity (msa) was directly related to the partition coefficient of the compound, highly lipophilic compounds such as propranolol being very effective local anaesthetics.

VII.   STRUCTURE–ACTIVITY RELATIONSHIPS OF EARLY β-BLOCKERS

Considering the fundamental structure (17) for arylethanolamines (X = direct link) and aryloxypropanolamines (X = OCH$_2$) one can identify two functions which are essential for β-blockade, namely the β-aminoethanol chain and the aromatic ring. Experience with the arylethanolamine series had shown that optimum β-antagonist activity resided with branched alkylamine substituents, the best of which were isopropyl and t-butyl. This was also found to be true for the aryloxypropanolamines and in all the early work on β-blockers the isopropyl- or t-butyl-amino substituents were retained. The insertion of additional groups between the amine and carbinol group, removal or alkylation of the hydroxyl group or acylation of the amine all led to a substantial or total loss of β-blocking activity. With the exception of X = OCH$_2$, all other linking groups tried have given compounds with little or no activity (X = CH=CH, SCH$_2$, —CH$_2$CH$_2$—) although modest activity was obtained when X = NHCH$_2$.

Methyl substitution at the α, β or γ carbon atom resulted in a reduction in β-

(17)

Biologically active
enantiomer of 17

TABLE II

Comparison of the Potencies of ortho, meta and para
Substituted Phenoxypropanolamines (**18**)[a]

(**18**)

R	ortho	meta	para
Cl	5	0.52	0.085
NO$_2$	2	0.39	0.028
CH$_3$	1.71	0.66	0.09
OCH$_3$	1.71	0.91	0.54
OC$_6$H$_5$	2	0.3	0.001

[a] Potency values related to propranolol = 1.

blocking activity which was least for α-substitution. The β-antagonist activity resides with one enantiomer, the (R)-ethanolamine and the (S)-aryloxypropanolamine, both of which have the same absolute configuration. Most commercially available β-blockers are sold as the racemates.

With some minor exceptions all β-blockers have an aromatic ring which need not necessarily be benzenoid but can be heterocyclic [e.g., timolol (**16**)], or benzheterocyclic [e.g., pindolol (**14**)] (Table I). The nature and position of the substituents in the aromatic ring have a crucial effect on the potency and overall pharmacological profile of the molecule. For the series of positional isomers listed in Table II it is clear that the order of β-antagonist potency is ortho > meta > para. In addition the ortho position can accommodate large substituents and retain β-antagonist activity whereas the para position is very sensitive to group size. This is clearly demonstrated by the isomers of the phenoxy analogue. Polysubstitution of the aromatic ring yielded compounds with a variety of potencies, except for 2,6-disubstitution which resulted in an almost complete loss of β-antagonist activity.

The size of the ortho substituent plays an important part in governing the levels of isa exhibited by the molecule. The larger the ortho substituent, the less is the isa observed. In an attempt to explain (*13*) this phenomenon, the effect of the ortho substituent on the conformation of the ethanolamine chain was computed and related to the isa observed for a series of aryloxypropanolamines. In another approach (*14*) Taft's steric factor for the ortho substituent was plotted against isa. Both approaches gave a straight line relationship.

A graphic example of the influence of the aromatic ring substituent on pharmacological profile is provided by the hydroxy substituent. The aryloxypropanolamine analogue of isoprenaline (**19**) has been shown (*15*) to be a potent β-agonist. The corresponding 3,5-dihydroxy analogue (**20**) is a partial agonist, as is the *meta*-hydroxy (**21**) and *para*-hydroxy analogue (**22**) [the laevorotatory isomer of which, prenalterol (*16*), has been under development as a cardiac stimulant for the treatment of heart failure]. The ortho analogue, however, is a β-blocker. The interesting heterocyclic derivative tazolol (**23**) is also a partial β_1-agonist, which contrasts markedly with timolol (**16**) which is devoid of isa.

(**19**) $R^1 = R^2 = $ OH
(**22**) $R^1 = $ OH; $R^2 = $ H

(**20**) $R^1 = R^2 = $ OH
(**21**) $R^1 = $ OH; $R^2 = $ H

(**23**) Tazolol

VIII. CARDIOSELECTIVE β-BLOCKADE

Propranolol (**8**) is a lipophilic compound, that is, it has a high partition coefficient, favouring transfer from aqueous to lipid media. This is known to facilitate transfer across the blood–brain barrier and could, perhaps, be part of the reason for the CNS side effects of certain β-blockers. It was felt that these effects could be reduced by making more hydrophilic compounds, and in 1964 the first reports of sotalol (**7**) prompted Crowther, Howe and Smith (*17*) to carry out the synthesis of the oxypropanolamine analogue (**24**). The synthesis of this compound was not trivial, and while this was underway Smith prepared the corresponding acetamido compound from the readily available *para*-acetamido-phenol. This compound, practolol (**25**), was not as potent as propranolol, and in addition it had some isa. The sulphonamide (**24**), prepared very soon afterwards, had similar properties. It was later found that practolol blocked cardiac β-receptors (β_1) without blocking vascular receptors (β_2), that is, it was cardioselective. It was urgently tested against bronchial β-receptors (β_2) and shown to be without effect

(7) Sotalol   (24)   (25) Practolol

here also. The sulphonamide was similarly selective.

Selectivity is usually defined by the ratio

$$\frac{ED_{50} \text{ vasodilation}}{ED_{50} \text{ heart rate}}$$

for antagonism of isoprenaline responses in animals, and by ratios of K_B values for β_1 and β_2 responses *in vitro*. All cardioselective β-blockers have a value for this ratio greater than 1, but it must be emphasised that the compounds are cardioselective not cardiospecific, that is, if enough drug is given (greater than the cardiac $ED_{50} \times$ this selectivity ratio) β_2 effects will be seen.

Practolol has a log P of 0.79 (i.e., a partition coefficient of 6:1 in favour of octanol versus water) compared with propranolol 3.65 (i.e., partition coefficient of 4500:1). It achieved the goal of less CNS side effects, and could be given with greater (though not absolute) safety to asthmatics. It also caused a smaller reduction of cardiac output than propranolol (due to its isa). Practolol, the first cardioselective β-blocker, was launched in 1970 and was used in the treatment of angina, hypertension, and also immediately post-infarction. Unfortunately, after several years of clinical use practolol-related toxicity was recognised in a small percentage of patients receiving the drug. The skin rashes, eye problems (sometimes leading to blindness) and a severe form of peritonitis (fatal in some cases) led to withdrawl of practolol from the market. The reasons for this toxicity are still neither known nor predictable from animal studies, and appear to be unique to practolol.

IX. STRUCTURE–ACTIVITY RELATIONSHIPS OF CARDIOSELECTIVE β-BLOCKERS

The discovery of practolol resulted in widespread chemical activity aimed at introducing other amidic groups into aryloxypropanolamines to achieve a practolol-like profile of activity. The structure–activity relationships described earlier still hold for this type of compound, with one exception: *para*-amidic substituents now give β-blockers which are more potent than their ortho counterparts.

TABLE III
Isomers of Amide-Substituted β-Blockers

(18)

R	Potency[a]	Selectivity	isa[b]
o-NHCOCH$_3$	0.075	−	+
m-NHCOCH$_3$	0.13	−	?
p-NHCOCH$_3$ (practolol)	0.36	+	+

[a] Propranolol = 1.
[b] isa, intrinsic sympathomimetic activity.

Only these para isomers are cardioselective (18) (Table III) and all compounds of this type, like practolol, have isa.

The next development came when Hull and co-workers (19) introduced a methylene group between the amide function and the aromatic ring. The first compound prepared, atenolol [(27), Table IV], was as potent as propranolol, cardioselective, but most surprisingly devoid of isa. It was found subsequently that this was a general phenomenon, and the related p-CH$_2$NHCOR and p-CH$_2$NHCONHR analogues were likewise cardioselective and without isa. Independently Carlsson (20) prepared the para-methoxy ethyl compound, metoprolol (28), and showed that this had the same profile.

The cardioselective β-blockers in clinical use are shown in Table IV. Compounds of all these series are considerably more hydrophilic than propranolol, and one school of thought attributed cardioselectivity to a relatively hydrophilic β$_1$-receptor and a more lipophilic β$_2$-receptor. However, Somerville (21) showed clearly that, in a series of isomeric meta and para compounds, selectivity resided with the para isomer only, although the log P values were identical in each case (Table V).

It is thought that cardioselectivity arises from an additional interaction of a para substituent, possibly via hydrogen bond formation with a complementary site on the β$_1$- but not β$_2$-receptor.

X.   β$_2$-SELECTIVE BLOCKADE

In β-antagonists and -agonists of the ethanolamine series introduction of an alkyl group on the carbon atom α to the amine resulted in an overall reduction in

TABLE IV
Cardioselective β-Blockers in Clinical Use

Structure	Name (manufacturer)	Relative potency[a]	isa[b]
	(25) Practolol (ICI)	0.25	+
	(26) Acebutolol (May & Baker)	0.4	+
	(27) Atenolol (ICI)	0.8	—
	(28) Metoprolol (Hassle)	0.8	—

[a] Propranolol = 1.
[b] isa, intrinsic sympathomimetic activity.

potency. The introduction of this alkyl group gives rise to two isomers, the erythro and threo, and in general the erythro isomers are more potent than the threo. The α-methyl analogue of dichloroisoprenaline (29) was found to block the vascular (β_2) receptors more effectively than the cardiac (β_1) receptors. Other substituted ethanolamines found to be β_2-selective were butoxamine (30) and H35/25 (31). However, they were not very potent and butoxamine exhibited non-specific cardiodepressant activity at doses slightly higher than those necessary for β_2-blockade, and H35/25 had marked β_2-agonist activity.

TABLE V
Cardioselectivity and Hydrophilicity

R	log P	K_D (heart, β_1)	K_D (corpus luteum, β_2)	β_2/β_1
p-NHCOCH$_3$	0.79	5.4×10^{-7}	7.2×10^{-5}	133
m-NHCOCH$_3$	0.74	8.2×10^{-7}	2.4×10^{-6}	2.9
p-CH$_2$CONH$_2$	0.23	3.7×10^{-7}	1.5×10^{-5}	40
m-CH$_2$CONH$_2$	0.22	5.9×10^{-7}	3.2×10^{-7}	0.5
p-CH$_2$NHCOCH$_3$	0.32	2.8×10^{-7}	4.6×10^{-6}	17
m-CH$_2$NHCOCH$_3$	0.34	8.0×10^{-7}	1.2×10^{-6}	1.5

In the aryloxypropanolamines too, α-methyl substitution results in an approximately 10-fold decrease in β-antagonist activity, and in the case of α-methylpropranolol (32) the erythro isomer is more potent than the threo by a factor of 2. *threo*-α-Methylpropranolol has been much studied for its β_2 effects, often with conflicting results largely attributable to the fact that some experiments were carried out *in vitro*, some *in vivo* and often different β-agonists were used. However, like propranolol itself, both erythro and threo α-methyl derivatives of propranolol are β_2-selective.

In 1977 it was reported (22) that the novel fluorene oximinopropanolamine, IPS 339 (33), was a potent β_2-antagonist with a selectivity ratio of 155:1 measured *in vitro* for trachea (β_2) versus atria (β_1) and a ratio of 23:1 *in vivo* in the dog. (Comparative data for butoxamine *in vitro* using the same system was 13:1). Other workers (23) have confirmed the β_2-selectivity of IPS 339 but were unable to confirm the high $\beta_2:\beta_1$ ratios, reporting selectivity ratios as low as 3:1.

O'Donnell (24) has shown that for a series of β_2-antagonists the selectivities observed *in vitro* are critically dependent on the agonist used and has recommended the use of a β_2-agonist to stimulate the β_2 tissue (usually trachea or uterus).

Tucker (25) showed that α-methyl substitution in aryloxypropanolamines does not necessarily confer β_2-activity, the main effects being a considerable reduction in β-antagonist activity. However, in the course of this work a β_2-selective and potent antagonist, ICI 118551 (34), was discovered, which has a β_2-selectivity of between 50 and 120:1 *in vitro* (depending on tissue and agonist used) and >250:1 *in vivo* (26). The corresponding threo analogue is likewise β_2-selective but less so. Clinical trials have confirmed that 118551 is a β_2-antagonist in man and it should be a useful agent for examining the role of β_2-adrenoreceptors in physiological control mechanisms and in disease states.

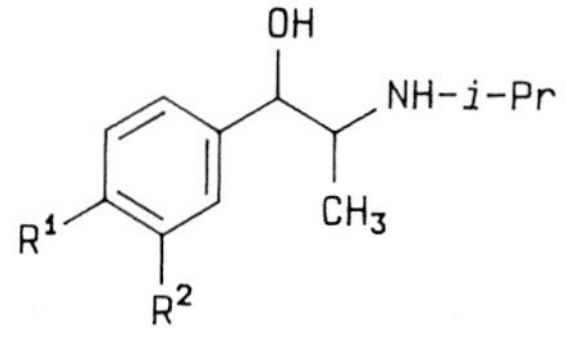

(29) R^1 = R^2 = Cl
(31) R^1 = CH$_3$; R^2 = H; H35/25

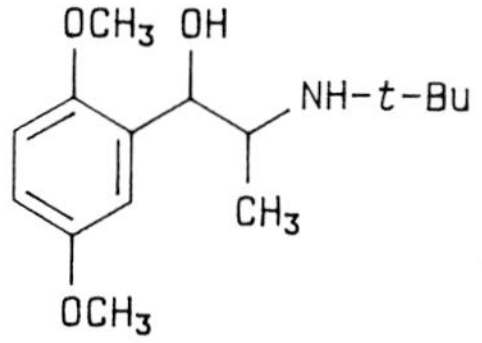

(30) Butoxamine

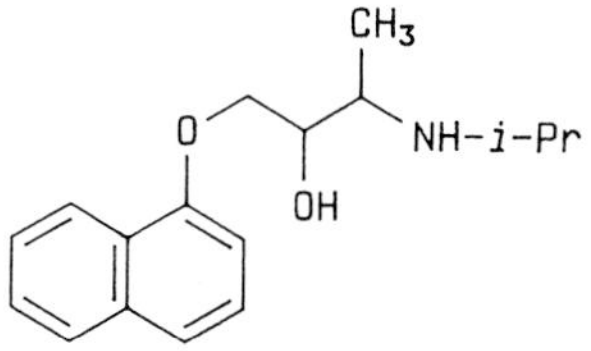

(32)

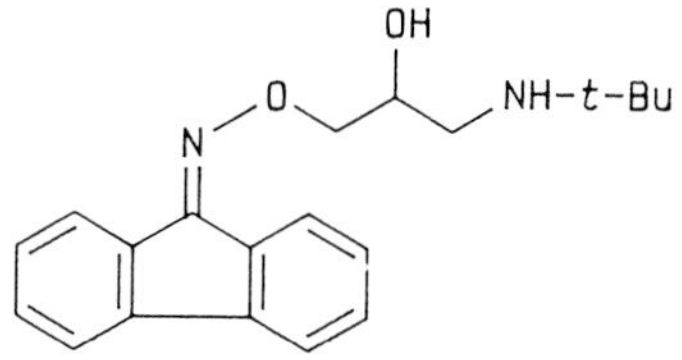

(33) IPS 339

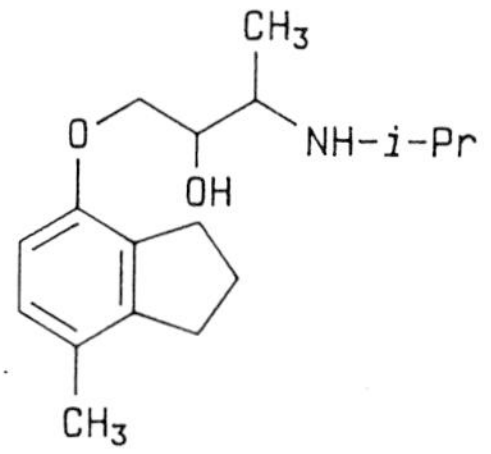

(34) ICI 118551 erythro

XI. "THIRD GENERATION" β-BLOCKERS

Early work on β-blockers had established that optimum potency resided with the isopropyl- or *t*-butylamino substituents, as compounds listed in Tables I and IV demonstrate. Hoefle (*27*), however, reported, on the basis of *in vitro* experiments, that compounds (e.g., **35**) containing the 3,4-dimethoxyphenethylamino group were cardioselective. Augstein's group (*28*) had reported previously that tolamolol (**36**), which contains an amide-substituted phenoxyethylamino group, was cardioselective, and suggested that this might be due to hydrogen bonding of the amide to the receptor. Smith and Tucker (*29*) showed that compounds containing non-amidic phenoxy- and thiophenoxy-substituted amine groups were also cardioselective, as were simple alkoxy- and alkylthio-ethylamine analogues (**37**) (*30*). This led them to conclude that there was an additional interaction at this part of the molecule with the β$_1$-receptor.

Smith (*31*) followed up this work with an extensive series of compounds in

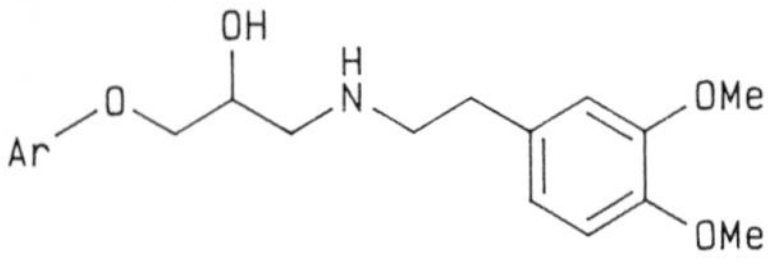

(35)

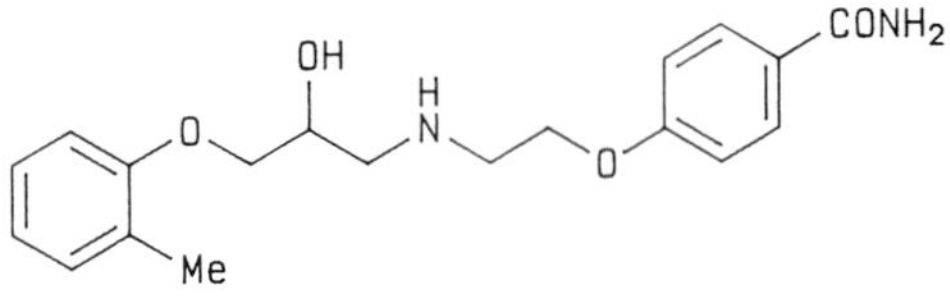

(36) Tolamolol

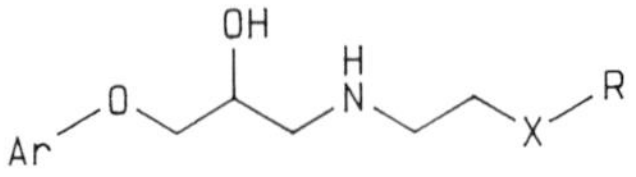

(37) X = O, S
      R = aryl, alkyl

      X = —NHSO$_2$—
          —CONH—   ⎫ increasing
          —NHCO—   ⎬ selectivity
          —NHCONH—   ⎭

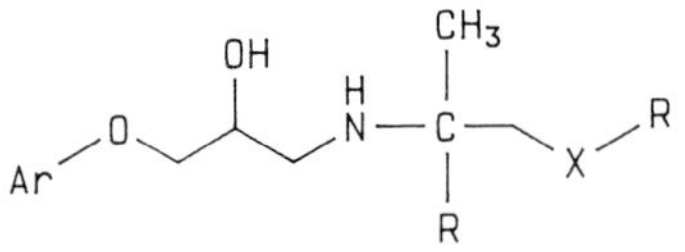

(38)

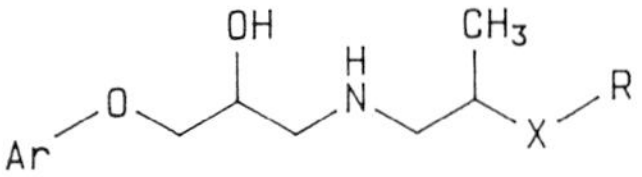

(39)

R = H or CH$_3$

which the (thio) ether group, X in (37), was replaced by a variety of amidic alternatives. These compounds proved to be both potent and cardioselective and strongly suggested a specific drug–receptor interaction at the amide site. The group R may be varied widely without losing activity, but the length of the alkylene chain is critical; thus extension to —NH(CH$_2$)$_3$—X—R caused a reduction in potency, and branching of the chain, as in compounds 38, tends to lessen cardio-selectivity. (Note: For 38, R = H also gives rise to inconvenient diastereoisomers.) Branching adjacent to the amide, as in compound 39, also reduced activity. It is important to note that, in this type of compound, amide substitution of the aryl ring (i.e., practolol-like compounds) either is unnecessary for cardioselectivity or actually decreases potency.

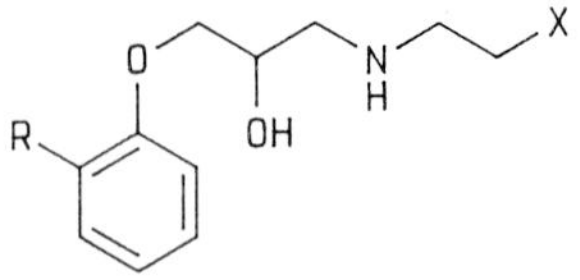

(40) ICI 89406   R = CN;   X = —NHCONHPh

(**41**)   ICI 141292   R = CN;   X = —NHCOCH₂ —⟨benzene ring⟩— OH

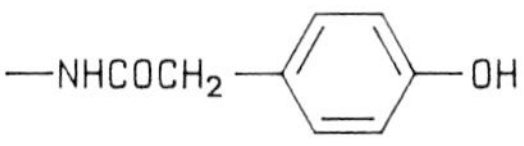

(**42**)   Primidolol   R = CH₃;   X = —N ⟨pyrimidinedione ring with Me⟩

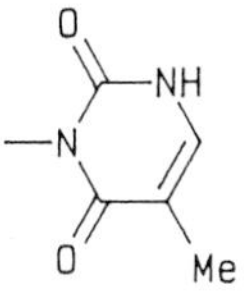

Several cardioselective agents have been selected from this class of compound for clinical study, for example, ICI 89406 (**40**), ICI 141292 (**41**) and Pfizer's primidolol (**42**).

XII.   CHEMISTRY OF β-BLOCKERS

β-Blockers of the ethanolamine series are prepared by the routes described earlier for the synthesis of arylethanolamine β-agonists. β-Blockers of the aryloxypropanolamine series are commonly prepared by base-promoted reaction of the corresponding phenol with epichlorohydrin which, depending on the reaction conditions employed, can give either the epoxide (**43**) or chlorohydrin (**44**) or mixtures of both which are then reacted with the appropriate amine (Scheme 1). The production of side products such as the bis-ether (**45**) and the tertiary

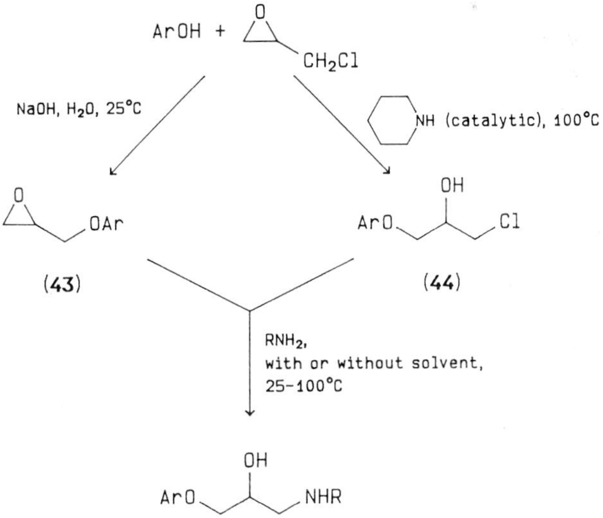

ArOH + ⟨epoxide⟩ CH₂Cl

NaOH, H₂O, 25°C   ⟨ring⟩NH (catalytic), 100°C

⟨epoxide⟩ OAr   OH
                                   ArO. CHCH₂ .Cl

(**43**)   (**44**)

RNH₂,
with or without solvent,
25–100°C

OH
ArO. CHCH₂ .NHR

Scheme 1   Synthesis of aryloxypropanolamines.

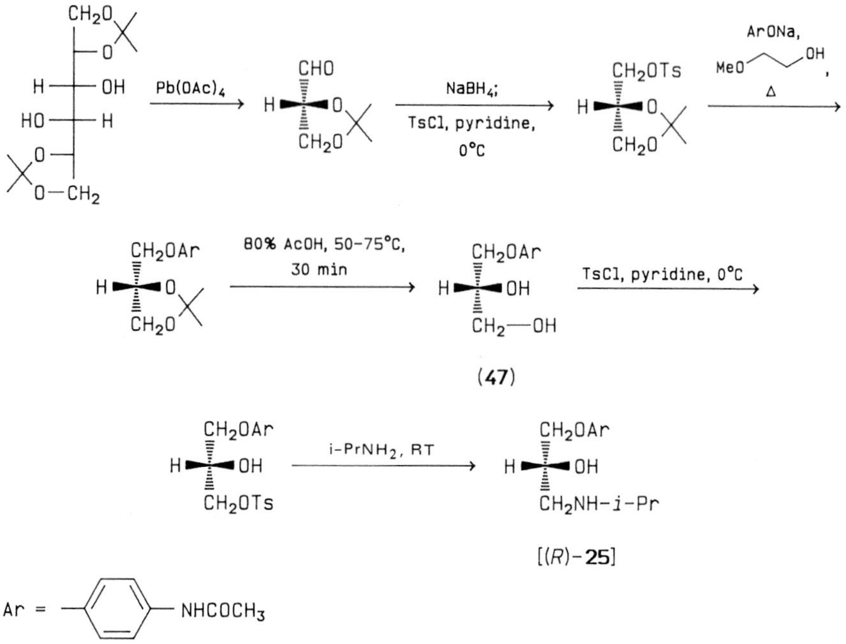

Ts = *p*-toluenesulphonyl

Scheme 2 Preparation of (*R*)-practolol.

amine (**46**) can be minimised by using an excess of epichlorohydrin and amine, respectively.

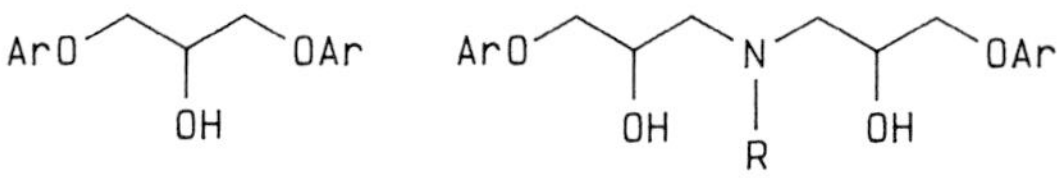

(**45**) (**46**)

The β-antagonist activity of the aryloxypropanolamines resides with one enantiomer which was shown in the case of propranolol to have the (*S*) absolute configuration by relating (+)-propranolol to (+)-lactic acid (*32*). The normal resolution techniques using optically active acids were found to be time-consuming and unpredictable, and much effort has been devoted to devising a general asymmetric synthetic route which would furnish both enantiomers reliably. In the first of these approaches a Pfizer group (*33*) prepared the (*R*) (less active) enantiomer of practolol from D-mannitol using the route outlined in Scheme 2. Success of this route was critically dependent on cleanly monotosylating the primary hydroxyl group of diol (**47**). The synthesis of the more active (*S*) enan-

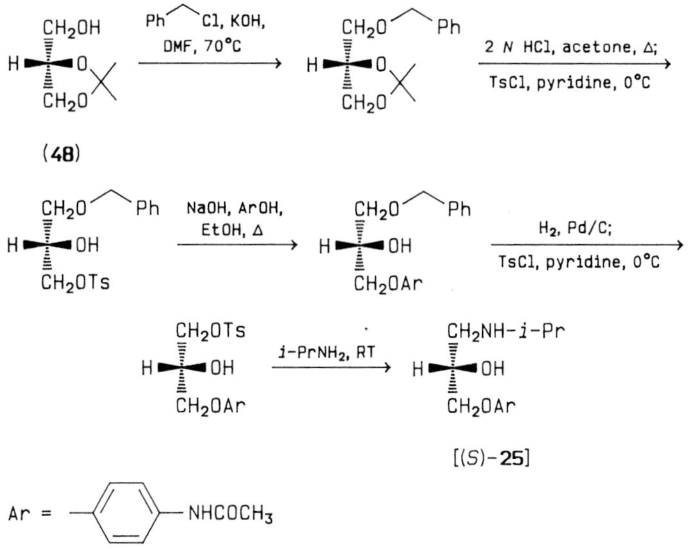

Scheme 3 Synthesis of (S)-practolol.

tiomer using an analogous route was not attractive because L-mannitol is not readily available.

The glycerol acetonide route, however, has been refined to enable the (S) enantiomer to be prepared (*34*). This involved protecting the primary hydroxy group of the glycerol acetonide (48), removing the acetonide moiety and selectively monotosylating the newly unmasked primary hydroxy group so that attack by the phenolate now occurs at the opposite end of the three-carbon unit. Debenzylation, selective tosylation (or mesylation) followed by reaction with the amine yields the corresponding (S) enantiomer (Scheme 3).

Starting from the same chiral three-carbon unit, (S)-glycerol acetonide (48), workers at Merck, Sharp & Dohme (*35*) have devised an elegant route to both (R)- and (S)-epichlorohydrin (49) (Scheme 4). In the course of this work they were able to elucidate the course of the reaction of phenols with epichlorohydrin. In principle there are two possible modes of attack by phenoxide ion: (a) direct S_N2 attack with displacement of the chlorine atom or (b) nucleophilic attack on the epoxide carbon atom followed by S_N2 attack of the alkoxide anion so formed on the primary alkyl chloride with elimination of chloride. Using an optically active epichlorohydrin should differentiate between these two mechanisms; path (a) should result in retention of configuration and path (b) in inversion of configuration (Scheme 5).

Under a variety of conditions, phenol reacted with (S)-epichlorohydrin (49) to give predominantly the (R) epoxide (50), i.e., inversion of configuration, path

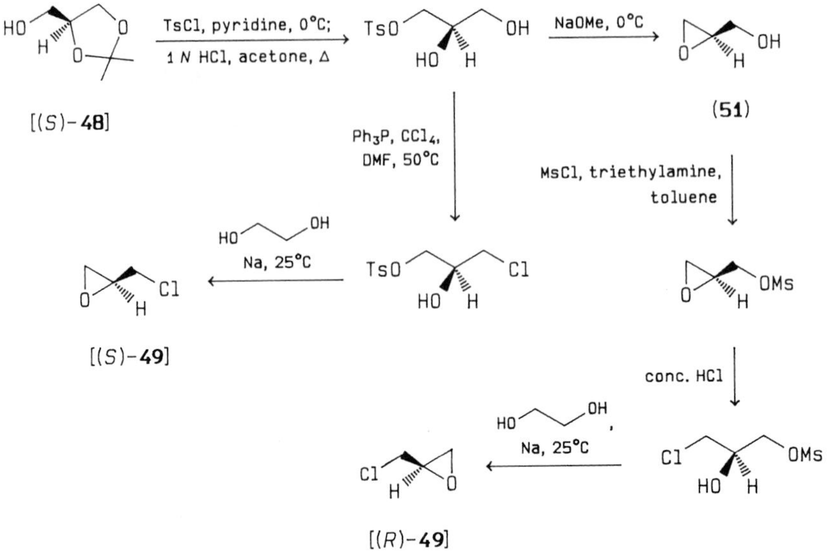

Ts = p-toluenesulphonyl
Ms = methanesulphonyl

Scheme 4   Synthesis of (R)- and (S)-epichlorohydrin.

(b). It was also discovered that for the preparation of the (S) enantiomers, synthesis of (R)-epichlorohydrin was unnecessary since the epoxy alcohol (51) could be converted into the corresponding triflate ester (52) which reacted with phenols by direct nucleophilic displacement of triflate anion, that is, pathway (a) (36).

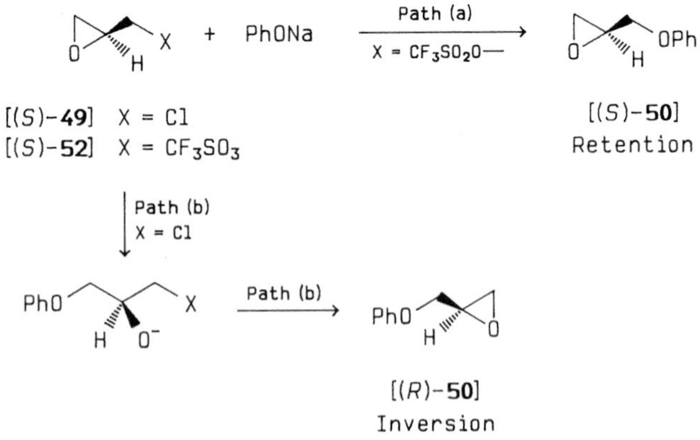

Scheme 5   Reaction of epihalohydrins with phenols.

XIII.   CLINICAL EFFECTS OF β-BLOCKERS

Black's original postulate that β-blockers would alleviate angina and control catecholamine-elicited arrhythmias was rapidly justified. Early observations that these agents would lower blood pressure were very unexpected, and in fact hypertension is now the main area of use. β-Blockers are used in a number of disease states in which raised sympathetic amine levels a e implicated. A discussion of these states follows.

Thyrotoxicosis.   An enlargement of the thyroid gland (due to iodine deficiency) causing palpitations and tremor due to over-production of catecholamines.

Phaeochromacytoma.   A tumour of the adrenal gland causing over-production of adrenaline.

Tremor.   Physiological tremor of the skeletal muscles may be due to the effects of an over-active sympathetic nervous system. It is readily treated by β-blockers (β_2-response). Perhaps related (though totally unexpected) is the ability of β-blockers to alleviate the trauma of alcohol and drug withdrawal, and also relieve the stress associated with examinations, race car driving, orchestral playing, public speaking etc., all of which are due to an inappropriate level of sympathetic activity.

Other indications for β-blockers where there is less obvious adrenergic involvement are as follows.

Glaucoma.   An eye disease characterised by an increase in intraocular pressure, and causing headache, visual disturbance and eventually blindness. It is effectively controlled by some β-blockers, and timolol (**16**), in particular, is widely used. The exact mechanism by which β-blockers control this disease is not yet known.

Anxiety.   Propranolol (**8**) is active in this condition, presumably because the peripheral (cardiac, tremor) symptoms are known to be mediated by the sympathetic nervous system. Whether propranolol has an action in the central nervous system as well is still debated.

Migraine.   Propranolol is used in the prophylaxis of migraine. The mode of action is not known, and the type of receptor has not yet been identified in this important area.

Myocardial Infarction ("Heart Attack").   Recent trials (*37*) have shown that some β-blockers are effective in preventing re-infarction in patients who have suffered heart attacks, for example, propranolol, timolol, oxprenolol (**13**). If these results are confirmed then β-blockers may become the first line of treatment for heart attack victims.

XIV. SIDE EFFECTS OF β-BLOCKERS

In common with all other classes of drugs β-blockers have side effects, the most important of which are as follows.

Bronchoconstriction in Asthmatics.   Asthmatic patients require continuous beta (β$_2$) stimulation to keep their bronchi dilated. β-Blockers, by preventing this bronchodilation, can cause (potentially fatal) bronchoconstriction in some sensitive patients.

Tiredness of the Limbs.   This is due to the reduction in cardiac output and is common to all β-blockers.

Effects on the Central Nervous System.   Dizziness, vivid dreams and sedation have been noted with β-blockers and are particularly common in those with a high partition coefficient [propranolol (**8**), pindolol (**14**), oxprenolol (**13**) etc.].

Heart Failure/Bradycardia.   All β-blockers produce a fall in resting heart rate (bradycardia) due to blockade of on-going sympathetic activity. Patients on the verge of heart failure are very dependent on the sympathetic nervous system, hence β-blockade may well push them into overt heart failure. Some authorities feel that drugs having isa will cause fewer problems as less sympathetic activity will be removed.

XV. CONCLUSION

The concept of β-adrenergic blockade was pioneered in the early 1960s. From modest beginnings in the treatment of angina pectoris, the clinical utility of this class of compound has progressed steadily to the present, where diverse disease states such as hypertension, anxiety and migraine are routinely treated with β-blockers. At present estimated world sales of β-blockers are approaching £1000 million, nearly two thousand patents have been filed, and approximately 20 major products are marketed. A figure of 100,000 might be a reasonable estimate of the number of compounds synthesised to get to the present position in this field of research.

REFERENCES

1. H. Konzett, *Arch. Exp. Pathol. Pharmakol.* **197**, 27 (1940).
2. R. P. Ahlquist, *Am. J. Physiol.* **153**, 586 (1948).
3. J. P. Arnold, T. G. Brown, A. M. Lands, F. P. Luduena, and J. P. McAuliff, *Nature (London)* **214**, 597 (1967).
4. K. Dickinson, S. R. Nahorski, and A. Richardson, *Mol. Pharmacol.* **19**, 194 (1981).
5. A. Levitzki *in* "Topics in Molecular Pharmacology" (A. S. V. Burgen and G. C. K. Roberts, eds), Vol. 1, p. 23. Elsevier, Amsterdam, 1981.
6. C. E. Powell and I. H. Slater, *J. Pharmacol. Exp. Ther.* **122**, 480 (1958).
7. N. C. Moran and M. E. Perkins, *J. Pharmacol. Exp. Ther.* **124**, 223 (1958).
8. J. W. Black and J. S. Stephenson, *Lancet* **2**, 311 (1962).
9. D. K. Phillips, *Handb. Exp. Pharmacol.* **54**, 3 (1980).
10. A. F. Crowther and L. H. Smith, *J. Med. Chem.* **11**, 1009 (1968).
11. V. Petrow, O. Stephenson, and A. J. Thomas, *J. Pharm. Pharmacol.* **8**, 666 (1956).
12. H. Grobecker, D. Hellenbrecht, and K.-F. Muller, *Eur. J. Pharmacol.* **29**, 223 (1974).
13. R. Clarkson, C. R. Ganellin, and W. G. Richards, *Philos. Trans. Roy. Soc. (London), Ser. B* **272**, 75 (1975).
14. B. G. Main, *J. Chem. Technol. Biotechnol.* **32**, 617 (1982).
15. W. D. Bowen, D. F. Colella, E. Garvey, T. Jen, C. Kaiser, and J. R. Wardell, *J. Med. Chem.* **20**, 687 (1977).
16. E. Carlsson, C-G. Dahloff, and A. Hedberg, *Naunyn-Schmiedebergs Arch. Pharmacol.* **300**, 101 (1977).
17. A. F. Crowther, R. Howe, and L. H. Smith, *J. Med. Chem.* **14**, 511 (1971).
18. L. H. Smith, *J. Appl. Chem. Biotechnol.* **28**, 201 (1978).
19. A. M. Barrett, J. Carter, R. Hull, and D. J. Le Count, *Br. J. Pharmacol.* **48**, 340P (1973).
20. B. Ablad, E. Carlsson, and L. Ek, *Life Sci.* **12**, 107 (1973).
21. A. J. Coleman, D. S. Paterson, and A. R. Somerville, *Biochem. Pharmacol.* **28**, 1011 (1979).
22. N. Bieth, G. LeClerc, A. Mann, J. Schwartz, and C-G. Wermuth, *J. Med. Chem.* **20**, 1657 (1977).
23. J. J. Baldwin, D. M. Gross, D. E. McLure, and M. Williams, *J. Med. Chem.* **25**, 931 (1982).
24. S. R. O'Donnell and J. C. Wanstall, *Nauyn-Schmiedebergs Arch. Pharmacol.* **308**, 183 (1979).
25. H. Tucker, *J. Med. Chem.* **24**, 1364 (1981).
26. A. J. Bilski, J. D. Fitzgerald, S. E. Halliday, and J. L. Wale, *J. Cardiovasc. Pharmacol.* **5**, 430 (1983).
27. R. M. Corey, S. G. Hastings, M. L. Hoefle, A. Holmes, R. F. Meyer, and C. D. Stratton, *J. Med. Chem.* **18**, 148 (1975).
28. J. Augstein, D. A. Cox, A. L. Ham, P. R. Leeming, and M. Sanrey, *J. Med. Chem.* **16**, 1245 (1973).
29. L. H. Smith and H. Tucker, *J. Med. Chem.* **20**, 1653 (1977).
30. J. F. Coope and H. Tucker, *J. Med. Chem.* **21**, 769 (1978).
31. M. S. Large and L. H. Smith, *J. Med. Chem.* **25**, 1286 (1982).
32. M. Dukes and L. H. Smith, *J. Med. Chem.* **14**, 326 (1971).
33. J. C. Danilewicz and J. E. G. Kemp, *J. Med. Chem.* **16**, 168 (1973).
34. W. L. Nelson, S. R. Sankar, and J. E. Wennerstrom, *J. Org. Chem.* **42**, 1006 (1977).
35. B. H. Arison, J. J. Baldwin, D. E. McClure, K. Menster, and A. W. Raab, *J. Org. Chem.* **43**, 4876 (1978).
36. B. H. Arison, J. J. Baldwin, and D. E. McClure, *J. Am. Chem. Soc.* **101**, 3668 (1979).
37. E. Braunwald and Z. G. Turi, *JAMA, J. Am. Med. Assoc.* **249**, 2512 (1983).

REVIEWS

PHARMACOLOGICAL ASPECTS

A. M. Barrett *in* "Drug Design" Vol. 111, (E. J. Ariens, ed.), p. 205. New York, London: Academic Press 1972.

CLINICAL ASPECTS

D. F. Weetman, *Drugs Today,* **13,** 261 (1977).
G. M. Lees, *Br. Med. J.,* **283,** 173 (1981).

STRUCTURE–ACTIVITY RELATIONSHIPS

See Ref. 9.

BIOCHEMICAL ASPECTS

See Ref. 5.
D. J. Triggle in "Burger's Medicinal Chemistry" 4th Edition, (M. E. Wolff, ed.), Part III, p. 225. Wiley, New York, 1981.

Discovery of Cimetidine

C. R. GANELLIN
Smith Kline & French Research Ltd.
Welwyn, England

I. BACKGROUND RATIONALE

A. PEPTIC ULCER DISEASE

Duodenal and gastric ulcers (collectively known as peptic ulcers) affect large numbers of people who are otherwise relatively fit. Peptic ulceration is the most common disease of the gastro-intestinal tract and it is estimated that approximately 10–20% of the adult male population in Western countries will experience a peptic ulcer at some time in their lives. It produces considerable illness and pain, and results in great economic loss to the patients and their communities; it can even be fatal. In 1970, for example, in the United States there were some 3.5 million peptic ulcer sufferers and 8600 deaths were attributed to this disease.

Duodenal and gastric ulcers are localised erosions of the mucous membrane of the duodenum or stomach, respectively, which expose the underlying layers of the gut wall to the acid secretions of the stomach and to the proteolytic enzyme pepsin. What causes acute peptic ulcer is still not properly understood but for many years the main medical treatment has been aimed at reducing acid production, based on the hope that neutralising gastric acid will reduce its irritating effects and also reduce the efficacy of pepsin, and so allow ulcers to heal.

The stomach contains many different types of highly specialised secretory cells controlled by the nervous system and hormones. For example, the parietal cells secrete hydrochloric acid. Prior to and during a meal, the volume of acid, pepsin, and mucus secretion increases to as much as 10 times the basal secretion rate, and the pH may fall to 1–2.

B.   Chemical Messengers

Secretion of gastric acid is initiated by the thought, sight, smell, or taste of food and is mediated by the autonomic nervous system via the vagus nerves which provide parasympathetic innervation to the stomach and small intestine (Fig. 1); the neurotransmitter released by stimulation of the vagus is acetylcholine (Fig. 11, Chap. 1).

Branches of the vagus, innervating the antral region of the stomach, stimulate the release of the peptide hormone gastrin from special gastrin-producing "G" cells. The presence of food in the stomach further stimulates release of gastrin,

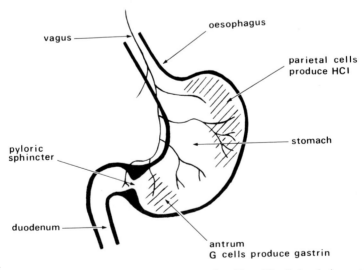

Fig. 1   Diagram of the stomach showing vagus nerve and position of G cells (producing gastrin) and parietal cells (producing HCl).

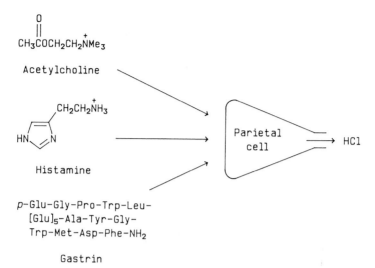

Fig. 2   Three chemical messengers stimulate the production of hydrochloric acid from the gastric parietal cell. The formulae show acetylcholine cation, histamine monocation (the most prevalent species at physiological pH of 7.4), and human gastrin I.

which passes into the blood stream and is carried to the parietal cells where it acts to stimulate them to secrete hydrochloric acid.

In addition to acetylcholine and gastrin, a third chemical secretagogue, histamine, is known to be involved (Fig. 2). As long ago as 1920, histamine was shown to stimulate gastric acid secretion when injected into the dog; subsequently it was found to be a natural constituent of the stomach lining and this led inevitably to the suggestion that it was involved in the physiological process of gastric secretion.

The presence of a hormone which stimulated secretion of gastric acid was inferred in 1905 by Edkins, who gave it the name gastrin, but the discovery by Popielski in 1920 that histamine was a potent stimulator of acid secretion led many to conclude that Edkins's gastrin and histamine were the same. It was not until 1938 that Komarov, working on the assumption that gastrin was a peptide, used chemical means to separate it from histamine.

The relationship between the three secretagogues acetylcholine, gastrin, and histamine has been a source of considerable controversy among physiologists for many years. When it was found (in the late 1940s and early 1950s) that the antihistamine drugs did not reduce acid secretion, the role of histamine was placed in serious question. By 1964, when gastrin had been isolated and sequenced at Liverpool University, most gastric physiologists were convinced that gastrin played the key role in the physiological control of gastric acid and considered histamine to be unimportant.

C.   Controlling Gastric Acid

For many years the main medical treatment for peptic ulcers relied on the use of antacids to neutralise the gastric acid; these come in various forms, for example, magnesium trisilicate, aluminium hydroxide, sodium bicarbonate, calcium carbonate. All, however, when taken in sufficient quantities may cause unpleasant side effects. For real neutralisation, very large quantities are required; for example, it has been calculated that 60 g of sodium bicarbonate daily would be required by intragastric drip to keep the pH of the stomach contents at 4.0 in patients with gastric ulceration.

Anticholinergic drugs (to block the acetylcholine transmission) can decrease gastric acid secretion, but their use in the treatment of peptic ulceration is limited by two factors: first, a dose high enough to decrease gastric acid secretion also blocks the action of acetylcholine at other receptor sites (Fig. 11, Chap. 1) and so causes "side effects" such as dryness of the mouth, urinary retention, and blurred vision; secondly, some of these drugs are quaternary ammonium salts and are poorly absorbed on oral administration so that patients may fail to receive an effective dose.

The alternative to drug treatment is surgery. This aims to cut out part of the acid secretory and gastrin producing regions of the stomach (e.g., partial gastrectomy) or to selectively cut the branches of the vagal nerve (e.g., selective vagotomy) that supply the acid-secretory region. This is a difficult and sometimes dangerous operation.

D.   The Search for New Anti-ulcer Drugs

With this background to treatment it is not surprising that most major pharmaceutical companies set up research programmes aimed at discovering anti-ulcer agents. For many years the main approach was to induce ulcer formation in rats, or to stimulate production of gastric acid in rats, and to screen compounds for their ability to protect against ulcer formation or to inhibit acid production. The record of success was pretty poor. One of the main problems is that acid secretion is a very active metabolic process which is easy to inhibit with metabolic poisons or via actions which reduce the metabolism but are not selective. Thus many agents were found to be active in laboratory animals but very few survived initial human trials.

In the 1960s, with increasing understanding of the physiology of gastric acid secretion, several companies established research programmes to discover specific inhibitors of the action of the chemical messengers. In the United Kingdom, ICI Pharmaceuticals initiated a search for a gastrin antagonist, and Pfizer and Smith Kline & French independently sought a histamine antagonist.

The idea that hormones and transmitter substances act at specific sites that we call receptors has been extremely valuable in the development of new drugs. These substances have a chemical individuality that is specifically recognised at the receptor sites; that is, the sites discriminate among different neurotransmitters, autocoids and hormones. This chemical control is a highly selective process. It follows that the design of compounds to act in competition with the natural substance for occupation of these sites is a potential way of attaining specificity of drug action. It also appears that the receptor sites for a particular chemical messenger are not necessarily homogeneous. Drugs have been discovered that appear to differentiate among sites for the same agonist, suggesting different populations of drug receptors. This allows further scope for introducing selectivity of drug action.

The two secretagogues, gastrin and histamine, therefore presented alternative targets for inhibiting acid production. If one of them has a controlling influence on acid secretion then blocking it might succeed in controlling acidity, but since blocking one site still leaves two others to act it is by no means certain that such an approach will be successful. Furthermore, as with acetylcholine, gastrin and histamine have other actions, and an agent that blocks their effects on acid stimulation may also block other sites leading to unacceptable side effects (as with the anticholinergics).

Thus, it can be appreciated that such an approach to drug discovery is highly speculative, and one certainly has no reason to presume that it will be successful in providing a new therapy. On the other hand it does have a scientific rationale founded on some working hypotheses which are capable of investigation and being put to the test. An important part of this analysis is provided by the pharmacologist's view of drug receptors.

E. HISTAMINE RECEPTORS

Histamine [2-(imidazol-4-yl)ethylamine] appears to be a locally acting transmitter substance that has very specific actions. In 1910 Dale and Laidlaw, working at the Wellcome Physiological Research Laboratories in London, published the first of a series of papers describing the pharmacological effects of histamine; in particular, they noted the powerful effect of histamine in stimulating contractions of smooth muscle and its potent action in lowering blood pressure (*1*).

The early studies on histamine indicated a similarity in some of its effects with the symptoms that appear during inflammation, and with symptoms characteristic of shock produced by trauma or allergic reactions. It became widely assumed that histamine was a principle mediator of inflammation and shock and this stimulated a search by Bovet in Paris for substances capable of counteracting these apparent injurious effects (2). His findings led to the development of the antihistamine drugs in the 1940s and to their introduction for the treatment of allergic conditions such as urticaria and hay fever.

(1) Mepyramine   (2) Diphenhydramine

Two typical antihistamine drugs, mepyramine (**1**) [Neoantergan (Rhone-Poulenc)] and diphenhydramine (**2**) [Benadryl (Parke-Davis)] were shown to be specific in antagonising histamine-stimulated contractions of the isolated ileum of the guinea-pig relative to other stimulants; they were effective at low concentrations and the antagonism they produced was surmountable and reversible. These antagonists came to be regarded as acting in competition with histamine for occupation of its specific receptor sites. Subsequently, they were also shown to antagonise actions of histamine on the vascular system, namely, the histamine-induced increase in capillary permeability and certain vasoconstrictor actions; however, it was also found that these antagonists reduced the intensity of, but did not abolish, vasodilator actions, and in 1948 it was suggested by Folkow, Haeger and Kahlson that there may be ''two types of receptor sensitive to histamine only one of which can be blocked by Benadryl and related compounds'' (3).

These antihistamines were used to compare receptors in different tissues and species; for example, mepyramine had similar antagonist potency when tested against histamine on the perfused lung of the guinea-pig, on the isolated ileum and the trachea of the guinea-pig, and on human bronchi. The results indicated a homogeneity for the histamine receptors in these tissues.

Several actions of histamine had been noted that could not be specifically antagonised by these drugs: for example, stimulation of gastric acid secretion in the rat, cat, or dog; stimulation of isolated atria of the guinea-pig; inhibition of rat uterus contractions; and the vasodilator effects of large doses of histamine.

Some pointers to the differentiation of histamine receptors had been obtained by considering the selectivity of action of agonists on different tissue systems. For example, Ash and Schild made quantitative estimates of the relative activities of different histamine congeners on the isolated guinea-pig ileum, on the isolated rat uterus, and in vivo as stimulants of rat gastric acid secretion; they obtained a correlation in activity ratios suggesting that the same type of receptor might be involved in rat gastric acid secretion and inhibition of contraction of rat uterus (*4*).

Such considerations led Ash and Schild to propose in 1966 that the actions of histamine blocked by the antihistamine drugs characterised one type of histamine receptor, which they named the H_1-receptor. They suggested that other actions of histamine not specifically antagonised were probably mediated by other histamine receptors, but the characterisation of these receptors awaited the discovery of specific antagonists; in the meantime they were to be regarded as non-H_1.

II. THE SEARCH FOR A HISTAMINE ANTAGONIST

A. THE BIOLOGICAL APPROACH

The inability of the antihistamine drugs (H_1-receptor antagonists) to inhibit histamine-stimulated gastric acid secretion has been known for many years and there have been a few published reports of efforts to discover a specific antagonist to this action of histamine. In the 1950s in collaboration with the Eli Lilly Company in the United States, Grossman reported on an extensive study of compounds, chemically related to histamine, that were examined for their action on acid secretion and also tested as possible inhibitors of histamine stimulation, but Grossman did not uncover a histamine antagonist (*5*).

A similar analysis by Dr. J. W. (now Sir James) Black led him to establish at the Smith Kline & French Research Laboratories in Welwyn Garden City, in 1964, the test procedures needed to detect antagonists of these other effects of histamine. It was hoped that the work would lead to a new type of pharmacological agent with possible clinical utility. It was argued that at the very least, such an agent ought to provide a valuable scientific tool that would assist investigation of the physiological role of histamine. But the prize, seen at the outset, was a possible means for selective pharmacological control of gastric acid secretion with the potential for treating peptic ulcer disease.

Compounds were tested for ability to inhibit histamine-stimulated gastric acid secretion in anaesthetised rats. Routinely, the stomach of an anaesthetised rat [starved and pretreated with atropine (anticholinergic) and urethane (as anaesthetic)] was perfused with glucose solution at 37°C. The perfusate was introduced via a tube placed in the oesophagus and collected via a funnel placed in the non-secretory lumen of the stomach; the perfusate was then passed through a micro-flow type glass electrode system and changes in gastric pH were recorded continuously on a potentiometric pen recorder.

Initially, compounds were administered as a constant intravenous infusion in the middle of a series of fixed-dose histamine responses (given by rapid intravenous injection). Subsequently, the system was modified and a plateau of gastric acid secretion was established by continuous intravenous infusion of histamine (at a dose high enough to produce a near maximal response) and potential inhibitors were then given by rapid intravenous injection. Since other types of inhibitors of gastric secretion could also be picked up by this test, compounds found to be active were also tested on isolated tissue systems to provide additional criteria for specific antagonism to histamine.

Two *in vitro* test systems were set up, namely, histamine-induced stimulation of the guinea-pig right atrium (which continues to beat spontaneously *in vitro* because it contains the pacemaker and histamine increases the rate of beating) and inhibition by histamine of evoked contractions of the rat uterus.

It is worth reiterating that the atmosphere prevailing in gastroenterological science at that time was far from conducive to the search for a histamine antagonist as a means of controlling gastric acid secretion. In the 1960s many researchers turned their attention to seeking specific inhibitors of gastrin-induced acid secretion. The import of histamine was difficult to prove and there was a widely held view that histamine had no place in the physiological maintenance of gastric acid secretion. The concerted but unsuccessful effort by researchers at Eli Lilly in the 1950s to find an antagonist of histamine-stimulated acid secretion added further to the general feeling that the approach was "played out". However, there were still some adherents to the view that histamine played a key role in gastric acid secretion, although they were very much in a minority.

B.   THE CHEMICAL APPROACH TO AN ANTAGONIST

Once the problem of obtaining a competitive antagonist was posed in biological terms it was necessary to then consider how to approach it chemically. How could one obtain such a compound? Where should one start, given no obvious "lead" compound? Nothing was known chemically about the physiological site of action of histamine.

Returning to first principles, the structure of histamine (Fig. 2) was used as a chemical starting point. The simple-minded view was taken that since the search was for a molecule that would compete with histamine for its receptor site, such a molecule would have to be recognised by the receptor and then bind more strongly than histamine, but not trigger the usual response. It therefore seemed worthwhile to retain in potential antagonist structures some chemical features of histamine to aid receptor recognition, and to include chemical groups that might assist binding.

Many different approaches were tried, including the use of analogies derived from known examples of chemical–biological relationships between other types of receptor agonists and antagonists, or enzyme substrates and inhibitors, or antimetabolites. The structure of histamine was modified to deliberately alter its chemical properties, while retaining some definite aspect of its structure or chemistry. Some examples have been discussed elsewhere by Ganellin *et al.* (6).

Many compounds were made, based on the structure of histamine. In the first 4 years some 200 compounds were synthesised and tested, without providing a blocking drug. The problem for the chemist is that there are too many possible compounds for synthesis. Even small modifications of the natural stimulant histamine introduce many variables.

Towards the end of this time many doubts were expressed about whether it really would prove possible to block the action of histamine on gastric acid secretion and, indeed, there was considerable pressure within the company to abandon the project. The scientists involved in the project were, however, firmly resolved to continue, and during this period the test system was refined and chemical ideas began to crystallise.

A most important aspect of research is to conduct the work in such a way as to learn from negative results. Even a list of inactive compounds is informative if they have been selected for particular reasons. Having tested many compounds

TABLE I

Structure and Antagonist Activities[a]
of Some Simple Imidazolylalkylisothioureas,
-Guanidines, and -Amidines

Number	n	Substituent	Activity[a]
3	2	X = NH	+
4	2	X = S	+ +
5	3	X = NH	+ + +
6	3	X = S	±
7	2	Z = SMe	±
8	2	Z = Me	±
9	3	Z = SMe	+ + +
10	3	Z = Me	+ + +

[a] Tested for inhibition of histamine-stimulated gastric acid secretion in the lumen-perfused anaesthetised rat. Results represented semiquantitively as: ±, detectable; +, $ID_{50} > 500$ μmol/kg; + +, $ID_{50} \sim 200$ μmol/kg; + + +, $ID_{50} = 100$–50 μmol/kg. ID_{50} is the intravenous dose which reduces a near maximal secretion to 50%.

with lipophilic substituents without seeing antagonism, the pharmacologists re-examined some of the early hydrophilic compounds, one of which showed some blocking activity. It was very weak but provided the vital lead. It was missed originally because this compound also acted as a stimulant; in fact it is a partial agonist. The compound is a histamine derivative in which a guanidine group replaces the amino group in the side-chain, namely, N^{α}-guanylhistamine (**3**) (Table I). It was selected for synthesis by Dr. Graham Durant based on an analogy with guanidine structures, which have a high affinity for catecholamine storage sites. Ironically, N^{α}-guanylhistamine was first synthesised by van der Merwe in 1928 and was reported to be "devoid of interesting physiological activity." Clearly, biological activity may be present, but its discovery depends on the way one looks for it!

C. DEVELOPMENTS BASED ON THE FIRST LEAD COMPOUNDS

The appearance of antagonism, albeit weak, provided a much needed lead and within a few days an analogous compound was retested and found to be more active, namely, (*S*)-[2-(imidazol-4-yl)ethyl]-isothiourea (**4**) (Table I). However, a much more active compound was required.

An immediate question to be answered was whether activity was due to the presence of the guanidine or isothiourea groups (amidines) *per se* or to the structural resemblance to histamine. Structure–activity studies suggested that for these structures the imidazole ring was important; antagonism did not appear to be a property of amidines in general. It was also necessary to identify the particular chemical properties that conferred antagonist activity in order to make analogues of increased potency.

The amidine groups are strong bases and are protonated and positively charged at physiological pH. Thus the molecules resemble histamine monocation, but also differ in several ways; the amidinium group is planar (whereas the ammonium group of histamine is tetrahedral) and the positive charge is distributed over three hetero atoms. It was noted that the distance between ring and terminal nitrogen is potentially greater than in histamine, and that there are several nitrogen sites for potential interactions instead of one, thereby affording more opportunities for intermolecular bonding.

It was envisaged that amidines might act as antagonists through additional binding being contributed by the amidine group. A type of bidentate hydrogen bonding between ion pairs can occur with an amidinium cation and an oxyacid anion, for example, carboxylate, phosphate, or sulphate, which might be part of the receptor protein (see Fig. 3).

Structural variables therefore identified for study initially were the amidine groups, amidino N-substituents, side-chain length, and alternatives to imidazole.

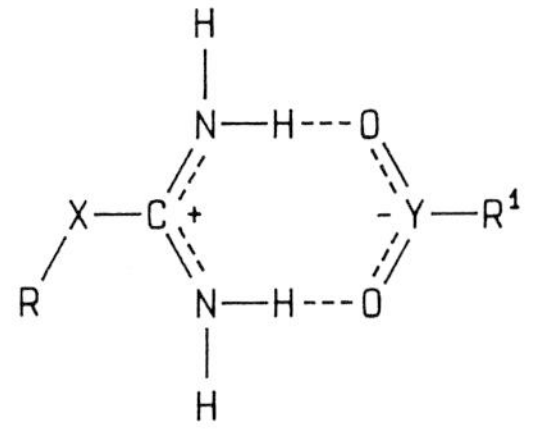

Fig. 3   Bidentate hydrogen-bonding envisaged between ions pairs formed between amidinium cations and oxyacid anions.

Many analogues of compounds **3** and **4** were made but most turned out to be less active; at that time, unsubstituted imidazole appeared to be the best ring; alkyl substitution on the amidine N gave inconsistent results; and lengthening the side chain gave another breakthrough but threw up an apparent contradiction.

For the guanidine structure, increasing the chain length led to a compound (**5**) showing an increase in antagonist activity. However, for the isothiourea, the reverse result was obtained; i.e., increasing the chain length gave a compound (**6**) of reduced antagonist activity (*8*).

Thus, although the first two compounds discovered [guanidine (**3**) and isothiourea (**4**)] appeared to be closely related in structure in simply being isosteric nitrogen and sulphur analogues, the results with the homologues suggested that the situation was more complex. In an attempt to rationalise these differences, various related amidines were examined (Fig. 4). The activities of some of these compounds are expressed semiquantitatively in Table I, reflecting the data available at the time. It was found that the reversed isothioureas (**7, 9**) (side chain on N instead of S) resembled the guanidines in chain-length requirements, as did carboxamidines (e.g., **8** and **10**).

The above results indicated that it was necessary to reappraise the view of amidine interactions. The initial analysis had suggested hydrogen-bonding of the terminal NH groups; in the reversed isothiourea and carboxamidine, hydrogen-bonding would include an NH within the side chain.

The apparent non-additivity between structural change and biological effect posed a typical problem familiar to all practising medicinal chemists: with so many structural variables to study (e.g., ring, side-chain length, amidine system, amidine substituents), there are many thousands of structures incorporating different combinations of these variables, and one cannot make and test them all. What then should govern the selection?

An essential feature of the discipline in medicinal chemistry is to find logical bases for defining the boundary conditions for the selection of structures for synthesis. In the case under study there was a continuous search for useful physicochemical models for studying the chemistry of these compounds, and the inconsistencies in the structure–activity pattern were used to challenge the model

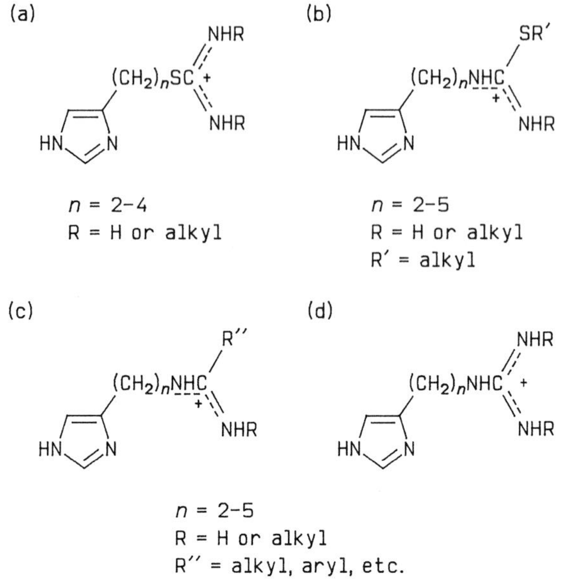

Fig. 4   Imidazolylalkylisothioureas, -amidines, and -guanidines synthesised and tested as potential antagonists of histamine stimulated gastric acid secretion. The structures are shown as side-chain cations. (a) Isothioureas. (b) "Reversed" isothioureas. (c) Amidines. (d) Guanidines.

or to reexamine the meaning of the biological test results. This dialogue, a search for self-consistency between the chemistry and biology, is vital to a new drug research where no precedent exists.

To explore structure–activity relationships further, it became desirable to increase the side chain length still more, but problems of chemical synthesis were experienced and new synthetic routes were required.

Exploration of amidines and substituents continued but it became clear that progress had become very slow. The problem seemed to be that the compounds had mixed activities, although to varying degrees. In the main they acted both as agonists and as antagonists; that is, they appeared to be partial agonists. This meant that although the compounds antagonised the action of histamine, they were not sufficiently effective inhibitors of gastric acid secretion because of interference from their inherent stimulatory activity. This appeared to impose a limitation on the potential of this type of structure for providing antagonists and seemed to be hindering progress.

Thus a critical stage was reached in the need for selectivity: it was necessary to achieve a separation between agonist and antagonist activities. It seemed that these compounds might act as agonists by mimicking histamine chemically, since like histamine, they have an imidazole ring and, being basic amidines, the side chain at physiological pH is protonated and carries a positive charge. It also seemed likely that these features would permit receptor recognition and provide binding for a competitive antagonist. This posed a considerable dilemma because the chemical groups that appeared to be required for antagonist activity were the same groups that seemed to confer the agonist effect.

In an attempt to separate these activities, the strongly basic guanidine group was replaced by non-basic groups that, though polar, would not be charged. Such an approach furnished analogues that indeed were not active as agonists; however, the first examples were also not active as antagonists. Eventually, one example, the thiourea derivative (SK&F 91581, **11**), that did not act as a partial agonist exhibited weak activity as an antagonist. Thioureas are essentially neutral in water because of the electron-withdrawing thiocarbonyl group. Conjugation forces the nitrogen atoms into a planar form and limits the availability of the nitrogen lone electron pairs, as in amides.

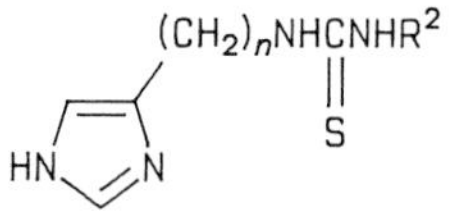
$(CH_2)_nNHCNHR^2$
S
HN
N

(**11**) SK&F 91581 $n = 3, R^2 = H$
(**12**) SK&F 91863 $n = 4, R^2 = H$
(**13**) Burimamide $n = 4, R^2 = Me$

At this time the higher homologous amine (with the four carbon atom chain length) was synthesised and further exploration revealed that with this type of structure, extension of the alkylene side chain resulted in a marked increase in antagonist potency. It was not until the side chain had been lengthened that the significance of the result with SK&F 91581 became clear and the desired aim was achieved, that is, a pure competitive antagonist without agonist effects. This compound (**12,** SK&F 91863) paved the way for the synthesis of substituted analogues, and in a short while the *N*-methyl analogue was obtained, which was given the name burimamide (**13**).

A synthesis of burimamide (Scheme 1) from lysine ethyl ester dihydrochloride

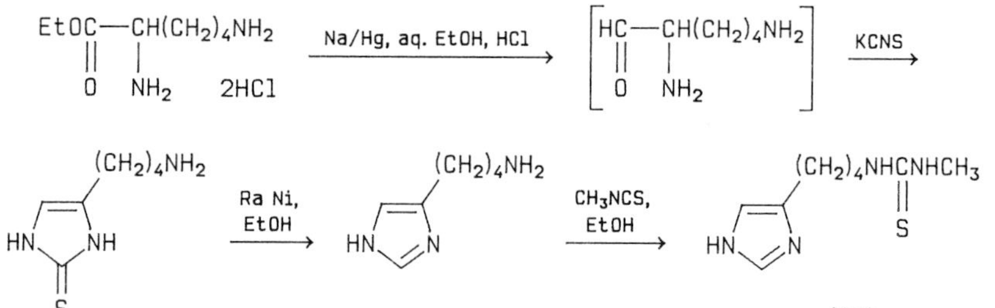
$EtOC—CH(CH_2)_4NH_2$
O
NH_2
2HCl
Na/Hg, aq. EtOH, HCl
$HC—CH(CH_2)_4NH_2$
O
NH_2
KCNS
$(CH_2)_4NH_2$
HN
NH
S
Ra Ni,
EtOH
$(CH_2)_4NH_2$
HN
N
CH_3NCS,
EtOH
$(CH_2)_4NHCNHCH_3$
S
HN
N

(**13**)

Scheme 1 Laboratory syntheses of burimamide (**13**).

involves reduction with sodium amalgam under carefully controlled conditions to generate an α-aminoaldehyde which, on being heated *in situ* with potassium thiocyanate, cyclises to the imidazol-2-thione. Desulphurisation to the imidazole followed by treatment with methyl isothiocyante gives the required thiourea, burimamide (**13**).

D.   BURIMAMIDE, THE FIRST CHARACTERISED H_2-RECEPTOR HISTAMINE ANTAGONIST

Burimamide (**13**) was an extremely important compound, and it provided a vital breakthrough. It was highly selective, showed no agonist activity, and antagonised the action of histamine in a competitive manner on the two *in vitro* non-H_1 systems, namely, guinea-pig atrium and rat uterus (Table II). It fulfilled the criteria required for characterising the existence of another set of histamine receptors, namely, the H_2-receptors. Thus, it allowed the above tissue systems to be defined as H_2-receptor systems, and thereby burimamide was defined as an H_2-receptor antagonist. This discovery was announced in 1972; the work had taken 6 years (*7*).

Burimamide also antagonised the action of histamine as a stimulant of gastric acid secretion in the rat, cat, and dog, and it was the first H_2-receptor antagonist to be investigated in man. Given intravenously, it blocked the action of histamine as a stimulant of gastric acid secretion in man, thereby confirming that burimamide behaves in humans as it does in animals. However, its one drawback was that it was not sufficiently active to be given orally. Thus, although burimamide was selective enough to define H_2-receptors, it was not active enough to permit proper drug development.

The activity of burimamide posed a structure–activity problem. If the amidine antagonists acted by ion pairing and H bonding, where did non basic thioureas fit in? A search of the literature revealed that thiourea will form crystalline salts with some carboxylic acids, for example, oxalic and trichloroacetic. Furthermore, with HNO_3, the nitrate will even crystallise out from water, suggesting that the molecular interaction is sufficiently strong to permit desolvation. In the crystal, protonation occurs on sulphur, and the conjugate cation then hydrogen-bonds to the oxyanion, just as with amidinium oxy-acid salts. Thus, in principle the amidines and thiourea groups might resemble one another when undergoing a bidentate hydrogen-bonding interaction.

E.   SULPHUR–METHYLENE ISOSTERISM, IMIDAZOLE TAUTOMERISM, AND THE DEVELOPMENT OF METIAMIDE

Various ways to alter the structure of burimamide were examined in an attempt to increase potency. One approach that proved successful resulted from two lines of exploration that merged. On one hand, attempts were being made to overcome

TABLE II

Structures and H$_2$-Receptor Histamine Antagonist Activities of Burimamide, Metiamide, Cimetidine and Isosteres

$$\text{R}^5\text{—CH}_2\text{XCH}_2\text{CH}_2\text{NHCNHMe}$$

Number	Compound Trivial name	Structure R^5	Structure X	Structure V	H$_2$-Receptor activities In vitro Atrium[a] K_B (95% limits) $\times 10^{-6}\ M$	H$_2$-Receptor activities In vitro Uterus[b] K_B (95% limits) $\times 10^{-6}\ M$	In vivo Acid secretion[c] ID$_{50}$ (μmol/kg)
13	Burimamide (thiourea)	H	CH$_2$	S	7.8 (6.4–8.6)	6.6 (4.9–8.3)	6.1
14	Thiaburimamide	H	S	S	3.2 (2.5–4.5)	3.2 (2.5–4.5)	5
15	Oxaburimamide	H	O	S	28 (13–69)	6.6 (4.9–8.3)	d
16	Metiamide (thiourea)	Me	S	S	0.92 (0.74–1.15)	0.75 (0.40–1.36)	1.6
17	Urea isostere	Me	S	O	22 (8.9–65)	7.1 (1.6–30)	27
18	Guanidine isostere	Me	S	NH	16 (8.1–32)	5.5 (2.8–13)	12
19	Nitroguanidine isostere	Me	S	N·NO$_2$	1.4 (0.79–2.8)	1.4 (0.72–3.2)	2.1
20	Cimetidine (cyanoguanidine)	Me	S	N·CN	0.79 (0.68–0.92)	0.81 (0.54–1.2)	1.4
21	Guanylurea derivative	Me	S	N·CONH$_2$	7.1 (4.0–14)	6.9 (4.1–12)	7.7

[a] Activities determined against histamine stimulation of guinea-pig right atrium *in vitro*. The dissociation constant (K_B) was calculated from the equation $K_B = B/(x - 1)$, where x is the respective ratio of concentrations of histamine needed to produce half maximal responses in the presence and absence of different concentrations (B) of antagonist.

[b] Activities determined against histamine inhibition of electrically evoked concentrations of rat uterus *in vitro*.

[c] Activities as antagonists of histamine stimulated gastric acid secretion in the anaesthetised rat as indicated in Table I, footnote *a*.

[d] Not determined.

the problem of synthesising the side chains by inserting a thioether link. Meanwhile, a study was being made of the pK_a characteristics of burimamide, since it was realised that burimamide in aqueous solution is a mixture of many chemical species in equilibrium. At physiological pH there are three main forms of the imidazole ring, three planar configurations of the thioureido group (a fourth is theoretically possible but is disfavoured by internal steric hindrance), and various trans and gauche rotamer combinations of the side chain CH_2-CH_2 bonds (Fig. 5). This means that at any given instant only a small proportion of the drug molecules would be in a particular form.

The existence of a mixture of species leads one to question which may be biologically active and whether altering drug structure to favour a particular species would alter drug potency [dynamic structure–activity analysis (DSAA)] (8). There are substantial energy barriers to interconversion between the species of burimamide so that it is quite likely that a drug molecule, presenting itself to the receptor in a form unfavourable for drug–receptor interaction, might diffuse away again before having time to rearrange into a more favourable form. The relative population of favourable forms might therefore determine the amount of drug required for a given effect.

The various species of burimamide do not interconvert instantaneously, but whereas the rotamers of the side chain and thioureido groups are interconverted simply by internal rotation of a C–C or C–N bond, interconversion of the ring forms probably involves a water-mediated proton transfer. If a molecule presents itself to the receptor with the ring in an unfavourable form it might not readjust, unless there were suitably oriented water molecules (or other hydrogen donor-acceptors) present. The form of the ring therefore merits special consideration.

The above arguments led to a study of the population of imidazole species in burimamide in comparison with histamine. At physiological pH the main species are (Fig. 5) the cation (13c) and two uncharged tautomers (13a and 13b), and their populations were estimated qualitatively from the electronic influence of the side chain using pK_a data and the Hammett equation (9):

$$pK_{a(R)} = pK_{a(H)} + \rho\sigma_m$$

where p is the Hammett reaction constant and σ_m the Hammett substituent constant.

For burimamide, the ring pK_a (7.25 at 37°C) is greater than that of unsubstituted imidazole (6.80), indicating that the side chain is mildly electron releasing. In contrast, for histamine the ammonium ethyl side chain was seen to be electron withdrawing, since it lowered the pK_a of the imidazole ring (pK_a 5.90). Thus, although both histamine and burimamide are monosubstituted imidazoles, the structural similarity is misleading in that the electronic properties of the respective imidazole rings are different.

If the active form of burimamide was tautomer 13a, the form most preferred for histamine, then increasing its relative population might increase activity; for

For burimamide:

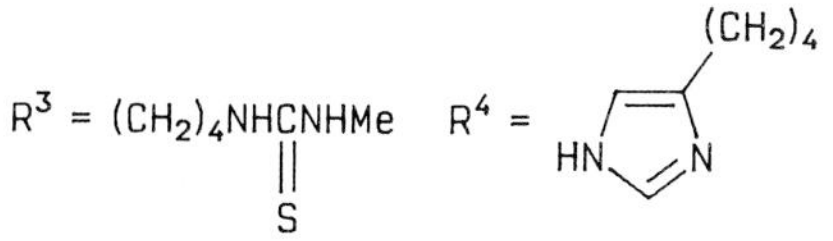

$$R^3 = (CH_2)_4NHCNHMe \quad R^4 = \quad V = S$$

(a) Imidazole ring (ionisation and tautomerism)

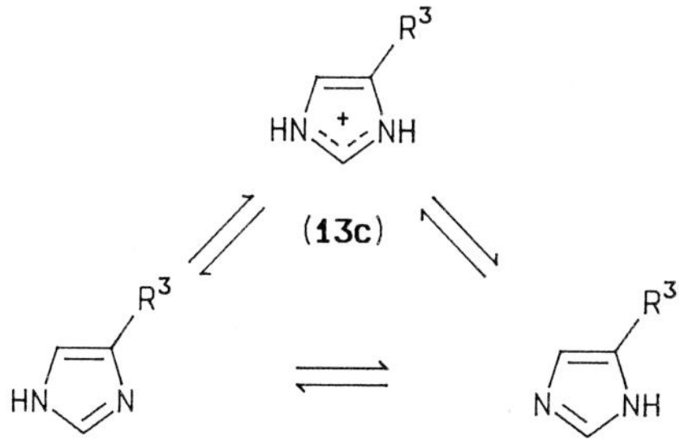

(13c)

(13a)   (13b)

(b) Alkane chain (C—C bond rotation gives trans and gauche conformers)

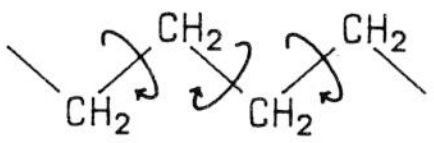

(c) Thiourea group (V = S) (configurational isomerism)

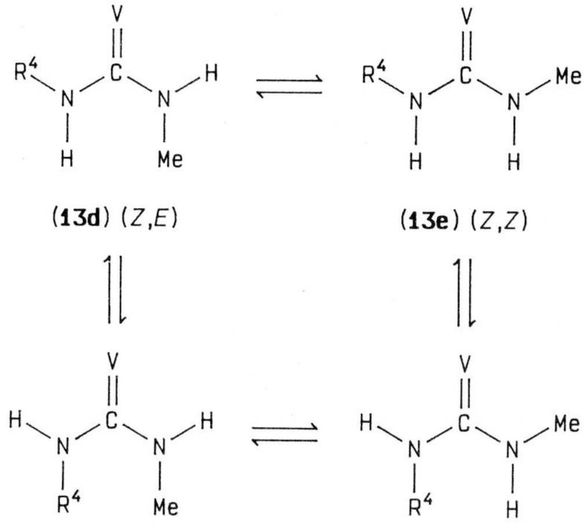

(13d) (*Z,E*)   (13e) (*Z,Z*)

(13f) (*E,E*)   (13g) (*E,Z*)

Fig. 5 Burimamide species equilibria in solution.

example, incorporating an electronegative atom into the antagonist side chain should convert it to an electron-withdrawing group and favour species **13a**. This would not be the only requirement for activity and it would be necessary to minimise disturbance to other biologically important molecular properties such as stereochemistry and lipid–water interactions. For reasons of synthesis, the first such substitution to be made was the replacement of a methylene group (—CH$_2$—) by the isosteric thioether linkage (—S—) at the carbon atom next but one to the ring, to afford "thiaburimamide" (**14**) (Table II), which was found to be more active as an antagonist.

It was argued that a further stabilisation of tautomer **13a** in thiaburimamide might be obtained by incorporating an electron-releasing substituent in the vacant 4(5) position of the imidazole ring. A methyl group was selected, since it was thought that it should not interfere with receptor interaction, 4-methylhistamine having been shown to be an effective H$_2$-receptor agonist. This approach was successful, and introduction of a methyl group into the ring of the antagonist furnished a more potent drug, which was named metiamide (**16**) (*10*) (Table II). Metiamide is synthesised from methyl isothiocyanate and the requisite amine, 4-[(2-aminoethyl)thiomethyl]-5-methylimidazole, the synthesis of which is outlined in Scheme 2.

Although the above molecular manipulations were made through consideration of the electronic effects of substituents, evidence has subsequently accrued to suggest that conformational effects are probably more important. Crystal structure studies indicate that the thioether linkage may increase molecular flexibility and the ring-methyl group may assist in orientating the imidazole ring (*11*). Furthermore, the oxygen (ether) analogue [oxaburimamide (**15**), Table II] which should fulfill the electronic requirements is less potent than burimamide, possibly by encouraging a different conformation through intramolecular hydrogen-bonding (e.g., Fig. 6).

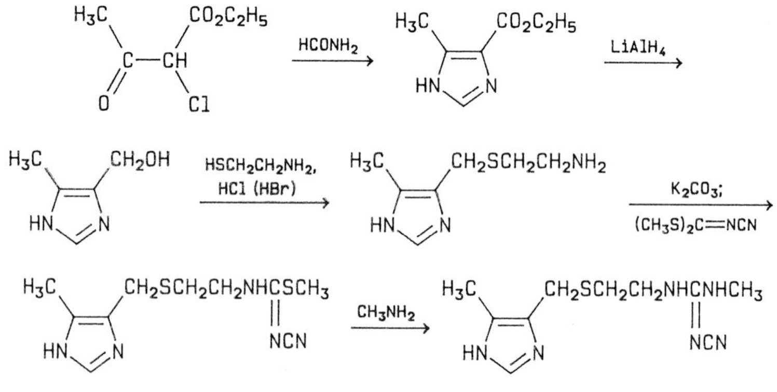

(**20**)

Scheme 2   Laboratory synthesis of cimetidine (**20**).

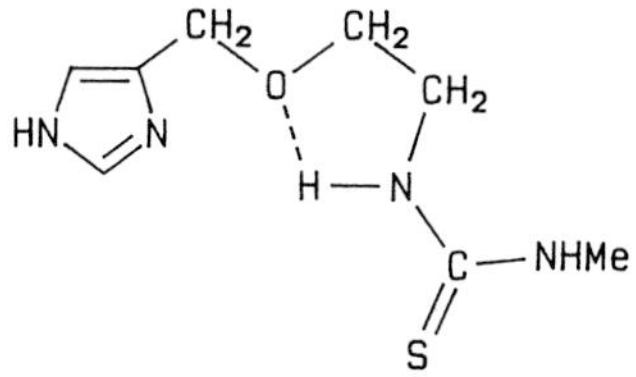

Fig. 6   Possible intramolecular hydrogen-bonding by oxaburimamide (**15**) (Table II).

Metiamide represented a major improvement, being 10 times more potent than burimamide *in vitro* and a potent inhibitor of stimulated acid secretion in man. It was investigated for potential use in peptic ulcer therapy and was shown to produce a significant increase in the healing rate of duodenal ulcers and marked symptomatic relief. However, out of 700 patients treated there were a few cases of granulocytopenia (causing a reduction in the number of circulating white cells in the blood and leaving patients open to infection). Although reversible, this severely limited the amount of clinical work.

F.   ISOSTERES OF THIOUREA, GUANIDINE EQUILIBRIA,
    AND THE DISCOVERY OF CIMETIDINE

The possibility existed that the granulocytopenia associated with metiamide was caused by the thiourea group in the molecule and this led to the need to examine another compound. Fortunately, exploration had continued with other possible structures and, in particular, with alternatives to the thiourea group. One approach taken was to examine isosteric replacement of the thiourea sulphur atom (=S) of metiamide. Replacement by carbonyl oxygen (=O) gave the urea analogue (**17**), but this was much less active. The idea of guanidine derivatives which had provided the original breakthrough was also reexamined; replacement by imino nitrogen (=NH) afforded the guanidine (**18**) which, interestingly, was not a partial agonist but a fairly active antagonist. However, *in vitro,* the urea and guanidine isosteres were both approximately 20 times less potent than metiamide, and other ways were investigated for removing the positive charge on the guanidine derivative.

An observation that nitroguanidine was not basic led to further investigation and revealed a publication by Charton on the Hammett relationship between σ and pK_a for substituted amidines and guanidines (*12*). Guanidine basicity is markedly reduced by electron-withdrawing substituents, and Charton demonstrated a high correlation between the inductive substituent constant σ_I and pK_a for a series of monosubstituted guanidines (Fig. 7). The cyano and nitro groups are sufficiently electron withdrawing to reduce the pK_a by over 14 units, to values <0; indeed, the ionisation constants of cyanoguanidine ($pK_a = 0.4$) and nitroguanidine ($pK_a = 0.9$) approach that of thiourea ($pK_a = -1.2$).

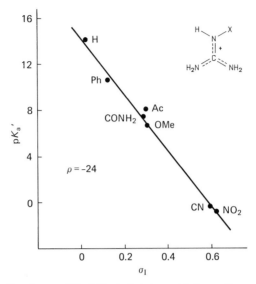

Fig. 7   Apparent pK_a values at 25° of N-substituted guanidinium cations versus σ_I substituent constants. Data from Charton (*12*). The line corresponds to the equation $pK_a' = 14.20 - 24.1\sigma_I$. (Reproduced from Burland and Simkins (*15*), with permission of the publisher.)

The nitroguanidine (**19**) and cyanoguanidine (**20**) analogues of metiamide were synthesised and found to be active antagonists comparable with metiamide (*13*). Of these two compounds, the cyanoguanidine (**20**) is slightly more potent and was selected for development (*14*), being given the non-proprietary name "cimetidine".

A laboratory synthesis of cimetidine is outlined in Scheme 2. 4-Carboethoxy-5-methylimidazole, made from ethyl α-chloroacetoacetate by condensation with formamide in the Bredereck procedure, is reduced by lithium aluminium hydride to give 4-hydroxymethyl-5-methylimidazole. This carbinol is then condensed with cysteamine in the presence of HCl or HBr, and the resulting amine salt is collected and neutralised with aqueous potassium carbonate. The liberated amine is treated with dimethylcyanodithioimidocarbonate and then with methylamine. Many variations of this synthesis have been developed.

The guanidinium cation can lose a proton from each of the three nitrogen atoms to give three different forms of the conjugate base (Fig. 8). Powerful electron-withdrawing substituents favour the imino-tautomer over the amino-tautomers, since the proton on the adjacent nitrogen in the cation is more acidic than the protons on the more distant terminal nitrogen atoms. Thus, cyanoguanidines exist predominantly in the cyanoimino form and, in cimetidine, the cyanoimino group ($=NCN$) replaces the thione ($=S$) sulphur atom of metiamide.

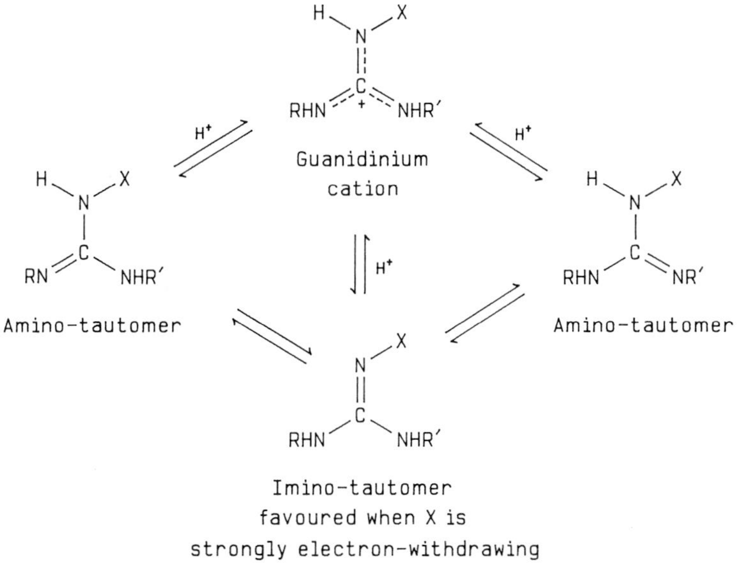

Fig. 8   Equilibria between guanidinium cation and the three conjugate bases.

Cyanoguanidine and thiourea have many chemical properties in common. They are planar structures of similar geometries; they are weakly amphoteric (very weakly basic and acidic), so that in the pH range 2–12 they are un-ionised; they are very polar and hydrophilic. The similar behaviour of cimetidine and metiamide as histamine H_2-receptor antagonists and the close similarity in physicochemical characteristics of thiourea and cyanoguanidine permit the description of the thiourea and cyanoguanidine groups in the present context as bioisosteres (*13*). Nitroguanidine may also be considered to be a bioisostere of thiourea in this series of structures. Bioisosterism is not a universally applicable property, however, and for other biological actions cyanoguanidine and thiourea may be non-equivalent. One important chemical difference between these groups is their conformational behaviour. Three conformations of a disubstituted thiourea group are energetically accessible, namely, **13e**, **13f**, and **13g** (Fig. 5, V = S) but, due to steric effects, only two conformations of a disubstituted cyanoguanidine are similarly accessible, namely, **13f** and **13g** (Fig. 5, V = NCN).

Cyanoguanidines and thioureas also differ sufficiently in chemical reactivity (e.g., in oxidative and hydrolytic reactions) for differences to be expected in the rates and products of biotransformation of drug molecules containing these groups. In the presence of excess dilute hydrochloric acid, cimetidine is slowly hydrolysed to the guanylurea (**21**, Table II, Scheme 3) and on being heated in acid, the latter is further hydrolysed and decarboxylated to give the guanidine

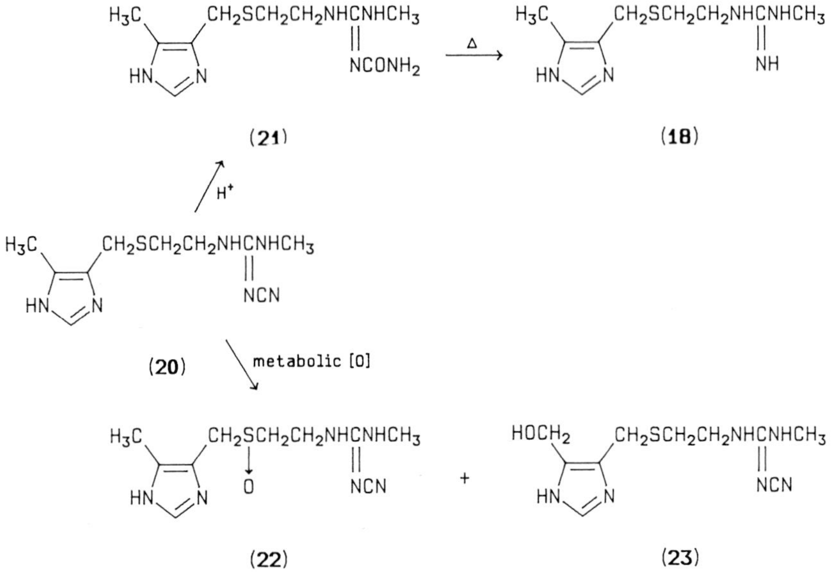

Scheme 3   Transformation products of cimetidine (**20**). (a) Hydrolysis gives the guanylurea (**21**) and thence the guanidine (**18**). (b) Metabolic oxidation gives the sulphoxide (**22**) and hydroxymethyl derivative (**23**).

(**18**). The guanylurea is also an H_2-receptor antagonist but it is less active than cimetidine.

The cyanoguanidine group in cimetidine is metabolically stable and cimetidine is largely excreted unchanged. The main metabolite is the sulphoxide (**22**) produced by oxidation of the side-chain thioether sulphur atom, together with lesser amounts of the hydroxymethyl oxidation product (**23**) of the ring CH_3 (Scheme 3).

III.   CIMETIDINE, A BREAKTHROUGH IN THE TREATMENT OF PEPTIC ULCER DISEASE

Cimetidine has been shown to be a specific competitive antagonist of histamine at H_2-receptors *in vitro,* and to be effective *in vivo* at inhibiting histamine-stimulated gastric acid secretion in the rat, cat, and dog (Table III). The ID_{50} values determined in the rat, cat, and dog were not significantly different from each other. Cimetidine has also been shown to be active when administered orally, and a dose of 20 μmol/kg (approximately 5 mg/kg) produced a mean inhibition of 90% of maximal histamine-stimulated secretion in the dog.

TABLE III
Inhibition of Gastric Acid Secretion *in vivo* by Intravenous Cimetidine

Animal	Preparation	Stimulant	Intravenous ID_{50} (μmol/kg)
Rat[a]	Lumen-perfused stomach	Histamine	1.37
		Pentagastrin	1.40
Cat[a]	Lumen-perfused stomach	Histamine	0.85
		Pentagastrin	1.45
Dog[b]	Heidenhain pouch	Histamine	1.70
		Pentagastrin	2.00

[a] Anaesthetised.
[b] Conscious.

Cimetidine is also an effective inhibitor of pentagastrin-stimulated acid secretion. (Pentagastrin is a synthetic, biologically active analogue of gastrin which contains the terminal four aminoacid residues of gastrin, namely, N-*t*-BOC-β-Ala-Trp-Met-Asp-Phe-NH$_2$.) The ID_{50} values shown in Table III indicate that the potency of cimetidine against pentagastrin-stimulated secretion is very similar to its potency against histamine-stimulated secretion. Cimetidine is also effective against food-stimulated acid secretion but is less active against cholinergically stimulated secretion.

The finding that H$_2$-receptor antagonists such as cimetidine effectively inhibit pentagastrin-stimulated secretion clearly indicates that gastrin and histamine are somehow linked in the gastric secretory process. The results with these antagonists firmly establish that histamine has a physiological role in gastric acid secretion.

Cimetidine has been extensively studied in man and its safety and efficacy have been established in the acute treatment of peptic ulcer. Cimetidine given orally as 1–1.2 g/day has been shown to relieve symptoms and promote healing of lesions in a majority of patients with peptic ulcer disease. Much of the seminal work with the new drug is published in the proceedings of an International Symposium held in London in October 1976 (*15*). Cimetidine was marketed first in the United Kingdom in November 1976, and was marketed in the United States in August 1977; by 1979 it was sold in over 100 countries under the trademark Tagamet, representing all the major markets with one important exception—it was not granted approval for use in Japan until 1982.

Cimetidine changed the medical management of peptic ulcer disease and became a very successful product (*16*). In 1983 its annual world-wide sales reached the level of nearly $1,000,000,000, and in several countries (including Canada and the United States) it was the number one selling prescription product.

IV. SUMMARY AND FURTHER OBSERVATIONS

The long-term nature of pharmaceutical research and development and the need for tenacity to continue in the face of considerable difficulty and disappointment is well illustrated by this case history of drug discovery (see Fig. 9).

The research project was initiated in 1964, and it took 6 years (to 1970) to obtain burimamide, which was used to characterise pharmacologically histamine H_2-receptors and verify the basic concept, and was examined in human volunteers. The next drug, metiamide, a more potent and orally active compound, was investigated clinically, but its use was severely restricted.

Cimetidine followed on from metiamide; it was first synthesised in 1972. Much work had to be done to evaluate the potential of cimetidine in animals, establish its safety in animals, and then investigate its behaviour in man. Finally, many clinical studies had to be undertaken to prove its value as a drug therapy before it could be made generally available in 1977. An overall time of 13 years had elapsed!

It is self-evident that any account of drug discovery must be incomplete and certainly only a small proportion of the total studies made have been described in this chapter. Many avenues examined during structure–activity analysis turned out to be ineffective and since, in the main, these are not mentioned here, the net effect may be to make the work appear to be more rational and more perceptive than is warranted.

In order to limit the scale of the problem the early work concentrated on

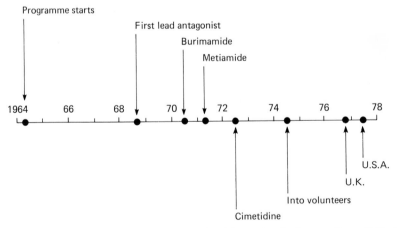

Fig. 9   Thirteen years to discover and develop cimetidine and make it generally available for therapeutic use.

$$(CH_3)_2NCH_2 \quad O \quad CH_2SCH_2CH_2NHCNHCH_3$$
$$\underset{CHNO_2}{\overset{\|}{}}$$

(24) Ranitidine

imidazole derivatives. However, it was soon demonstrated that other heterocycles such as pyridine and thiazole could be effectively used in place of imidazole. Later on, researchers at Glaxo demonstrated that it was not even necessary to have a nitrogen heterocycle, and they synthesised a furan derivative, ranitidine **(24)**, which became the second H_2-receptor histamine antagonist to be introduced clinically (under the trademark Zantac) for treatment of peptic ulcer disease (*17*).

ACKNOWLEDGEMENT

The work described here was a collaborative effort among Sir James Black, F.R.S., Dr. G. J. Durant, Dr. J. C. Emmett, Dr. C. R. Ganellin, Dr. M. E. Parsons, and Dr. G. R. White. Major contributions were also made by R. C. Blakemore and A. C. Rasmussen (pharmacology), M. J. Graham, Dr. R. C. Mitchell and Dr. E. S. Pepper (physicochemical studies), and Dr. R. C. Young (correlation studies). More than 50 chemists contributed to the work of actually making the compounds over the years. The success of the project attests to their skill. Substantial technical contributions were made by Dr. M. E. Footit, A. J. Hayter, D. W. Hills, D. R. Hollyman, R. J. King, J. M. Loynes, P. D. Miles, H. D. Prain, W. Tertiuk, and C. S. Whyatt.

REFERENCES

1. H. H. Dale and P. P. Laidlaw, *J. Physiol. London* **41,** 318 (1910).
2. D. Bovet, *Ann. N.Y. Acad. Sci.* **50,** Art. 9, 1089 (1950).
3. B. Folkow, K. Haeger, and G. Kahlson, *Acta Physiol. Scand.* **15,** 264 (1948).
4. A. S. F. Ash and H. O. Schild, *Br. J. Pharmacol. Chemother.* **27,** 427 (1966).
5. M. I. Grossman, C. Robertson, and C. E. Rosiere, *J. Pharmacol. Exp. Ther.* **104,** 277 (1952).
6. C. R. Ganellin, G. J. Durant, and J. C. Emmett, *Fed. Proc., Fed. Am. Soc. Exp. Biol.* **35,** 1924 (1976).
7. J. W. Black, W. A. M. Duncan, G. J. Durant, C. R. Ganellin, and M. E. Parsons, *Nature (London)* **236,** 385 (1972).
8. C. R. Ganellin, *J. Med. Chem.* **24,** 913 (1981).
9. M. Charton, *J. Org. Chem.* **30,** 3346 (1965).
10. J. W. Black, G. J. Durant, J. C. Emmett, and C. R. Ganellin, *Nature (London)* **248,** 65 (1974).
11. K. Prout, S. R. Critchley, C. R. Ganellin, and R. C. Mitchell, *J. Chem. Soc., Perkin Trans. 2,* 68 (1977).
12. M. Charton, *J. Org. Chem.* **30,** 369 (1965).
13. G. J. Durant, J. C. Emmett, C. R. Ganellin, P. D. Miles, H. D. Prain, M. E. Parsons, and G. R. White, *J. Med. Chem.* **20,** 901 (1977).

14. R. W. Brimblecombe, W. A. M. Duncan, G. J. Durant, J. C. Emmett, C. R. Ganellin, and M. E. Parsons, *J. Int. Med. Res.* **3,** 86 (1975); R. W. Brimblecombe, W. A. M. Duncan, G. J. Durant, J. C. Emmett, C. R. Ganellin, G. B. Leslie, and M. E. Parsons, *Gastroenterology* **74,** 339 (1978).
15. W. L. Burland and M. A. Simkins, eds., "Cimetidine—Proceedings of the 2nd International Symposium on Histamine H$_2$-Receptor Antagonists". Excerpta Medica, Amsterdam, 1977.
16. J. W. Freston, *Ann. Intern. Med.* **97,** 573 (1982); D. H. Winship, *Gastroenterology* **74,** 402 (1978).
17. J. Bradshaw, M. E. Butcher, J. W. Clitherow, M. D. Dowle, R. Hayes, D. B. Judd, J. M. McKinnon, and B. J. Price, *in:* "Chemical Regulation of Biological Mechanisms" (A. M. Creighton and S. Turner, eds.), pp. 45–57. Special publications No. 42. Royal Society of Chemistry, London, 1982.

CHAPTER 7

Discovery of Buprenorphine, a Potent Antagonist Analgesic

J. W. LEWIS
Pharmaceutical Division
Reckitt & Colman
Kingston-upon-Hull, England

I. INTRODUCTION

Pain is a universal and distressing experience of all human beings, but it is difficult to define and quantify. The sensations experienced with headache, gout, rheumatoid arthritis, broken ankle, kidney stones and bone carcinoma may differ widely but all are easily recognised as pain. The problems of definition, measurement, and significance of pain have occupied the minds of scientists, philosophers and theologians for centuries, but the sufferer has no difficulty in recognising it and wanting relief from it. The relief of pain has always been a matter of major concern to the medical profession, and in many cases where the disease process can neither be cured nor arrested, as, for example, in terminal carcinoma, it becomes the only real service that the doctor can give his patient.

From earliest recorded times the principal drug for the relief of more severe pain has been opium and substances derived from opium. Although opium appears to have been unknown in ancient times in India and China, it was well known in ancient Mesopotamia, and Assyrian herb lists and medical texts translated from the cuneiform make reference to it.

119

Thomas Sydenham, regarded by many as the real father of English medicine, introduced laudanum, a tincture of opium, into England, and towards the end of his life was able to say "few would be willing to practice medicine without opium".

Opium is the dried latex exuded by incised seed capsules of the poppy *Papaver somniferum*. This is a showy annual plant widely cultivated for opium production and for oilseed in the Balkans, Asiatic Turkey, India, Burma, China, parts of Russia and Mexico.

Opium has a place in the pharmacopeias of the world as powdered opium, dry and liquid extracts, tinctures, mixtures, linctuses, syrups, solutions and pastilles. It is a complex mixture of substances and contains morphine (9–17%), narcotine (now known as noscapine) (2–9%), codeine (0.3–4%), thebaine (0.1–0.8%), papaverine (0.5–1%), other alkaloids (0.1%), triterpenes (e.g., cyclolaudenol) and steroids (e.g., glycosides of sitosterol) but its pharmacological effects are produced only by the alkaloids. The first of these alkaloids, indeed the first alkaloid from any source to be obtained in a pure state, was morphine, named after Morpheus, the god of sleep. The French chemist Sertürner is generally credited with its isolation in 1805 (*1*), but Séguin had already described the isolation to the Academy of Sciences in 1804 though his report was not published until 10 years later (*2*). Morphine subsequently became available in reasonable quantities to the medical profession as the result of a process developed in 1833 by William Gregory (*3*), who treated an extract of opium with a concentrated solution of calcium chloride. This precipitated calcium meconate, lactate and sulphate, which were removed by filtration and the filtrate was evaporated to give "Gregory Salt", a mixture of morphine and codeine hydrochlorides. This salt was recrystallised, dissolved in water, and morphine was precipitated from solution with ammonia. This process, which results in a good recovery of morphine from the opium, was first operated commercially in 1833 by J. F. Macfarlan and Co. of Edinburgh and later by T. and H. Smith, also of Edinburgh, until a more efficient process was introduced in 1960.

It was quickly recognised that morphine is the component of opium responsible for its pain-relieving properties, and the alkaloid rapidly established its place in medicine as an analgesic. In the non-tolerant patient, 10–15 mg of morphine sulphate is effective against pain of all but the utmost severity. However, although it remains the most widely prescribed drug for the relief of severe pain it is by no means the ideal analgesic, since it has several undesirable effects. It causes marked respiratory depression, a lowering of the blood pressure, some nausea and vomiting, and constipation. The most serious disadvantage, however, is that on continued administration of the drug, patients develop not only tolerance, which means that more drug is required to produce the same effect, but also dependence, manifested as an overwhelming craving for the drug.

Anyone who has become dependent on morphine, or a similar narcotic, as a result of medical or illicit use of the drug requires its continued administration for normal functioning of the body (physical dependence). If for any reason the drug is withdrawn the most distressing physiological symptoms follow, commencing about 8 hours after the last dose. The "withdrawal syndrome" comprises a characteristic complex of symptoms, the most important of which are extreme agitation, severe and long-lasting abdominal cramps, profuse watering of eyes and nose, long-lasting diarrhoea and often nausea and vomiting. These effects, which increase in severity and finally die away, may last for 10–14 days and are not such as will be voluntarily endured. Since further administration of morphine or a similar narcotic results in their complete suppression there is a virtually irresistable impulse to take further doses of the drug and voluntary abandonment of the habit becomes impossible. Illicit users of narcotics establish the habit because they like the psychological effects of the drug, particularly the sense of tranquillity and euphoria, but it is the withdrawal symptoms that perpetuate addiction.

Addiction to narcotic drugs is a world-wide problem which has increased dramatically during the past 20 years. Narcotic addiction can be established by the use of pure morphine but is most likely to involve heroin, morphine's di-acetyl derivative, which has a stronger euphoric effect. Opium smoking was unknown until after the discovery of America and the use of tobacco.

The addictive properties of opium were well known long before morphine was isolated from it, and once the alkaloid was available it was hoped that this pure substance, which was a highly effective analgesic, might be free of the addictive property. Similar hopes were subsequently held for other derivatives of morphine, only to be shown to be unfounded. In those days addiction potential could not be assessed except on the basis of practical use, and the development of reliable methods of assessment of this potential has been a very important feature of work in this field in the last 40–50 years.

When morphine was first isolated the science of organic chemistry was in its infancy, and the elucidation of the chemical structure of the alkaloid presented a formidable challenge. Progress in this study was at first very slow, depending as it did upon the growth of an understanding of organic reactions; indeed the progress of this structural problem, culminating in the successful synthesis of morphine in 1952, represents in many ways a history in miniature of organic chemistry.

The correct composition of morphine (**1**) was determined in 1847 (*4*) and of codeine (**2**) in 1842 (*5*). In 1881 morphine was shown to be a phenol (*6*) and was methylated to its methyl ether which was found to be identical with codeine (*7*). Morphine was shown to contain two hydroxy groups in 1874 by the production of a diacetyl ester by the action of acetic anhydride on the alkaloid (*8*). Diacetyl morphine, also known as diamorphine or heroin, was thought to be a superior analgesic to morphine and was soon introduced into medicine, but since heroin

Morphine (1)   R = Me
Nalorphine (13)   R = CH₂CH=CH₂

Codeine (2)

produces a greater degree of euphoria it is substantially more attractive to the illicit user. Indeed the drug is by far the most widely used and greatly demanded narcotic among illicit users. Heroin is regarded by many as a drug whose undoubted medicinal value is outweighed by its addictive potential and likelihood of abuse, and many countries have banned its production, importation and use.

Unlike the diacetyl ester, morphine methyl ether, which is codeine, has only about one-tenth of the analgesic potency of morphine,* produces little if any euphoria and is of relatively low addiction potential and has, as a result, been for many years a widely used oral analgesic. Codeine has the advantage that, compared with morphine which is usually administered by injection, it has good oral bioavailability which enables it to be administered in tablet form, usually in combination with aspirin or paracetamol.

One of the minor alkaloids of opium, thebaine (3), was shown in 1906 to be closely related to codeine (9), and the results of chemical studies of all three alkaloids could thus be combined in studies of the structural problem. The solution of this problem was greatly complicated by the remarkable variety of structural rearrangements that the alkaloids undergo under different conditions (10).

Thebaine (3)

Shortly after the First World War, a programme of work was initiated in the United States, the aim of which was the development of a wholly synthetic agent that possessed the analgesic properties of morphine but was devoid of addiction potential. Parallel work on modifications of the three morphine alkaloids to produce a "semi-synthetic" agent with the same profile was also undertaken.

*Potency means the amount of drug required to produce a pharmacological effect. In this case 10 times more codeine is required to produce the same effect as morphine.

The principal aim of the work, however, was a wholly synthetic substance since it was argued that, if such a drug could be produced, the use of morphine could be discontinued, and cultivation of the opium poppy might then be banned by international agreement thus crippling at its source illicit traffic in opium alkaloids. Considerable progress has been made along these lines in the last 50 years, though not quite in the direction originally envisaged. It is appropriate to summarise the work done up to 1960, prior to the involvement of Reckitt & Colman in this field.

II. EARLY WORK ON THE PREPARATION OF MORPHINE ANALOGUES

The work of preparing new analgesics proceeded in three distinct phases: (i) modification of the morphine molecule, (ii) synthesis of simpler structures representing certain portions of the morphine molecule, and (iii) synthesis of morphine-antagonists of the *N*-allyl-normorphine (nalorphine) type.

A.   MODIFICATION OF THE MORPHINE MOLECULE (*11, 12*)

Morphine contains a number of modifiable centres, notably a phenolic hydroxy group, an alcoholic hydroxy group, a cyclic tertiary amino group and a double bond. Esterification of the two hydroxy groups to heroin (**4**) marginally

Heroin (**4**)

increases activity; it appears that heroin acts through the 6-monoacetyl derivative which has equal potency. Methylation of the alcoholic group also results in some increase of activity, but alkylation of the phenolic hydroxy group greatly reduces activity, codeine being only about one-tenth as active as morphine. Reduction of the double bond generally results in slightly higher activity; oxidation of the secondary alcohol to carbonyl and its replacement by hydrogen results in significantly greater activity.

Treatment of heroin with cyanogen bromide results in replacement of N-CH_3 by N-CN, and hydrolysis of the product yields the secondary base normorphine (*13*) from which a variety of derivatives may be obtained in which the N-CH_3

group of morphine is replaced by other alkyl, alkenyl and arylalkyl groups (*14*). The activity of the *N*-alkyl series decreases initially as the size of the N-substituent increases but then rises again reaching a peak at about C_6. The most active compound in this series is *N*-β-phenylethylnormorphine (**5**) which is about 14

N–β–Phenylethylnormorphine (**5**)

times as potent as the parent alkaloid and is the most active of all the simple morphine derivatives.

B.   SIMPLER FRAGMENTS OF THE MORPHINE MOLECULE (*15*)

When work on synthetic analgesics began in the early 1920s the structure of morphine had yet to be elucidated. Consequently it was chance that led to the discovery of the first totally synthetic opiate—pethidine (meperidine in the United States). This was identified during an investigation of a series of atropine-like agents. The drug has been widely used, particularly in obstetrics, although, as was soon discovered, it has a physical dependence liability similar to that of morphine. When drawn as in **6** the resemblance of the structure of pethidine to that of morphine can be readily seen.

Pethidine (**6**)

A more distant analogue of morphine, methadone (**7**) was introduced into medical use shortly after the end of the Second World War. Although somewhat more potent as an analgesic it is less euphorigenic than morphine and longer acting so that in the dependent state abstinence symptoms develop more slowly and in a milder form when the drug is withdrawn. For this reason it is used therapeutically to assist in recovery from opiate addiction (*16*). The treatment involves weaning the addict off heroin or morphine and transferring to methadone, the daily dose of which is controlled and gradually reduced.

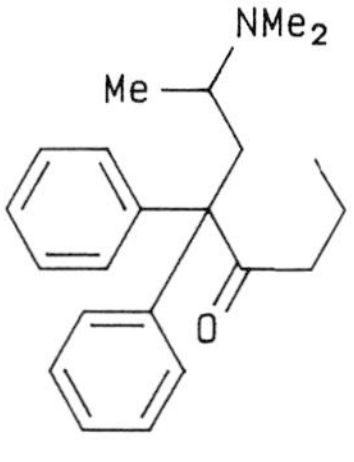

Methadone (**7**) 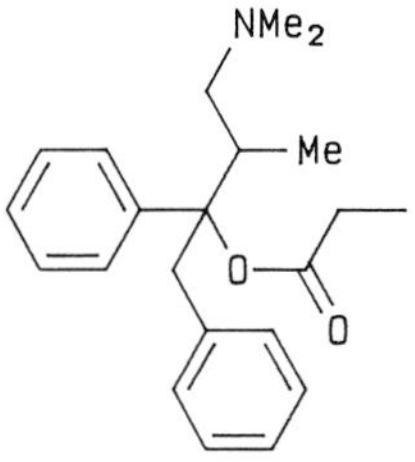   Propoxyphene (**8**)

Propoxyphene (**8**) is similar in chemical structure to methadone but considerably less potent. It has found very widespread use since its introduction in 1957 as an oral analgesic, particularly in combination with aspirin or paracetamol, for the treatment of moderate pain. The incidence of dependence on propoxyphene is low, mainly because injection of the drug (which is preferred by opiate addicts) is limited by deleterious effects at the site of injection. A serious problem with dextropropoxyphene is overdosage, which is too often fatal as a result of respiratory depression.

More closely related to the natural opiates are the morphinans which are bases having the main carbon skeleton of morphine without the 4,5-ether bridge. The simplest tertiary base in the series in which the ring B/ring C fusion is cis, is *N*-methylmorphinan (**9**), a weak analgesic. Greater activity is achieved by introduction of the phenolic hydroxy at C-3 and opiate activity resides in the laevorotatory enantiomer, as in the natural morphine series. Levorphanol (**10**) is more potent and longer acting than morphine, but the pharmacological profile is otherwise similar to that of morphine. The benzomorphans (e.g., **11**) are similar in struc-

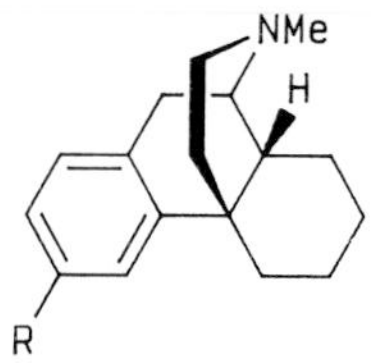

(**9**)   R = H
(**10**)   R = OH

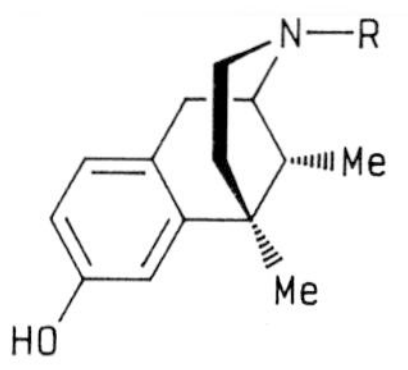

(**11**)   R = Me
(**12**)   R = CH$_2$CH$_2$Ph
(**14**)   R = CH$_2$—▷ 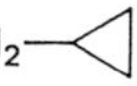
(**15**)   R = CH$_2$CH=CMe$_2$

ture to the morphinans but lack ring C. The *N*-phenylethyl derivative phenazocine (**12**) is 20 times more potent than morphine (*17*) but otherwise a typical opiate in man. It has found limited use as an oral analgesic for severe chronic pain.

C. ANTAGONIST ANALGESICS

Little or no progress in dissociating analgesic activity from physical dependence liability by modifications of the morphine structure or by the synthesis of novel structures had been made by 1954 when it was shown that nalorphine (**13**), despite being a specific antagonist of morphine, has analgesic properties in man (*18*). Nalorphine does not support morphine dependence and it is not a dependence-producing drug in its own right (*19*), but it is not a clinically useful analgesic since it causes dysphoric effects and often frightening hallucinations in an unacceptable proportion of patients. These findings with nalorphine, however, led to a major change of direction in analgesic research, where the emphasis shifted to a search for narcotic antagonists with analgesic properties. Since nalorphine did not show analgesia in the animal tests then in use, new test systems had to be developed and progress was slow. Tests for narcotic antagonism were, however, relatively simple, and it became apparent that antagonists were only to be found in the morphine, morphinan and benzomorphan series. The N-substituent groups which were found to confer antagonist properties in these series were *n*-propyl, allyl and substituted allyl, cyclopropylmethyl and cyclobutylmethyl (*20*). These groups appropriately substituted in the pethidine and methadone series failed to generate antagonists.

The benzomorphan series produced the first antagonist analgesics to receive serious attention. Two members, cyclazocine (**14**) and pentazocine (**15**), were selected for clinical evaluation. Cyclazocine is a very potent analgesic and an even more potent antagonist, whereas pentazocine has only low potency for both these effects. Cyclazocine was found in man to have a profile similar to nalorphine whereas pentazocine appeared to have an acceptable separation of analgesic from unwanted effects (*21*). It was shown to have a low addiction potential, was introduced into medicine in 1967 and has established a significant position in the group of strong analgesics.

III. INVOLVEMENT OF RECKITT & COLMAN IN OPIATE RESEARCH

Reckitt & Colman's interest in the opiate field started in 1958 when the company formed a joint research association with J. F. Macfarlan and Co. of Edinburgh, who had pioneered the industrial production of morphine in the nineteenth century. From 1960 the medicinal chemistry investigation was led by K. W. Bentley, who had become interested in the possibility of preparing compounds substantially more complex than morphine which might fit the analgesic receptor but be prevented from fitting the receptors which, it was then thought, might be responsible for the unwanted effects of morphine.

The starting point for this work was the alkaloid thebaine (**3**), a minor component of opium which has no pharmaceutical value, being primarily a convulsant. Thebaine is chemically the most reactive of the morphine alkaloids, and contains a reactive diene system that leads it to undergo the Diels–Alder reaction to produce, with different dienophils, a range of adducts in very high yield.

The first such compound to be prepared was the adduct with benzoquinone (**16**). This substance, which had been known since 1937 (*22*), is a convulsant like thebaine, but its dihydro compound was shown to be an analgesic with about one-seventh the potency of morphine. The structure of the dihydro compound can be drawn as in **17**, and when this is compared with a similar perspective view of morphine (**18**) it will easily be seen that the almost flat side of the morphine

(**16**)   (**17**)   (**18**)

molecule has been completely altered by the building on of a substantial additional section. Moreover, this new part contains chemically reactive groups that facilitate the attachment of other groups further to complicate that face of the molecule. The Diels–Alder reaction, therefore, generated compounds that not only met the original requirements of the approach but also were ideally constituted as intermediates from which a large number of further compounds could be produced by relatively simple reactions.

Since adduct **17** was almost insoluble, attention was turned to other Diels–Alder adducts, and the first of these to be examined was found to be the ideal compound for further study and was the basis of most of the future work. This was the adduct of thebaine and methyl vinyl ketone (**19**), which is an analgesic as potent as morphine. A full account of the exciting chemistry of this and analogous adducts was written by Bentley in 1971 (*23*).

The ketone (**19**) was converted, by reaction with Grignard reagents, into a series of homologous alcohols of general structure **20.** The Grignard reaction is

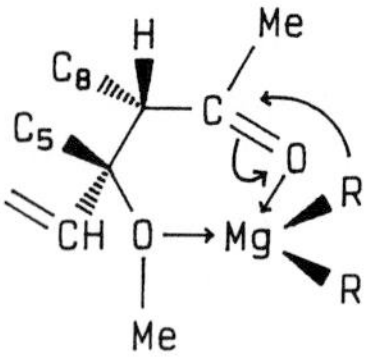

Fig. 1

stereospecific, being controlled by an intramolecular complex between the reagent and the oxygen atoms of the C-6 methoxy group and the C-19 carbonyl
which can deliver the alkyl group only to the less hindered face of the carbonyl
group to produce the tertiary alcohol (as shown in Fig. 1). Diastereoisomers of
20 in which the groups R and Me are interchanged can be prepared by reaction of
methyl magnesium bromide with ketones having structure **19** with the COR
group replacing $COCH_3$.

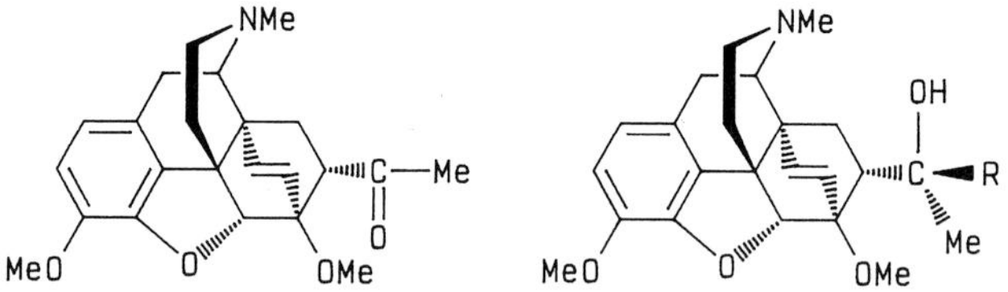

(19)   (20)

As shown in Table I the tertiary alcohols (**20**) had remarkable analgesic properties, in many cases far higher than any previously reported for derivatives of

TABLE I
Analgesic Potency
of Bases of Structure **20**
(Morphine = 1)
in Rat Tail-Pressure Test

R	Potency
CH_3	4.4
C_2H_5	13.3
C_3H_7	59
C_4H_9	56
C_5H_{11}	25
C_6H_{13}	10
Ph	0.04
CH_2Ph	75
$(CH_2)_2Ph$	300
$(CH_2)_3Ph$	1.1

TABLE II
Analgesic Potency for Bases of Structure **21**
in Rat Tail-Pressure Test (Morphine = 1)

	R^1		
R^2	CH_3	C_2H_5	C_3H_7
CH_3	4.4	0.39	0.71
C_2H_5	13.3	1.33	
C_3H_7	59	7.7	3.3
C_4H_9	56	5.9	

morphine (*24*). Potency rose sharply as the size of the alkyl group increased, reaching a maximum with *n*-propyl and thereafter declining gradually. With a phenyl group attached to the end of the alkyl chain the effect of lengthening the chain was even more pronounced (*25*). There was a 2000-fold increase in potency in changing phenyl to benzyl and a further fourfold increase to phenylethyl (300 times the potency of morphine) and then a 270-fold decrease to the phenylpropyl carbinol.

The effect of variation of alkyl group R^1 in structure **21** keeping R^2 constant on analgesic activity was not so substantial (Table II). Changing R^1 from methyl to ethyl resulted in a 10-fold reduction in potency but further increase to *n*-propyl had very little effect. As a result diastereoisomeric pairs show very pronounced differences. For example the two *n*-propyl methyl carbinols differ by a factor of over 80 (*24*).

(**21**)

All of these compounds are more closely related to codeine than to morphine, since they all bear a methoxy (OMe) rather than a hydroxy (OH) group at position 3. Codeine has only about one-tenth of the analgesic potency of morphine, so that O-demethylation of the alcohols (**20**) would be expected to lead to bases of even greater potency. This was achieved in good yield with sodium hydroxide in boiling diethylene glycol* and gave a series of phenols that in-

---

*Acid conditions could not be used since the tertiary alcohols undergo acid-catalysed rearrangements.

cluded analgesics of unprecedented potency, up to 10,000 times that of morphine in animal models of analgesia. These compounds have to be handled with great care, as certain chemists who were involved in their synthesis can testify: even extremely dilute solutions are readily absorbed through the skin. The increase in analgesic potency achieved by 3-O-demethylation of the bases of structure **21** ranged between 10- and 50-fold. When examined in detail it was found that all of these *N*-methyl compounds were fully opiate in character and no separation of desirable from undesirable effects had been achieved. It was obvious, however, that this chemical approach had uncovered a new and very extensive series of compounds with a different range, and in many cases a different order of potency from any previously encountered.

It was decided to select and investigate in greater detail one member of the extremely potent series of opiates. Etorphine (**22**) was found, in animal studies, to be 2000–10,000 times more potent than morphine, depending on the test. Although the dose of etorphine required to immobilise animals is greater than that required for analgesia, it is still small and the amount needed for even very large animals can be dissolved in very small volumes of solution.

(**22**) R = Me
(**23**) R = Ph

These properties make etorphine the ideal drug for the immobilisation and capture of wild animals. It was first used in this way in Africa in 1963, when it was very rapidly accepted by game conservationists and has since become the drug of choice for this purpose throughout the world. The small quantities of etorphine required to immobilise even the largest animals dissolve readily in less than 1 millilitre of water, easily contained in the shaft of a cross-bow dart, which can be used as a high velocity hypodermic syringe capable of penetrating the toughest hide.

IV. STEREOCHEMISTRY, ACTIVITY AND RECEPTOR THEORY OF COMPOUNDS RELATED TO MORPHINE

With all of the synthetic analgesics the biological activity is found in the enantiomer stereochemically related to natural morphine. The mirror image of morphine has been prepared from the alkaloid sinomenine (*26*) and has no

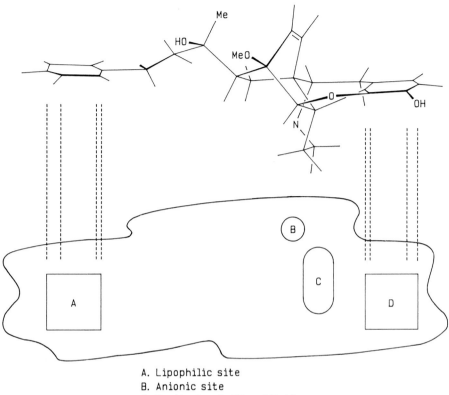

A. Lipophilic site
B. Anionic site
C. Cavity for C-15 and C-16
D. Flat surface for aromatic ring

Fig. 2   Diagrammatic representation of an analgesic receptor. A, lipophylic site; B, anionic site; C, cavity for C-15 and C-16; D, flat surface for aromatic ring.

analgesic properties. These findings were interpreted as indicating that morphine exerts its analgesic action by interaction with some three-dimensional surface (presumably of a protein) in the central nervous system.

By the mid-1950s a rough plan of such an analgesic receptor (Fig. 2, sites B, C and D) had been made by Beckett and Casy (27), following a study of the solid geometry of known analgesics. The flat surface was assumed to accommodate the aromatic nucleus, and the cavity part of the nitrogen-containing ring, with the piperidine N atom interacting with the "anionic site."

The magnitude of the effects on analgesic activity of very small changes of structure in the region of C-19 in the oripavine derivatives **22** and **23** strongly suggested that stereospecific receptor interactions additional to those postulated in the Beckett and Casy model were involved.

The C-19 alcoholic function appeared to exert a very specific influence on the interaction. It was first thought that a hydrogen-bonding interaction to the receptor surface protein was a requisite for the effect. Later when it was discovered that extremely high potency analgesics could exist in the oripavine series without OH groups attached to C-19, it was recognised that an alternative influence of the OH group was to fix the conformation about C-19 by hydrogen-bonding to the C-6 methoxy group (28). The interaction with the receptor which determines the extent of the analgesic and other opioid effects involves the lipophilic group represented by the group R in structure **21.**

Taking the peak of activity in the phenylethylcarbinol (**23**) as representing the most complete interaction with the receptor, it was deduced that the lipophilic site did not extend more than about 6 Å from C-7 and was also proximate to C-8 (*23*) (Fig. 2).

This discussion of the significance of the lipophilic site to analgesic activity was published in the early 1970s before unequivocal evidence for the existence of opiate receptors had been obtained. The subsequent identification and eventual isolation of the natural ligands (*29*) for these receptors, particularly the enkephalins, fully confirmed the important role of the lipophilic site. The enkephalins, both methionine and leucine types (**24**), have the phenyl group of the phenylalanine moiety oriented in relationship to the tyrosine residue to correspond almost exactly to the relationship of the side-chain phenyl group (**23**) to the phenolic aromatic ring of the oripavine nucleus (*30*).

Tyrosine   Glycine Glycine Phenyl-   R = SMe   Methionine
                                alanine   R = i-Pr Leucine

(**24**)

V.   ORIPAVINE ANTAGONISTS AND PARTIAL AGONISTS

The alcohols of structure **21–23** had their N-Me groups replaced by other alkyl groups, alkenyl groups, and cycloalkylmethyl groups using the nor-compound (N-H) as intermediate. The procedure involved the von Braun degradation with cyanogen bromide which gave the N-CN derivative and this was converted to the nor-compound by treatment with alkali at 180°C in diethylene glycol. The new N-substituent was introduced by direct alkylation of the nor-compound or by acylation followed by reduction of the amide (*31*).

TABLE III
Activity in Rat Tail-Pressure for Bases of Structure **25**

	R^1			
R^2	CH_3	C_2H_5	$n\text{-}C_3H_7$	$n\text{-}C_4H_9$
CH_3	0.34[b]	0.2[b]	IA[c]	0.22[a]
C_2H_5	0.05[b]	0.007[b]		
C_3H_7	6.7[a]			
C_4H_9	2.1[a]			

[a] Analgesia (morphine = 1).
[b] Morphine antagonism (nalorphine = 1).
[c] IA, inactive.

The test employed in the Reckitt & Colman laboratories to measure morphine antagonism was the reversal of the analgesic activity of morphine in the rat tail-pressure test. Using this test in which an individual compound shows either analgesic activity or morphine antagonist activity but not both, it was found that when morphine antagonism was evident it was in the *N-n*-propyl, *N*-allyl, and *N*-cyclopropylmethyl (*N*-CPM) series of bridged oripavine (3-OH) derivatives. In the corresponding thebaine (3-OMe) series, only when the N-substituent was cyclopropylmethyl (**25**) were any antagonists found (Table III). It was of particular interest that several of the *N*-allyl thebaines of structure **26** which were

(**25**) R = Me, R^3 = CPM
(**26**) R = Me, R^3 = —CH$_2$CH=CH$_2$
(**27**) R = H, R^3 = —CH$_2$CH=CH$_2$
(**28**) R = H, R^3 = CPM
(**29**) R = H, R^1 = Me, R^2 = *n*-Pr, R^3 = CPM
(**30**) R = H, R^1 = *n*-Pr, R^2 = Me, R^3 = CPM

CPM = cyclopropylmethyl

analgesic (agonist) in the tail pressure test (Table IV) were demethylated to oripavines (**27**) which showed no analgesia but were morphine antagonists (Table V). It had previously been thought that compounds related to codeine (i.e., having the 3-OMe group) owed their pharmacological action to metabolic

TABLE IV

Activity in Rat Tail-Pressure for Bases
of Structure **26**

R[2]	R[1]		
	CH_3	C_2H_5	$n\text{-}C_3H_7$
CH_3	0.018^a	IA^b	IA^b
C_2H_5	0.13^a	0.045^a	
$n\text{-}C_3H_7$	0.74^a		
$n\text{-}C_4H_9$	1.90^a		

[a] Analgesia (morphine = 1).
[b] IA, inactive.

TABLE V

Activity in Rat Tail-Pressure
for Bases of Structure **27**

R[2]	R[1]	
	CH_3	C_2H_5
CH_3	2.4^b	1.2^b
C_2H_5	0.12^b	1.04^b
$n\text{-}C_3H_7$	60.6^a	

[a] Analgesia (morphine = 1).
[b] Morphine antagonism (nalorphine = 1).

TABLE VI

Activity in Rat Tail-Pressure for Bases of Structure **28**

R[2]	R[1]			
	CH_3	C_2H_5	$n\text{-}C_3H_7$	$n\text{-}C_4H_9$
CH_3	50^b	8.33^b	0.96^b	5.71^a
C_2H_5	25^b	1.92^b		
$n\text{-}C_3H_7$	1000^a			
$n\text{-}C_4H_9$	77^a			

[a] Analgesia (morphine = 1).
[b] Morphine antagonism (nalorphine = 1).

demethylation to the corresponding morphine analogue. In the *N*-allyl series of thebaine and oripavine derivatives described above, the thebaine derivatives having qualitatively different activity from the oripavines are likely to exert their action through the intact molecule.

The influence of the size of the groups R^1 and R^2 on the analgesic (agonist)/morphine antagonist character and potency of the *N*-allyl and *N*-CPM bases is shown in Tables III–VI (*28*). The data refer to activity in the tail pressure test. For a fixed group R^1, with R^2 methyl or ethyl, morphine antagonism predominates whereas the corresponding *n*-propyl and *n*-butyl derivatives are analgesics. These changes are most strikingly demonstrated in the *N*-cyclopropylmethyl (*N*-CPM) oripavine group (Table VI) where the R^2 = ethyl member is a morphine antagonist 25 times more potent than nalorphine whilst the R^2 = *n*-propyl member is an agonist 1000 times more potent than morphine. For constant R^2, change of R^1 has a relatively small effect. Nevertheless it was demonstrated in both the *N*-CPM and *N*-allyloripavine series that, for R^2 = Me, there is a switch from antagonism to agonist at R^1 = *n*-butyl.

The difference of activity between diastereoisomers was, in certain cases very striking. *N*-CPM noretorphine (**29**) in the tail pressure test is an agonist 1000 times more potent than morphine whereas its diastereoisomer (**30**) is a morphine antagonist equipotent with nalorphine.

The pharmacological profiles of the *N*-CPM and *N*-allyl derivatives of structures **25–28** can be compared with the prototype antagonist analgesics which were known at that time, particularly nalorphine and pentazocine. These were not active as agonists in the tail pressure test. Both were identified as antagonists in this test though pentazocine had very low potency. Thus the Reckitt & Colman programme had eliminated from consideration as "low abuse" analgesic candidates compounds with significant agonist activity. Attention was focused on those members which were antagonists in the tail pressure test but showed analgesic activity in a second test, the mouse anti-writing test where the noxious stimulus is a chemical, usually *p*-phenylbenzoquinone, which causes mice to exhibit a writing motion which is inhibited by a wide range of analgesic compounds including aspirin and paracetamol. Both nalorphine and pentazocine were active in this test.

In the period 1963–1968 several candidates were selected from among the compounds included in Tables III–VI and each of these was examined in some depth in laboratory animals before being administered to patients or human volunteers. Each one was abandoned because, to a greater or less extent, it produced dysphoric and psychotomimetic effects which would have limited its utility as a clinical analgesic.

It was mentioned above that the members of the series which showed activity as agonists in the tail-pressure test were initially rejected as candidates for detailed evaluation. They had not been shown to have morphine antagonist activity,

and since agonist activity in the tail-pressure test had correlated well with tolerance and morphine-like physical dependence characteristics they were not considered interesting. The programme was held up for several years as a result. It
was eventually discovered that many of those *N*-allyl and *N*-cyclopropylmethyl
carbinols which did not show up as morphine antagonists in the tail-pressure test
were active as antagonists in the alternative tail-flick test, particularly in mice.
Moreover, the dose–response curves for a number of this latter group were bell-
shaped with the highest doses showing virtually zero analgesic effect. It appeared
that this phenomenon was an example of autoinhibition—the antagonism of a
drug's action mediated by interaction at one receptor by an opposing effect
mediated by a second receptor. This interpretation was consistent with developing theories of opiate drug action which recognised that there was more than one
opiate receptor. It was thus clear that these compounds had antagonist actions
and were unlikely to show a full morphine-like profile of tolerance and
dependence.

From amongst this group buprenorphine was eventually selected from a short
list of three. The other two were *N*-CPM noretorphine (**29**) and its 17,18-dihydro
analogue. These two were rejected since in the large-scale synthesis and development of pharmaceutical formulations each showed signs of dysphoric and psychotomimetic side effects. Despite use of face masks and rubber gloves, scientists handling the drugs on some occasions felt these rather unpleasant effects.
The drugs are extremely potent as analgesics (~1000 times morphine); only
extremely small quantities need to be absorbed to cause their pharmacological
effects. Such amounts can be absorbed easily through skin and other body
surfaces and this is facilitated by the high lipophilicity of the molecules.

VI.   BUPRENORPHINE

Buprenorphine (**31**), a 17,18-dihydro compound, was first synthesised and
tested early in 1966 but, for the reasons discussed above, it was not considered
seriously as a product candidate until 1969. It was first administered to man in
1971 and first marketed (in injection form in the United Kingdom) in 1978.

The synthetic route used for the first batches of buprenorphine is shown in
Scheme 1 (*31*). The thebaine methyl vinyl ketone adduct (**19**) is hydrogenated to
introduce the (saturated) ethano function at C-17–C-18. Later hydrogenation is
not possible since the tertiary alcohol function attached at C-7 shields the olefinic
function to the extent that it undergoes very few of the normal reactions of an
ethenic group. The CPM function was introduced by acylation followed by
lithium aluminium hydride reduction but in the commercial synthesis direct
alkylation with cyclopropylmethyl bromide is used.

A similar route is used to prepare the close analogue of buprenorphine, the

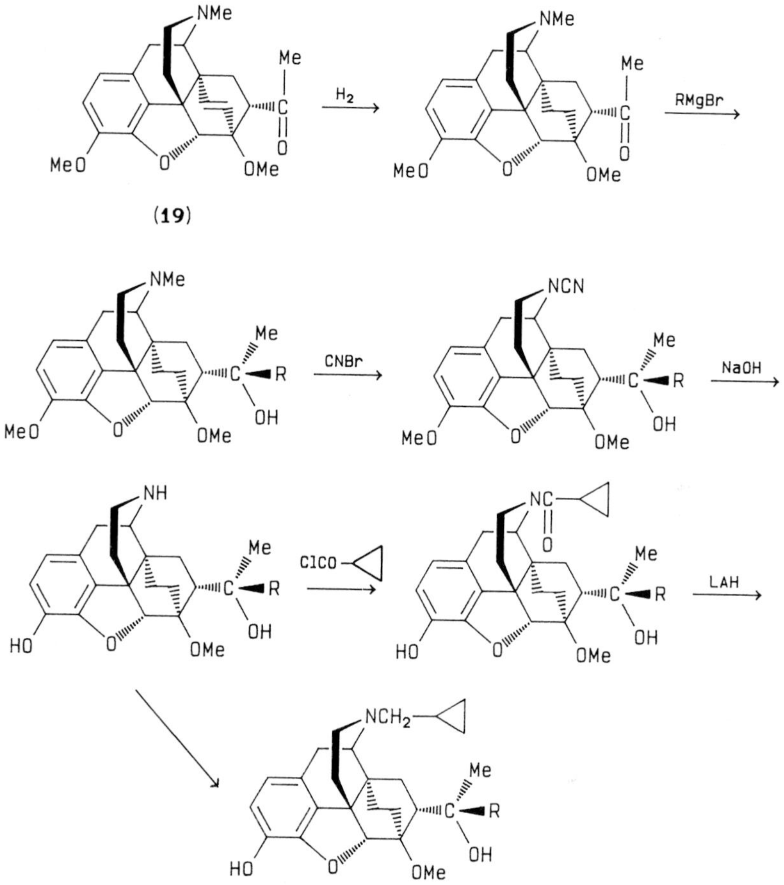

Scheme 1   Synthesis of diprenorphine and buprenorphine.

(31) R = t-Bu   Buprenorphine
(32) R = Me   Diprenorphine

pure antagonist diprenorphine (**32**). This antagonist is used to reverse the effects of etorphine used in immobilising both wild animals and domestic animals particularly dogs and horses, in the latter cases following surgery.

The structure–activity relationships in the series of which diprenorphine and buprenorphine are members were studied in some detail (*31*). Diprenorphine is a pure antagonist, that is, it has no analgesic activity. The analogue of structures **31** and **32** in which R is ethyl is also a potent antagonist but it shows strong analgesic activity in the anti-writhing test (Table VII). The *n*-propyl member (one of the short list from which buprenorphine was selected) was predominantly

TABLE VII

Relative Potencies of Compounds of Structural Type **31** and **32**

R	Rat tail-pressure agonism	(A) Mouse anti-writing agonism	(B) Mouse tail-flick antagonism	A/B
Me	<0.005	0.005	317	$<1.6 \times 10^{-5}$
Et	<0.005	6.8	67.9	0.10
n-Pr	225	213	0.17	1250
i-Pr	120	14.2	41.3	2.91
n-Bu	43.9	53.3	0.56	95.2
i-Bu	13.5	9.4	5.83	0.62
s-Bu	450	107	1.0	107
t-Bu	75	19.4	4.3	4.51
Nalorphine	<0.005	0.30	1	0.3
Morphine	1	1	<0.01	>100

agonist and extremely potent as was the n-butyl analogue. When the alkyl group R was branched, the balance of agonist to antagonist character shifted towards antagonism.

(**31**) R = t-Bu
(**32**) R = Me

Buprenorphine was shown to be about 50 times more potent than morphine in the tail-pressure test; it was inactive as an antagonist in this test but in the mouse tail-flick test it was a very potent antagonist (*32*). At its time of peak effect (which is somewhat delayed in comparison to nalorphine and morphine) buprenorphine was up to 50 times more potent than nalorphine as a morphine antagonist. This balance of powerful agonist and antagonist effects and the long duration of these effects were the basis of its selection as a product candidate.

A feature of the pharmacology of buprenorphine which has been mentioned earlier—bell-shaped dose–response curves—proved of great significance (*33*). It was shown that this type of relationship existed not only for various analgesic tests in animals but also for inhibition of gastro-intestinal motility (constipation) and, most importantly, for respiratory depression (*34*). The cause of death in overdosage of morphine and other opioids is depression of respiration leading to apnoea. In the case of buprenorphine at the very highest doses, the extent of respiratory depression is less than at some lower doses. This confers on buprenorphine a high level of safety.

The other feature of buprenorphine's profile which has proved important in determining its pharmacology is the slowness of its association with and dissociation from the specific opiate receptors in the brain. This accounts for its relatively slow onset and long duration of action, but more importantly it is a major factor in conferring on buprenorphine a unique freedom from the problems of physical dependence. The latter is manifested as an abstinence syndrome when a dependence-producing drug is removed from its receptor following a period of continuous or regular administration. In the case of buprenorphine the drug is removed from the receptor so slowly that the equilibrium in the biochemical system is never disturbed and an abstinence syndrome does not appear.

Buprenorphine is a very lipopilic drug (more soluble in lipid than in aqueous media) and as such would be expected to easily cross the blood–brain barrier for entry into the central nervous system (*35*). Such drugs normally have very rapid onset of action. In the case of buprenorphine the onset of action is slow and is controlled by the kinetics of its interaction with the opioid receptors in the brain rather than by the processes involved in giving it access to those receptors (*36*).

The opioid receptors in the central nervous system have been shown to be of several different subtypes which have been designated μ, κ and δ. The various opioid drugs have different affinities (binding power) and intrinsic activities (receptor activation leading to pharmacological response) at each of these receptors. Only μ and κ receptors would appear to be responsible for analgesia and respiratory depression. The physiological significance of the δ receptor, which is the primary receptor for the enkephalins, has not been determined.

The μ receptor is the primary receptor at which morphine exerts its actions. Buprenorphine has been shown to be a partial agonist at this receptor (*37*), which means that it produces a morphine-like agonist response but the maximum level of that response (however high the dose) is well below that of morphine. In other words, the intrinsic activity of buprenorphine at the μ receptor is considerably less than that of morphine, in contrast to the affinity which is very much higher. The latter is manifested in its much higher potency as an analgesic. Stated simply, a much lower dose of buprenorphine is required to produce a given level of analgesia than of morphine but there are very high levels of pain that morphine will counteract but buprenorphine will not. Buprenorphine also has extremely high affinity for κ and δ receptors but its intrinsic activity at these receptors is even lower than at μ receptors.

When the first human volunteer studies were undertaken we were naturally very concerned that buprenorphine, like the several earlier candidates from related series of oripavines, would cause dysphoria and psychotomimetic effects. The author received the first effective dose administered to a human subject and was greatly relieved not to see little purple men or other manifestations of nalorphine-like psychotomimetic effects. The lack of these side effects has carried through into patients in whom the prototype antagonist analgesic, pentazocine, occasionally does cause them.

During the later phases of the development of the injection formulation of buprenorphine, attention was turned to a solid dosage form for administration by mouth. It was found that buprenorphine's oral activity (swallowed) was much lower than its activity by injection. Only about 5% of the administered dose entered the blood stream, the rest being metabolised in the gut wall and on first pass through the liver before absorption into the systemic circulation. It thus appeared unattractive to develop a normal oral preparation of buprenorphine.

An alternative to swallowing a tablet is to dissolve it under the tongue so that it may be absorbed through the sublingual mucosa and directly enter the systemic circulation without first passing through the liver. It was found that buprenorphine is very well absorbed sublingually—at least 50% of the administered dose being absorbed. The rest escapes before absorption and is swallowed. The sublingual route proved to be extremely attractive to patients in clinical trials and sublingual buprenorphine was introduced into clinical practice, again in the United Kingdom, early in 1981. The sales to hospitals developed strongly, and by the end of 1982 buprenorphine was the leading strong analgesic in the hospital sector. It is used in hospitals particularly to treat the pain of carcinoma and following surgery, before and during which buprenorphine is also used as a premedicant and as an adjunct in anaesthesia (38).

Buprenorphine has thus become a successful drug—sold in many countries—and plays a useful part in therapy. It represents the nearest we have got so far to the ideal analgesic. It has good analgesic efficacy and very good safety in overdosage without producing physical dependence. It still shows morphine-like acute effects and some of these, (notably nausea and vomiting), though not serious, limit its utility, so we are continuing the quest. The story of the discovery and development of buprenorphine is like other stories in the field of drugs—it is one of frustration, perseverance, and a little luck such that in retrospect a story illustrating rational drug design and development can be told.

ACKNOWLEDGEMENT

The author is deeply grateful to Professor Kenneth W. Bentley who provided him with the opportunity to work in the Reckitt & Colman programme and gave inspiration and leadership to that programme. He specifically acknowledges the material from which the historical part of the chapter is derived.

REFERENCES

1. F. W. Sertürner, *Trommsdorff's J. Pharmazie* **13**, 234 (1805).
2. A. Seguin, *Ann. Chim.* **92**, 225 (1814).
3. W. Gregory, *Justus Liebigs Ann. Chem.* **7**, 261 (1833).
4. A. Laurent, *Ann. Chim, Phys.* **19**, Series 3, 359 (1847).
5. C. Von Gerhardt, *Justus Liebigs Ann. Chem.* **44**, 279 (1842).
6. P. Chastaing, *J. Pharm. (Antwerp)* **4**, 19 (1881).
7. M. E. Grimaux, *C. R. Acad. Sci. Paris* **92**, 1140 (1881).
8. C. R. A. Wright, *J. Chem. Soc.* **27**, 1031 (1874).
9. L. Knorr and H. Horlein, *Ber. Dtsch. Chem. Ges.* **39**, 1409 (1906).
10. J. M. Gulland and R. Robinson, *Mem. Proc. Manchester Lit. Philos. Soc.* **69**, 79 (1925).
11. P. O. Wolff, *Bull. W.H.0.* **2**, 193 (1949).
12. O. Braenden, N. B. Eddy, H. Halback, and P. O. Wolff, *Bull. W.H.0.* **14**, 353 (1949).
13. J. Von Braun, *Ber. Dtsch. Chem. Ges.* **47**, 2312 (1914).
14. E. L. McCawley, E. R. Hart, and D. F. Marsh, *J. Am. Chem. Soc.* **63**, 314 (1941).
15. J. H. Jaffe and W. R. Martin, *in* "The Pharmacological Basis of Therapeutics" (A. G. Gilman, L. S. Goodman and A. Gilman, eds), p. 513. Macmillan, New York, 1980.
16. W. R. Martin, *in* "Drug Addiction I" (W. R. Martin, ed.), p. 279. Springer-Verlag, Berlin, 1977.
17. W. R. Martin and D. R. Jasinski, *in* "Drug Addiction I" (W. R. Martin, ed.), p. 184. Springer-Verlag, Berlin, 1977.
18. L. Lasagna and H. K. Beecher, *J. Pharmacol. Exp. Ther.* **112**, 356 (1954).
19. H. Isbell, *Fed. Proc., Fed. Am. Soc. Exp. Biol.* **15**, 442 (1956).
20. S. Archer, L. S. Harris, N. F. Albertson, B. F. Tullar, and A. K. Pierson, *in* "Molecular Modification in Drug Design" (R. F. Gould, ed.), pp. 162–169. Am. Chem. Soc., Washington, D.C., 1964.
21. A. S. Keats and J. Telford, *in* "Molecular Modification in Drug Design" (R. F. Gould, ed.), p. 162. Am. Chem. Soc., Washington, D.C., 1964.
22. C. Schopf, K. von Gottberg, and W. Petri, *Justus Liebigs Ann. Chem.* **536**, 216 (1938).
23. K. W. Bentley, *in* "The Alkaloids, Chemistry and Pharmacology" (R. H. F. Manske and H. L. Holmes, eds), Vol. XIII, p. 75. Academic Press, New York, 1971.
24. K. W. Bentley and J. W. Lewis, *in* "Agonist and Antagonist Actions of Narcotic Drugs" (H. W. Kosterlitz, H. O. J. Collier, and J. E. Villareal, eds.), p. 7. 1972.
25. J. W. Lewis and M. J. Readhead, *J. Med. Chem.* **16**, 84 (1973).
26. K. Goto and I. Yamamoto, *Proc. Jpn. Acad.*, 769 (1954).
27. A. H. Beckett and A. F. Casy, *J. Pharm. Pharmacol.* **6**, 986 (1954).
28. J. W. Lewis, K. W. Bentley, and A. Cowan, *Annu. Rev. Pharmacol.* **11**, 241 (1971).
29. J. Hughes, T. W. Smith, H. W. Kosterlitz, L. A. Fothergill, B. A. Morgan, and H. R. Morris, *Nature (London)* **258**, 577 (1975).
30. A. F. Bradbury, D. G. Smythe, and C. R. Snell, *Nature (London)* **260**, 165 (1976).
31. J. W. Lewis, *in* "Advances in Biochemical Psychopharmacology" (M. C. Braude, L. S. Harris, E. L. May, J. P. Smith, and J. E. Villareal, eds), Vol. 8, p. 123. Raven, New York, 1974.
32. A. Cowan, J. W. Lewis, and I. R. Macfarlane, *Br. J. Pharmacol.* **60**, 537 (1977).
33. A. Cowan, J. C. Doxey, and E. J. R. Harry, *Br. J. Pharmacol.* **60**, 547 (1977).
34. J. C. Doxey, J. E. Everett, L. W. Frank, and J. E. Mackenzie, *Br. J. Pharmacol.* **75**, 118P (1982).

35. A. Herz and H. Teschemacher, *Adv. Drug Res.* **6,** 79 (1971).
36. R. Schultz and A. Herz, *in* "Opioids and Endogenous Opioid Peptides" (H. W. Kosterlitz, ed.), p. 319. Elsevier, Amsterdam, 1976.
37. W. R. Martin, C. G. Eades, J. A. Thompson, R. E. Hupler, and P. E. Gilbert, *J. Pharmacol. Exp. Ther.* **197,** 517 (1976).
38. R. W. Houde, *Br. J. Clin. Pharmacol.* **7,** 297S (1979).

CHAPTER 8

Atracurium: Design and Function

J. B. STENLAKE
Department of Pharmacy
University of Strathclyde
Glasgow, Scotland

I. INTRODUCTION

Neuromuscular blocking agents are used for skeletal muscle relaxation in surgery. They act by blockade of nervous transmission at the neuromuscular junction where they compete with acetylcholine (**1**) for specific acetylcholine

$$\overset{+}{Me_3}NCH_2CH_2OCOCH_3 \quad X^-$$

(**1**)

receptors on the post-synaptic membrane (Fig. 1). Such compounds are used in conjunction with general anaesthetics to provide a degree of muscle relaxation sufficient for effective surgery. Much deeper general anaesthesia would be required to achieve the same degree of muscle relaxation in the absence of a muscle relaxant. This anaesthetic-sparing effect therefore contributes to overall safety.

MEDICINAL CHEMISTRY

143

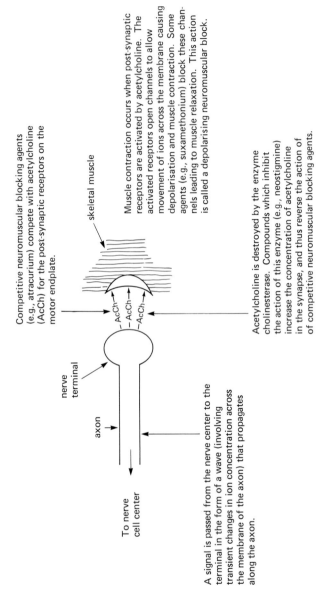

Competitive neuromuscular blocking agents (e.g., atracurium) compete with acetylcholine (AcCh) for the post-synaptic receptors on the motor endplate.

skeletal muscle

Muscle contraction occurs when post-synaptic receptors are activated by acetylcholine. The activated receptors open channels to allow movement of ions across the membrane causing depolarisation and muscle contraction. Some agents (e.g., suxamethonium) block these channels leading to muscle relaxation. This action is called a depolarising neuromuscular block.

nerve terminal

axon

To nerve cell center

A signal is passed from the nerve center to the terminal in the form of a wave (involving transient changes in ion concentration across the membrane of the axon) that propagates along the axon.

Acetylcholine is destroyed by the enzyme cholinesterase. Compounds which inhibit the action of this enzyme (e.g., neostigmine) increase the concentration of acetylcholine in the synapse, and thus reverse the action of of competitive neuromuscular blocking agents.

Fig. 1   Action of agents at the neuromuscular junction.

II.   FIRST GENERATION MUSCLE RELAXANTS

A.   DISCOVERY AND DEVELOPMENT

The site of action of skeletal muscle paralysing agents was first recognised in 1850 by Claude Bernard (*1*) when he showed that the South American arrow poisons known as curare block transmission of the nerve impulse at the neuromuscular junction. Not so very much later, Crum Brown and Fraser (*2*) showed that the methochlorides of various alkaloids including strychnine, brucine, codeine, thebaine, and morphine possessed similar properties. It was confirmed through the work of later investigators, notably Hunt and Renshaw (*3*) and Ing and Wright (*4*), that neuromuscular blockade was a characteristic property of most quaternary ammonium salts.

Interest in the neuromuscular blocking properties of the curare alkaloids was renewed when structural studies revealed that (+)-tubocurarine, the principal alkaloid of tube curare, was a quaternary ammonium salt. Shortly afterwards, Griffiths and Johnson (*5*) successfully used purified curare extracts for muscle relaxation clinically, heralding a new era in anaesthetic practice which allowed rapid advances in almost every area of general surgery.

The assignment of the bisquaternary structure **2** (R^1 = Me; R^2 = H) to tubocurarine (*6*), although later shown to be erroneous (*7*) and corrected to the monoquaternary bis cation **2** (R^1 = H; R^2 = H), sparked considerable interest in

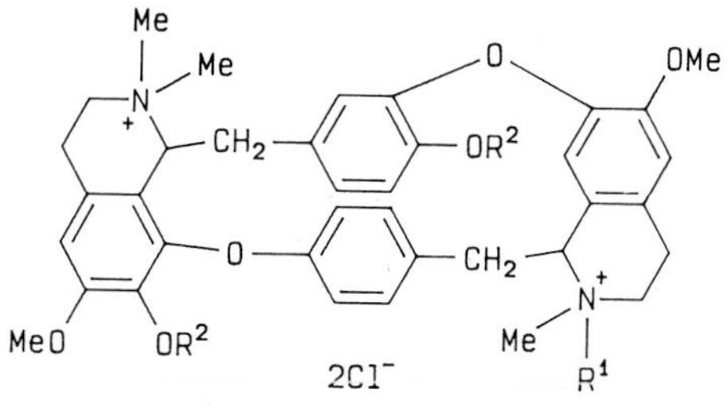

(2)

$$\overset{+}{Me_3}N(CH_2)_{10}\overset{+}{N}Me_3 \quad 2I^-$$

(3)

$$Me_3\overset{+}{N}CH_2CH_2OCOCH_2CH_2COOCH_2CH_2\overset{+}{N}Me_3 \quad 2Cl^-$$

(4)

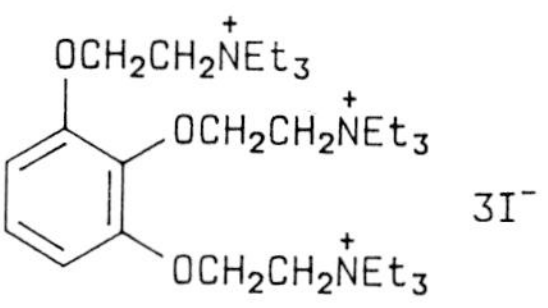

(5)

(6)

(7)   (8)

similar compounds. As a result, a number of synthetic bisquaternary ammonium salts were successfully introduced into clinical practice within a remarkably short period of time. These early compounds, decamethonium (3), suxamethonium (4), the trisquaternary compound gallamine (5), and their immediate successors, alcuronium (6), pancuronium (7), and fazadinium (8), all suffer from a number of defects which limit their usefulness.

B.   PROPERTIES AND LIMITATIONS

First generation neuromuscular blocking agents suffer from two major deficiencies: (i) lack of specificity for the neuromuscular junction, and (ii) undue dependence on renal and biliary mechanisms for termination of full block and recovery. The former gives rise to undesirable cardiovascular effects at full neuromuscular blocking doses, whilst the latter leads to prolongation of full block and recovery in patients with either renal impairment or diminishing drug metabolising activity, due for example to liver obstruction or damage, aging, or enzyme deficiencies such as those of the plasma pseudocholinesterases.

1. Specificity

Acetylcholine is not only responsible for nervous transmission at the motor endplates of neuromuscular junctions but is also released at synapses in both sympathetic and parasympathetic ganglia of the peripheral nervous system

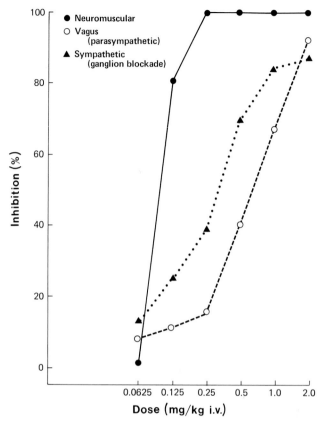

Fig. 2 Dose–response curve for tubocurarine showing neuromuscular, vagal and sympathetic blockade in monkeys (mean of four monkeys) (8).

(Chap. 1). Stimulation of the vagus nerves (the parasympathetic nerve fibres serving the heart) releases acetylcholine and, amongst other actions, slows heart rate and lowers blood pressure. It is not surprising, therefore, that neuromuscular blocking agents, which as quaternary ammonium salts resemble acetylcholine, also inhibit some of the other actions of acetylcholine in the peripheral nervous system. Due, however, to the strongly hydrophilic character of quaternary ammonium salts, they do not pass the blood–brain barrier and, for this reason, have no action on the central nervous system where acetylcholine also functions as a transmitter agent.

In general, monoquaternary compounds are more effective as ganglion blockers,* whereas compounds with two or more quaternary centres are predomi-

*Ganglion blockers are antagonists that act on the receptors attached to the ganglia in the sympathetic and parasympathetic nervous systems (see Fig. 11, Chap. 1).

nantly neuromuscular blockers. With the exception of suxamethonium, all first generation muscle relaxants show both vagal blockade and autonomic (ganglionic) effects with accompanying tachycardia (increase in heart rate) and fall in blood pressure. This is demonstrated in the dose–response curves of tubocurarine (Fig. 2) derived from simultaneous recording of neuromuscular, vagal, and sympathetic blockade. The percentage inhibition of vagal response at full paralysing doses of the first generation neuromuscular blocking agents in cats is

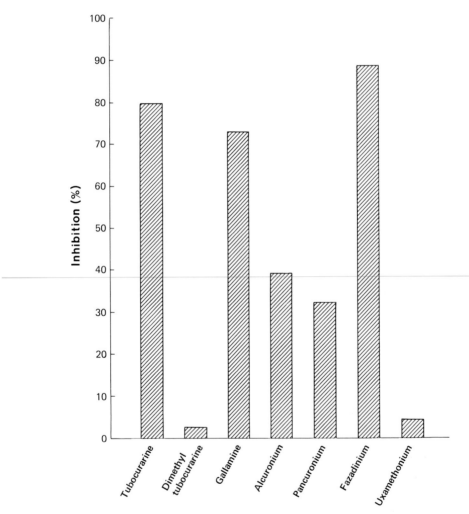

Fig. 3   Inhibition of vagal response at full paralysing doses of neuromuscular blocking agents in cats (*28*).

shown in Fig. 3. Similar responses are shown by the same agents in other mammalian species (dogs) and primates (rhesus monkey and man).

It is evident from the data shown in Fig. 3 that only suxamethonium (**4**) and metocurine [dimethyltubocurarine (**2**) $R^1 = R^2 = Me$] are virtually free from vagal blockade at full neuromuscular blocking doses, that substantial vagal blockade occurs with tubocurarine, gallamine, and fazadinium, and that it is by no means insignificant with alcuronium and pancuronium.

2. Duration and Recovery as a Function of Metabolism and Excretion

With regard to the recovery times, first generation agents fall broadly into two categories, (a) those that are of long duration of action (tubocurarine, metocurine, gallamine, and alcuronium) and (b) shorter acting agents such as suxamethonium, pancuronium, and fazadinium (8). Significantly, duration is related to metabolism and excretion, since the first group of compounds are metabolised slowly and only to a limited extent, and duration is largely a function of the excretion rate of the intact molecule. In contrast, the shorter acting compounds pancuronium and fazadinium are fairly quickly metabolised, whilst suxamethonium is rapidly metabolised.

The duration of action of compounds in the latter group is partly determined by the metabolic pathway and whether or not the essential bisquaternary structure is fragmented to inactive components. Thus, suxamethonium (**4**) is rapidly and extensively metabolised in normal subjects by pseudocholinesterases primarily to monosuccinylcholine (**9**) which has only about one-eightieth the potency of the parent compound (Scheme 1) (9).

Fazadinium (**8**) is also extensively metabolised (by azo reduction) rapidly in the rat and slightly less rapidly in the dog (10) with molecular fragmentation of

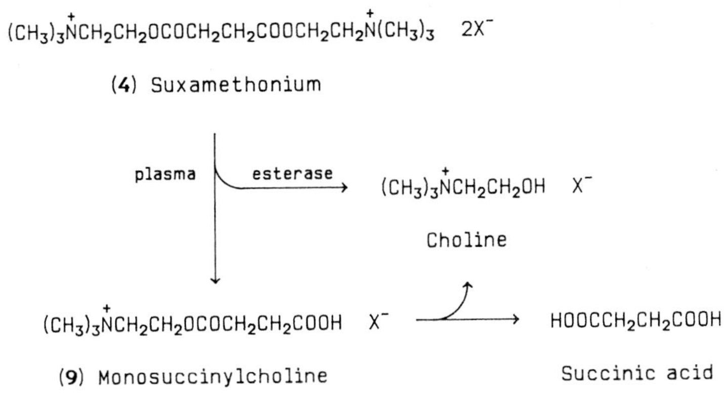

$(CH_3)_3\overset{+}{N}CH_2CH_2OCOCH_2CH_2COOCH_2CH_2\overset{+}{N}(CH_3)_3$ $2X^-$

(**4**) Suxamethonium

plasma | esterase → $(CH_3)_3\overset{+}{N}CH_2CH_2OH$ X^-

Choline

$(CH_3)_3\overset{+}{N}CH_2CH_2OCOCH_2CH_2COOH$ X^- ———→ $HOOCCH_2CH_2COOH$

(**9**) Monosuccinylcholine   Succinic acid

Scheme 1   Metabolism of suxamethonium.

its bisquaternary structure (Scheme 2). It is therefore relatively short-acting in these species. On the other hand, metabolism is very much slower in man. Hence, duration is longer in man and extended in kidney failure (*11*).

The contributory roles of excretion and metabolism as determinants of duration of action are well illustrated by comparison of the fate of tubocurarine and pancuronium. Thus, pancuronium has a significantly shorter duration of action than tubocurarine in man, while the rate of excretion of pancuronium and its metabolites is substantially less than that of tubocurarine. The more rapid recovery from pancuronium is therefore almost certainly due to the formation of the metabolites **10–12** (Scheme 3), which, despite the fact that they retain the bisquaternary structure, are significantly less potent than the parent compound (relative potency 50, 2, and 2% for compounds **10, 11,** and **12,** respectively).

3. Effects of Impaired Excretion and Metabolism

It is not really surprising that the action of all four of the longer acting agents (tubocurarine, metocurine, gallamine, and alcuronium) is prolonged in kidney failure, or that the action of both fazadinium and pancuronium is similarly affected due to retention of the parent compound and/or metabolites that retain the bisquaternary structure.

The duration of action of compounds that undergo deactivation by metabolism is, of course, influenced by factors which affect the rate of metabolism. Thus, some patients show genetically determined deficiencies in the biosynthesis of pseudocholinesterase that lead to reduced and, in a few cases, almost zero levels of plasma pseudocholinesterase (*12*). Metabolism of suxamethonium is markedly slowed in such patients (*13*), and prolonged neuromuscular blockade then results. This is, of course, highly undesirable, not only because of the unwelcome extension of full block but, more importantly, because the block is depolarising (Fig. 1) and not readily reversible by anticholinesterases such as neostigmine and edrophonium which, in contrast, readily reverse the competitive block of the other agents already discussed. Agents that are subject to hepatic metabolism are sensitive to liver disease or obstruction, and patients with such problems may

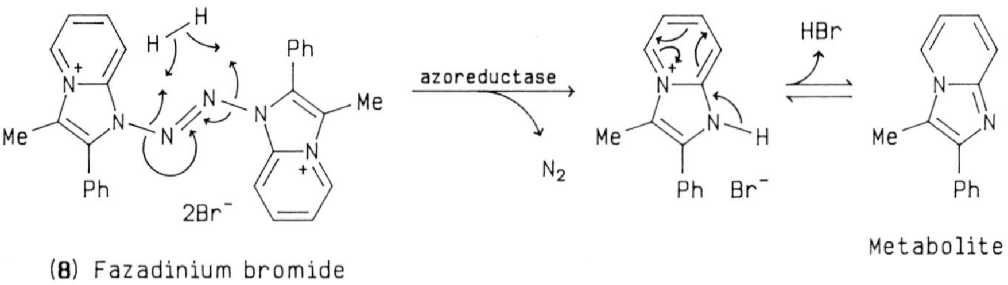

Scheme 2   Metabolism of fazadinium.

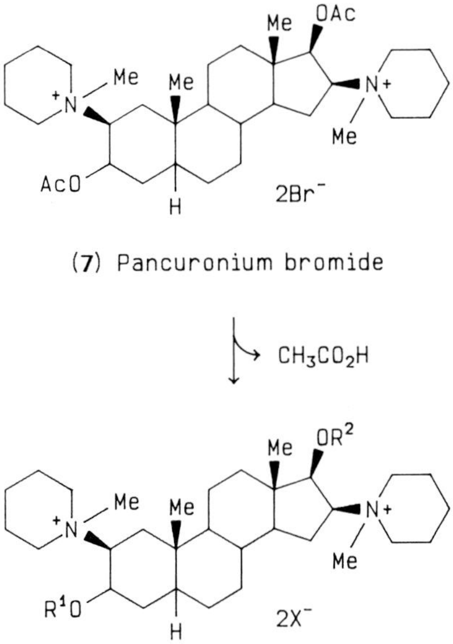

(7) Pancuronium bromide

CH₃CO₂H

(10) 3-Deacetylpancuronium R^1 = H, R^2 = Ac
(11) 17-Deacetylpancuronium R^1 = Ac, R^2 = H
(12) 3,17-Dideacetylpancuronium R^1 = R^2 = H

Scheme 3   Metabolism of pancuronium.

experience extended duration of blockade which may well be aggravated where there is accompanying kidney failure.

III. OBJECTIVES AND DESIGN CONCEPT

A. TARGET REQUIREMENTS

Studies leading to the development of atracurium were commenced with the objective of obtaining a relatively short-acting competitive neuromuscular blocking agent free from the major deficiencies of the existing agents. A substantial background knowledge and experience from earlier work (*14*) suggested that the required compound should possess the following features.

1. A bisquaternary structure with some 10 or 12 atom units separating the two quaternary nitrogens to achieve an adequate level of neuromuscular blocking potency.

2. Relatively large quaternary nitrogen substituents to ensure that the compound would have a competitive antagonistic action, denying access of acetylcholine to the cholinergic receptors at the motor endplate. We now know that

long slender molecules with small quaternary nitrogen substituents such as decamethonium and suxamethonium are channel blockers (*15*), that is, they block the channels opened by acetylcholine that allow the rapid and massive movement of ions across the membrane, causing depolarisation and triggering the excitation which normally causes muscle contraction (Fig. 1; Fig. 5, Chap. 1). There is also now some evidence to suggest not only that the cholinesterase inhibitor neostigmine fails to reverse the action of channel blockers but also that blockade is actually accentuated by such agents—a further reason for seeking a compound with competitive action.

3. A quaternary ammonium structure which would favour specific actions at the neuromuscular junction and minimise effects at other cholinergic centres. Little information on the structural features to ensure such specificity was available, apart from the fact that shorter interquaternary chains (five and six atom units) and small substituents on nitrogen appear to favour ganglion blockade (*16*). Structural features favouring vagal blockade were unknown.

4. A molecular structure which would assist rapid degradation *in vivo* independently of enzymic control, thereby ensuring relatively short action and speedy recovery.

B. HOFMANN ELIMINATION

An unrelated study of the chemical structure of a natural product suggested a novel approach to the problem. The alkaloid designated petaline, isolated from the plant *Leontice leontopetalum* L., was found to be a simple quaternary ammonium salt (**13**) derived from tetrahydroisoquinoline. Significantly, it was degraded unexpectedly readily by Hofmann elimination to yield a tertiary base, leonticine (**14**). This suggested the possibility of using such a reaction to produce a neuromuscular blocking agent which would degrade non-enzymatically to inactive and innocuous components at physiological pH (7.4) and temperature (37°C).

(**13**)   (**14**)

The Hofmann elimination of quaternary ammonium salts was first reported by A. W. Hofmann in 1851 within a few months of the discovery by Claude

Bernard of the action of curare in the neuromuscular junction. As first described, the reaction occurs under strongly alkaline conditions (pH 12–14) and at relatively high temperatures (~100°C). It results in decomposition of the quaternary compound with the formation of water, a tertiary amine and an olefin [Eq. (1)].

$$HO^- H\!-\!CH_2\!-\!CH_2\!-\!\overset{+}{N}R_3 \xrightarrow[100°C]{pH\ 12-14} H_2O + CH_2\!=\!CH_2 + NR_3 \tag{1}$$

Extensive studies of the reaction have demonstrated its mechanism and shown that the pathway and rate of the reaction are controlled by both electronic and steric factors (*17*). The positively charged nitrogen atom attracts electrons, weakening adjacent bonds, and functions as an electron sink. Nucleophilic attack occurs preferentially at the least hindered β-hydrogen atom with the formation of water and the breaking of C—H and C—$\overset{+}{N}$ bonds.

The presence of a second electron attracting group (X) attached directly to the β-carbon atom weakens the β-CH bond still further, so that the reaction is promoted at lower pH and temperature, and hence should be feasible within the normal physiological range (pH 7.4 and 37°C) [Eq. (2)].

$$HO^- H\!-\!CH\!-\!CH_2\!-\!\overset{+}{N}R_3 \xrightarrow{pH\ 7.4,\ 37°C} H_2O + CH\!=\!CH_2 + NR_3 \tag{2}$$
$$\qquad\quad | \qquad\qquad\qquad\qquad\qquad\quad |$$
$$\qquad\quad X \qquad\qquad\qquad\qquad\qquad\quad X$$

The reaction is inhibited by depletion of base. It follows, therefore, that it should be possible to prepare injection solutions which are stable at low pH and temperature (pH ~3–4 and 5°C).

C. MOLECULAR OBJECTIVES

In summary, the molecular target was a bisquaternary compound with large onium groups spaced some 10 or 12 atom units apart, incorporating electron withdrawing substituents β to the quaternary centres to facilitate ready decomposition under physiological conditions to inactive and, ideally, innocuous breakdown products.

IV.   DEVELOPMENT OF ATRACURIUM

A. APPROACH TO THE LEAD COMPOUND

In all, four series of compounds were prepared in pursuit of the objective. All were based on tetrahydroisoquinoline, many derivatives of which were already known to produce competitive neuromuscular blocking agents.

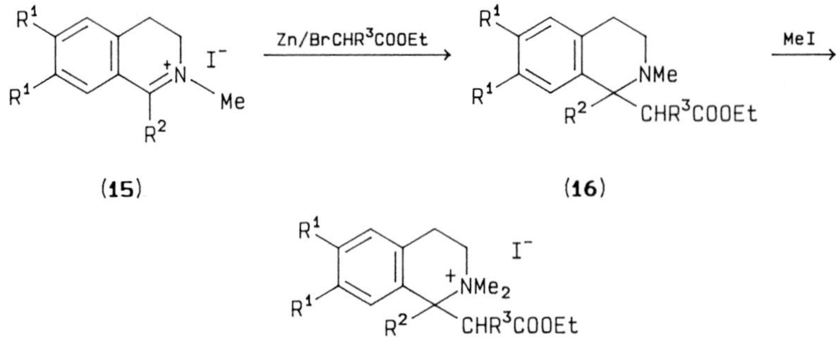

(15)   (16)

(17)

Scheme 4   Preparation of ester (17).

The nucleophilic addition of Reformatsky and Grignard reagents to 3,4-di-hydroisoquinolinium salts (15) and quaternisation of the product amines (16) with methyl iodide provided a flexible synthetic route to a range of model compounds (17–19) (Scheme 4). All these compounds were of very low neuromuscular blocking potency, the most active (18) having only 14% of the potency of tubocurarine in the cat (*18*).

Study of the quaternary ester (20) and its elimination product (21) in buffer pH 7.4 at ambient temperature showed that Hofmann elimination is incomplete and reversible under these conditions. This unexpected reversibility was attributed to the retention of the product amine and olefin in one and the same molecule thereby favouring re-quaternisation in a retro-Hofmann reaction.

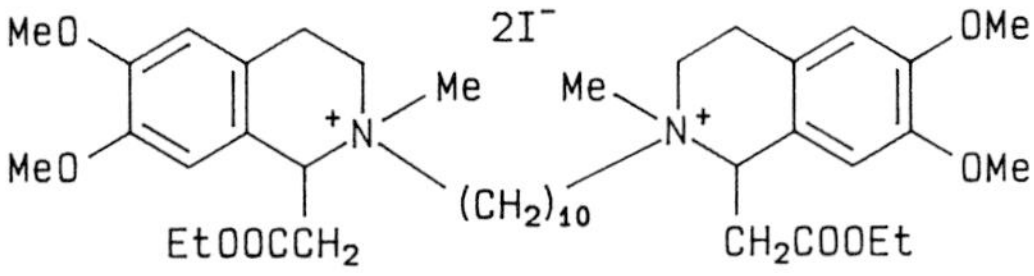

(18)

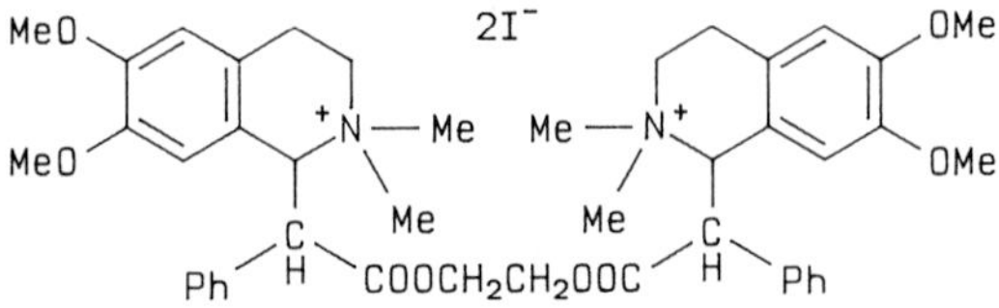

(19)

MeO, ... I$^-$ ... MeO, ... NMe$_2$

MeO ... $\overset{+}{N}$—Me   MeO   +   HI

EtOOCCH$_2$ Me   CHCOOEt

(**20**)   (**21**)

A second series of monoquaternary (**22**) and bisquaternary (**23**) 1-phenacyl-1,2,3,4-tetrahydroisoquinolinium compounds were also of very low neuromuscular blocking potency (*19*). They demonstrated, however, that the *rate* of elimination was largely governed by electronic effects in the phenacyl ring. Thus electron donating groups (OMe) retarded elimination, whereas electron withdrawing substituents (Cl) increased the rate of elimination to such a degree that, had other structural requirements to ensure potency been satisfied, duration of action would have been very short. The *extent* of elimination was dependent on steric factors, increasing with increasing bulk of the N-substituents due to greater relief from steric strain in the elimination products.

MeO ... $\overset{+}{N}$—R^3 MeO ... $\overset{+}{N}$—R^3

MeO   R^4 MeO   (CH$_2$)$_5$

CH$_2$ CH$_2$

I$^-$ CO   I$^-$ CO

R^2 R^2

R^1 R^1]$_2$

(**22**)   (**23**)

The importance of achieving complete molecular fragmentation to ensure irreversible Hofmann elimination focused attention on a third series of compounds (**24**) capable of degradation to the bases (**25**) and methyl acrylate (Scheme 5) (*20*).

The compounds **24**, where n = 6, 8, or 10 were considerably more potent (~20% that of tubocurarine) than those of the first two series but, unfortunately, they showed an unacceptably high level of vagal blockade in the cat. A fourth series of compounds with analogous degradation potential provided one compound (**26**) with about 60% of the potency of tubocurarine and a wide separation between neuromuscular and vagal blocking doses when tested in the cat.

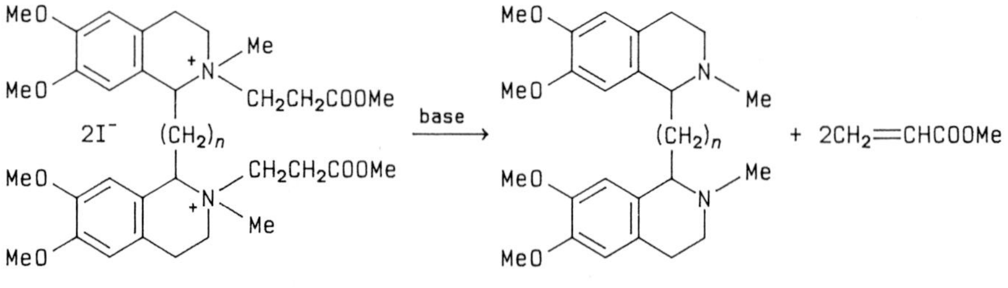

Scheme 5   Hofmann elimination of methyl acrylate from bisquaternary ammonium compound (24).

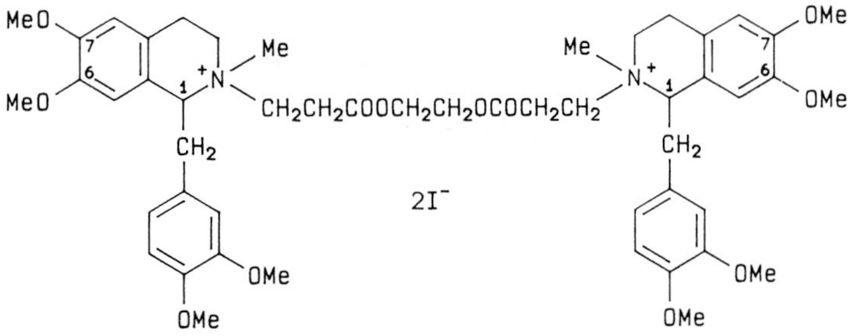

(26)

B.   DEVELOPMENT OF THE BISQUATERNARY COMPOUND (26) TO ATRACURIUM

Development was concentrated on structural variations to enhance potency and reduce vagal blockade. These centred principally on two aspects: (a) altering the ring substituents and (b) extending and modifying the interquaternary chain (21). Replacing the N-methyl substituents by larger alkyl groups was known to be counterproductive and, therefore, was not attempted. The two-carbon separation of ester groups and quaternary nitrogen was also sacrosanct to retain the capability of performing the Hofmann elimination (see later).

1. Ring Substituents

Replacement of the 6,7-dimethoxy substituents in compound 26 by a 6,7-methylenedioxy group (OCH_2O) (which in other series is favourable to increasing potency and reducing vagal blockade) actually reduced the relative potency and increased vagal blockade.

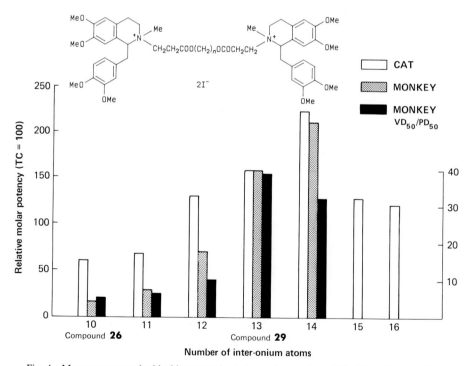

(27) R^1 = Br, R^2 = H, R^3 = R^4 = OMe
(28) R^1 = R^4 = H, R^2 = R^3 = Cl

Variation of the substituents in the 1-benzyl ring showed that the unsubstituted ring compound is the least potent compound. Methoxy groups enhance potency, but their number, position, and arrangement are critical; the 3,4-dimethoxy compound (26) was the most potent of the compounds studied. Two halogenated compounds, the 2-bromo-4,5-dimethoxy (27) and 3,4-dichloro (28) compounds,

Fig. 4   Mean neuromuscular blocking potencies (cat, monkey) and vagal blocking effect (monkey) of atracurium (29) and its homologues (28).

with potential for more rapid Hofmann elimination had relatively low potency. Further development was therefore concentrated on compounds with the same substituent pattern as the lead compound (26).

2. The Interquaternary Chain

Two aspects were considered: firstly chain length, and secondly chain structure. As anticipated, potency increased in both cats and monkeys with extension of the polymethylene chain up to a maximum in the compound with 14 atom units separating the two quaternary centres (Fig. 4). There was, however, little change in the duration of action on modifying the chain length. The separation between neuromuscular and vagal blocking potencies (VD_{50}/PD_{50}, i.e., dose to cause 50% vagal block divided by dose to cause 50% neuromuscular block) also increased with increasing chain length up to a maximum in compound 29 with 13 interquaternary atom units. This compound showed the optimum combination of potency and vagal blockade and was provisionally ear-marked as a potential candidate for clinical trial.

A group of compounds in which the central pentamethylene chain of compound 29 was modified showed that the introduction of an ether oxygen substituent, an aromatic ring, or chain branching in all cases reduced potency.

(29)

3. Pharmaceutical Development

Although the bisquaternary iodide (29) possessed a favourable pharmacological profile, its water solubility was too low for clinical use (a suitable compound must be sufficiently soluble to permit injection of a standard paralysing dose in a volume no greater than 1–2 ml). The solution of this seemingly simple problem, however, was complicated by the competing economic objective of not unnecessarily increasing the number of steps in the synthetic pathway. An additional, final, ion-exchange step to provide a more hydrophilic anion, which is feasible experimentally, was therefore not the ideal approach. A more satisfactory method would comprise the replacement of methyl iodide in the final quaternisation step by an alternative alkylating agent capable of generating the hydrophilic anion directly. Also, because of the potential carcinogenicity of all alkylating agents, any excess of the appropriate reagent must be capable of easy and complete removal from the product.

In the event, the problem was solved by a series of experiments with a range of sulphonic acid methyl esters. The methanesulphonate, benzenesulphonate (besylate), toluenesulphonate (tosylate), and 1- and 2-naphthalenesulphonates were prepared. Both naphthalenesulphonates had lower solubilities than the methiodide. The methanesulphonate had reasonable solubility but was hygroscopic

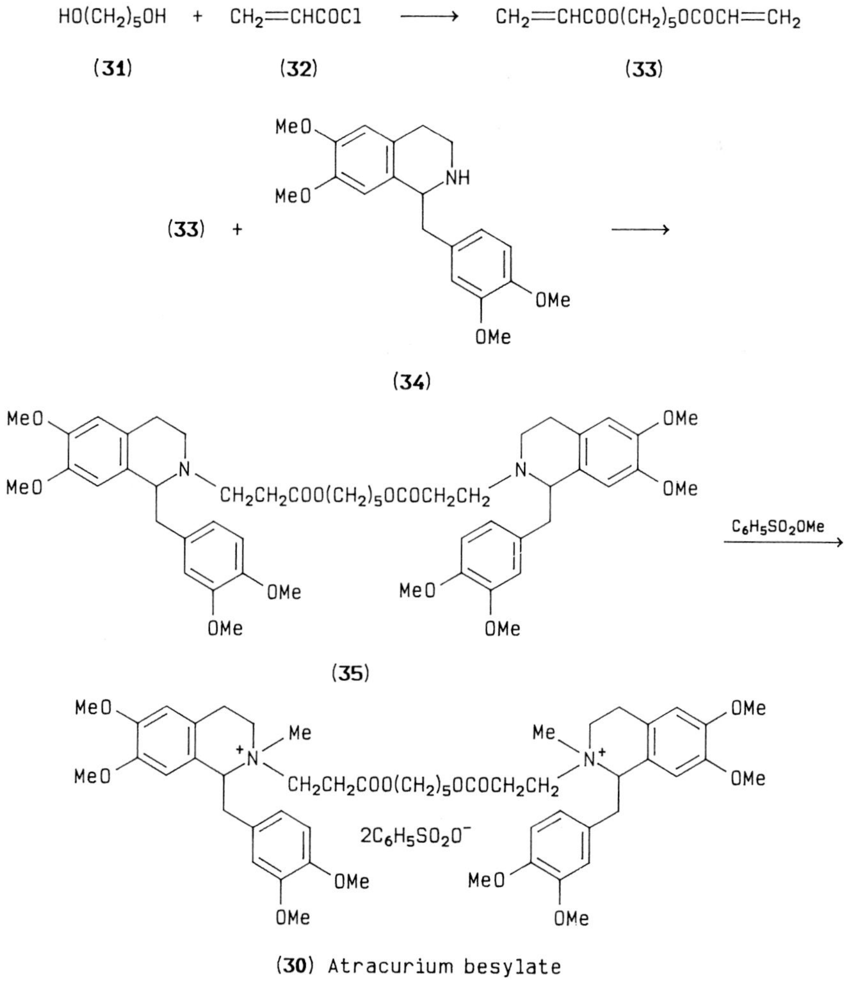
HO(CH2)5OH + CH2=CHCOCl → CH2=CHCOO(CH2)5OCOCH=CH2
(31)
(32)
(33)
(33) +
MeO
MeO
NH
OMe
OMe
(34)
CH2CH2COO(CH2)5OCOCH2CH2
C6H5SO2OMe
(35)
Me
Me
2C6H5SO2O⁻
(30) Atracurium besylate

Scheme 6 Synthesis of atracurium.

and there were doubts about its stability. The besylate and tosylate were more stable than the mesylate and readily soluble in water to the extent of about 60 and 35 mg/ml at 25°C, respectively. Accordingly, the besylate salt (**30**), designated Atracurium Besylate (British Approved Name), became the clinical trial candidate compound.

4. Synthesis

Despite its molecular complexity, atracurium besylate (**30**) is readily synthesised in just three steps from relatively cheap and easily available components (Scheme 6). The acylation of 1,5-pentanediol (**31**) with acryloyl chloride (**32**) to form the diacrylate (**33**) is followed by Michael addition of tetrahydropapaverine (**34**) to yield the ditertiary base (**35**). The final step is the quaternisation of the base (**35**) with methyl benzenesulphonate to form atracurium besylate (**30**).

V. PHARMACOLOGICAL AND CLINICAL PROPERTIES

Atracurium is a potent neuromuscular blocking agent in cats, dogs, monkeys, and man (*22*). Its action is competitive and hence readily reversed by the anticholinesterases neostigmine and edrophonium (*23*). Also it shows a wide separation in doses required to block neuromuscular and autonomic (vagal, ganglionic) mechanisms so that appreciable vagal blockade occurs only at some 8–16 times the full paralysing dose in the cat and monkey, respectively. Full block with a half-life of 20 ± 3 min is readily achieved in man at doses of 0.25–0.30 mg/kg with minimal effects on arterial blood pressure and heart rate, even at much higher doses. Full block was achieved in all the species examined with very similar doses (relative to body weight) and can be sustained as long as may be required by any number of incremental doses (0.1 mg/kg) without increase of recovery time.

VI. METABOLISM AND PHARMACOKINETICS

The consistency of response to atracurium is a feature which almost certainly results from the predominance of its purely chemical rather than enzyme-catalysed breakdown *in vivo*. The two-carbon separation between the positively charged quaternary nitrogen and electron attracting ester groups promotes mutual activation of Hofmann elimination and ester hydrolysis (Scheme 7). Metabolic studies in cats (*24*) have confirmed that breakdown occurs to furnish laudanosine

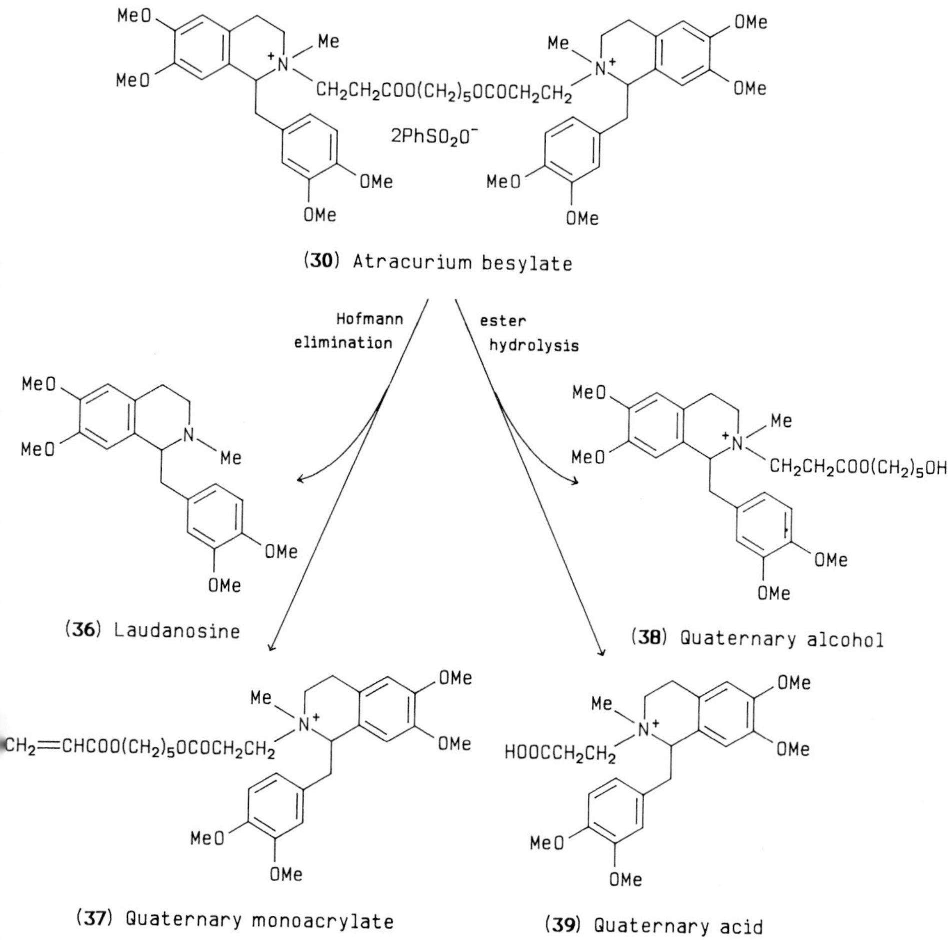

(30) Atracurium besylate

Hofmann elimination / ester hydrolysis

(36) Laudanosine

(38) Quaternary alcohol

(37) Quaternary monoacrylate

(39) Quaternary acid

Scheme 7   Metabolism of atracurium benzoate (29).

(36) and the quaternary monoacrylate (37) and, by concurrent ester hydrolysis, the quaternary alcohol (38) and the quaternary acid (39), all of which are not only virtually inactive at the neuromuscular junction but also innocuous. The plasma elimination half-life of atracurium was shown to be 19 ± 3 min, which is consistent with the observed duration of muscle paralysis.

The importance of Hofmann elimination as determinant of duration has been demonstrated by comparison of atracurium with analogue 40. This compound is structurally identical to atracurium (30) in all respects except the interquaternary chain which is modified to $\overset{+}{N}(CH_2)_3COO(CH_2)_3OCO(CH_2)_3\overset{+}{N}$ (21). Therefore it has the same overall interonium chain length as atracurium, and, accordingly, potency and vagal inhibition are not significantly different from those of atracurium. The composition of the chain, however, is different, with three methylene groups (instead of two in atracurium) between each quaternary nitrogen and its adjacent ester carbonyl, and three (instead of five) such groups separating the two ester groups. The greater separation of quaternary nitrogen and ester groups lowers the potential for both Hofmann elimination and ester hydrolysis, so that in contrast to atracurium, compound **40** shows a significant increase from 22.2 ± 2.9 min to 51.4 ± 5.2 min in recovery time from the onset of full neuromuscular block in the cat.

(40)

Experiments in human plasma from normal subjects and patients with virtually zero pseudocholinesterase activity demonstrate that this enzyme is not involved in the breakdown of atracurium (25). Thus, the mean half-life of suxamethonium was extended from 2.6 min in patients with normal pseudocholinesterase levels to more than 4 hours in plasma from patients with virtually zero enzyme activity. In contrast, no significant difference was observed in the half-life of atracurium in atypical and normal plasma samples.

In view of this striking evidence in support of chemical rather than enzyme-catalysed metabolism *in vivo*, it is not surprising to find that the duration of action of atracurium is independent of renal function. Thus, no extension in the duration of full block is observed in patients with renal failure or with deficiencies resulting from increasing age (26).

VII.   STABILITY: pH AND TEMPERATURE DEPENDENCE

The rates of Hofmann elimination and ester hydrolysis have distinctly different pH- and temperature-dependent profiles, which control the stability and life of the intact molecule both *in vivo* and *in vitro*.

Since both Hofmann elimination and ester hydrolysis are base catalysed, the breakdown and the duration of action of atracurium is pH dependent. This has been clearly demonstrated in cats following standard doses of atracurium (27). During respiratory and metabolic acidosis when the blood pH was reduced from 7.35 to 6.82, neuromuscular blockade by atracurium was increased and prolonged. Conversely, when the blood pH was increased from 7.29 to 7.66 during respiratory and metabolic alkalosis, neuromuscular paralysis was significantly shortened. This emphasises the sensitivity of atracurium to alkali and the need for care in manipulative procedures in the operating theatre where it may be used following solutions of agents which are distinctly alkaline.

Ester hydrolysis is also acid catalysed, but, in contrast, Hofmann elimination is increasingly inhibited with decrease in pH. Optimum stability for the molecule as a whole is therefore achieved at about pH 3.5. Inactivation of atracurium by both Hofmann elimination and ester hydrolysis is slowed by cooling, and injection solutions (pH ~3.5) stored in a refrigerator at 2–8°C have a shelf-life which is adequate for normal distribution and storage.

VIII. CONCLUSION

In summary, the muscle paralysing action of atracurium, like that of most other neuromuscular blocking agents, is dependent on its molecular structure, which is based on two suitably spaced quaternary ammonium groups. It differs, however, from other such agents in the exceptional instability of its quaternary ammonium groups. Thus, atracurium is reasonably stable in acid media, sufficient to permit the production of injection solutions, but is unstable under the mildly alkaline conditions that exist at physiological pH (7.4) and temperature (37°C). As a result, the onset of neuromuscular blockade following intravenous injection is followed rapidly by a controlled decomposition with destruction of the quaternary ammonium centres and formation of inactive and innocuous metabolites. This chemical (non-enzymatic) breakdown of atracurium with the loss of its quaternary structure ensures that the duration of full neuromuscular blockade is purely dose related and that recovery from paralysis is rapid, consistent, and independent of dosage.

Other advantages stem from the spontaneous degradation of atracurium *in vivo*. Quaternary ammonium salts generally are reasonably stable chemical entities and are not normally metabolised in the human body. They are also strongly hydrophilic. As a result, quaternary ammonium compounds are normally excreted via the kidneys with their quaternary structure still intact. In consequence, the excretion of most neuromuscular blocking agents is delayed in patients with impaired kidney function and the duration of full block is increased in older patients. In contrast, the spontaneous chemical destruction of the quaternary ammonium structure of atracurium *in vivo* ensures that the duration of neuromuscular blockade is unaffected by excretion kinetics and is not increased in kidney failure or in older patients. Also, since its degradation is virtually independent of enzymic activity, its duration of action is similarly unaffected by the status of hepatic (liver) function. Thus, atracurium represents a very significant addition to the range of compounds that act as neuromuscular blocking agents.

ACKNOWLEDGEMENTS

The author wishes to thank the respective publishers, authors, and editors for permission to reproduce Figs. 2, 3, and 4, and Scheme 7.

REFERENCES

1. C. Bernard, *C. R. Soc. Biol.* **2,** 195 (1851).
2. A. Crum Brown and T. R. Fraser, *Trans. R. Soc. Edinburgh* **25,** 151 (1867).
3. R. Hunt and R. R. Renshaw, *J. Pharmacol.* **25,** 315 (1925).
4. H. R. Ing and W. M. Wright, *Proc. R. Soc. Edinburgh* **109B,** 337 (1932); *idem, ibid,* **114B,** 48 (1934).
5. H. R. Griffiths and G. E. Johnson, *Anaesthesiology* **3,** 418 (1942).
6. H. King, *J. Chem. Soc.* 1381 (1935); *idem, ibid,* 265 (1948).
7. A. J. Everett, A. Lowe, and S. Wilkinson, *J. Chem. Soc. Chem. Commun.,* 1020 (1970).
8. R. Hughes and D. J. Chapple, *Br. J. Anaesth.* **48,** 59 (1976).
9. F. F. Foldes, P. G. McNall, and J. H. Birch, *Br. Med. J.* **1,** 967 (1954); V. P. Whittaker and S. Wijesundera, *Biochem. J.* **52,** 475 (1952).
10. L. Bolgar, R. T. Brittain, D. Jack, M. R. Jackson, L. E. Martin, J. Mills, D. Poynter, and M. B. Tyers, *Nature (London)* **238,** 354 (1972).
11. R. Duvaldestin, J. C. Bertrand, D. Concina, D. Henzel, L. Lareng, and J. M. Desmonts, *Br. J. Anaesth.* **51,** 943 (1979).
12. F. T. Evans, P. W. S. Gray, H. Lehman, and E. Silk, *Br. Med. J.* **1,** 136 (1953); M. Whittaker, *Anaesthesia* **35,** 174 (1980).
13. W. Kalow and D. R. Gunn, *Ann. Hum. Genet.* **23,** 239 (1959).
14. J. B. Stenlake, *Prog. Med. Chem.* **3,** 1 (1963).
15. P. R. Adams and B. Sakman, *Proc. Natl. Acad. Sci. U.S.A.* **75,** 2994 (1978).
16. W. D. M. Paton and E. J. Zaimis, *Br. J. Pharmacol.* **4,** 381 (1949); *idem, ibid,* **6,** 155 (1951).
17. C. K. Ingold, *Proc. Chem. Soc., London,* 265 (1962), and references therein.
18. J. B. Stenlake, J. Urwin, R. D. Waigh, and R. Hughes, *Eur. J. Med. Chem.-Chim. Ther.* **14,** 77 (1979).
19. J. B. Stenlake, J. Urwin, R. D. Waigh, and R. Hughes, *Eur. J. Med. Chem.-Chim. Ther.* **14,** 85 (1979).
20. J. B. Stenlake, R. D. Waigh, J. Urwin, J. H. Dewar, R. Hughes, and D. J. Chapple, *Eur. J. Med. Chem.-Chim. Ther.* **16,** 508 (1981).
21. J. B. Stenlake, R. D. Waigh, G. H. Dewar, R. Hughes, D. J. Chapple, and G. G. Coker, *Eur. J. Med. Chem.-Chim. Ther.* **16,** 515 (1981).
22. R. Hughes and D. J. Chapple, *Br. J. Anaesth.* **52,** 238P (1980).
23. G. G. Coker, G. H. Dewar, R. Hughes, T. M. Hunt, J. P. Payne, J. B. Stenlake, and R. D.

Waigh, *Acta Anaesthesiol. Scand.* **25,** 67 (1981); T. M. Hunt, R. Hughes, and J. P. Payne, *Br. J. Anaesth.* **52,** 238P (1980).

24. E. A. M. Neill and D. J. Chapple, *Xenobiotica* **12,** 203 (1982).
25. R. A. Merrett, C. W. Thompson, and F. W. Webb, *Br. J. Anaesth.* **55,** 61 (1983).
26. J. M. Hunter, R. S. Jones, and J. E. Utting, *Br. J. Anaesth.* **55,** Suppl. 1, 129S (1983); D. E. Rowlands, *Br. J. Anaesth.* **55,** Suppl. 1, 123S, 125S (1983); B. C. Weatherby, S. G. Williams, and E. A. M. Neill, *Br. J. Anaesth.* **55,** Suppl., 47S (1983).
27. R. Hughes and D. J. Chapple, *Br. J. Anaesth.* **53,** 31 (1981).
28. J. B. Stenlake, *Pharm. J.* **229,** 116 (1982).
29. J. B. Stenlake, R. D. Waigh, J. Urwin, G. H. Dewor, and G. G. Coker, *Br. J. Anaesth.* **55,** Suppl. 35 (1983).

CHAPTER 9

Discovery of a Family of Potent Topical Anti-inflammatory Agents

J. ELKS
The Ridgeway
London, England

G. H. PHILLIPPS
Department of Medicinal Chemistry
Glaxo Group Research Ltd.
Greenford, England

I. INTRODUCTION

In this chapter we wish to trace the development of the use of steroids as potent anti-inflammatory agents.

It has been known for many years that women suffering from rheumatoid arthritis often experience a remission of symptoms (i.e., relief from pain and inflammation) during pregnancy. As progesterone levels are high in pregnancy this was considered a possible cause of the remission, but that steroid proved to have no such activity and it seemed probable that another hormone was responsible. In 1949, the dramatic effects of cortisone in alleviating the symptoms of rheumatoid arthritis were announced by Hench, Kendall, Slocumb and Polley of the Mayo Clinic. Cortisone had been known for some 10 years as one of the many steroidal compounds (corticoids) isolated from the adrenal cortex. The compound had been synthesised on a substantial scale in the United States

167

because of the mistaken wartime belief that the Germans were using it to enhance the performance of their pilots, and a sufficient quantity was therefore available for test in rheumatoid arthritis (elaborate pre-clinical toxicology was not at that time a necessity). The successful outcome of that test made it urgently necessary to develop other syntheses of cortisone (**1**) capable of producing large quantities economically.

A particularly difficult aspect of the syntheses was the need to introduce the sterically hindered ketonic oxygen at C-11. Desoxycholic acid (**2**), available from ox bile, has an α-hydroxy group at the neighbouring C-12 and was used as starting material in the first methods of synthesis; improvements in the method by Sarett and his colleagues at Merck were accompanied by a reduction in the price from \$200/g in 1949 to \$10/g in 1951. However, the method still entailed more than 20 chemical stages (Scheme 1) (*1*).

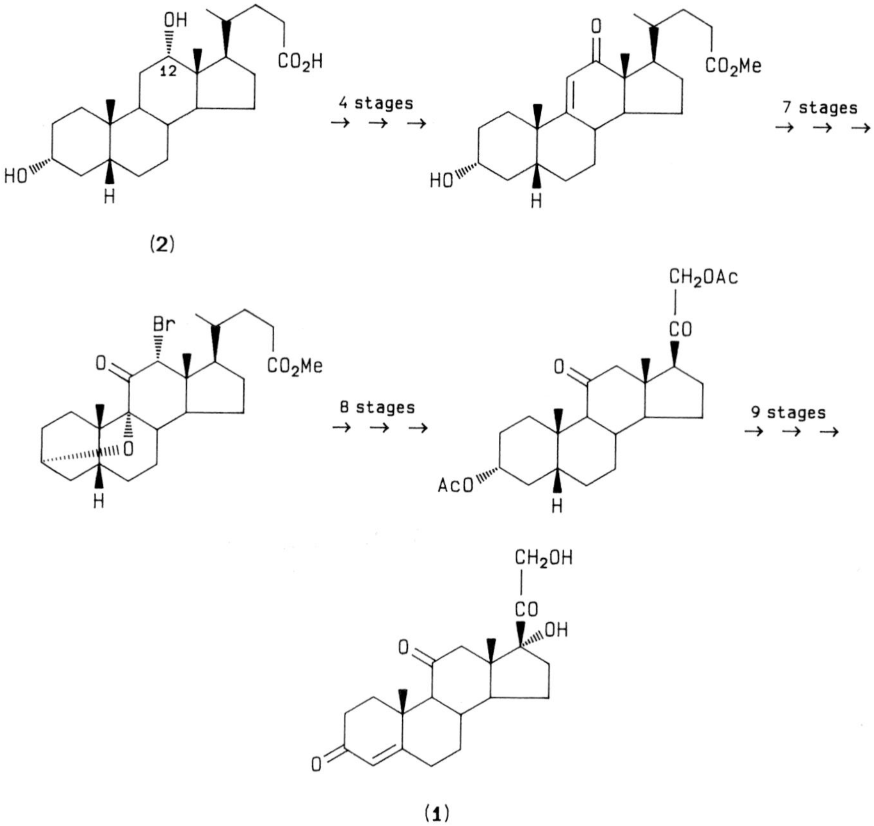

Scheme 1

(3) Progesterone   (4) 11α-Hydroxyprogesterone

(5) Stigmasterol

There was no easy chemical method for the introduction of an 11-oxygen function into the more freely available sterols such as cholesterol, stigmasterol and diosgenin, so the Upjohn Company mounted an effort to find a micro-organism that would perform this conversion, which was already known to occur in the adrenal cortex. Success came quickly using a strain of *Rhizopus arrhizus* that literally landed on their windowsill; this mould converted progesterone (3) into 11α-hydroxyprogesterone (4). Subsequent improvements involved different microorganisms and controlled conditions of growth; higher concentrations of progesterone could then be 11α-hydroxylated in almost quantitative yield. The substrate progesterone could be obtained from stigmasterol (5), a cheap by-product of processing the soya-bean, or from diosgenin (6), at that time readily available from Mexican yams. A route from 11α-hydroxyprogesterone to cortisone was quickly developed (Scheme 2) and the price dropped further to $3.50/g.

In 1950, the only identified naturally occurring steroid (other than the adrenal corticoids themselves) with an oxygen function at C-11 was sarmentogenin (7), which had been isolated from the seeds of a poorly identified African plant. Expeditions were sent to Africa from Switzerland, the United Kingdom and the United States, and the source of sarmentogenin was properly identified. Although a route to cortisone was devised, it never became a practicable one and a more important outcome of the British expedition was the identification of hecogenin (8), formerly a rare steroid, as a constituent of the widely cultivated *Agave sisalana,* the sisal plant (2). It occurs, in the form of its glycosides, in the

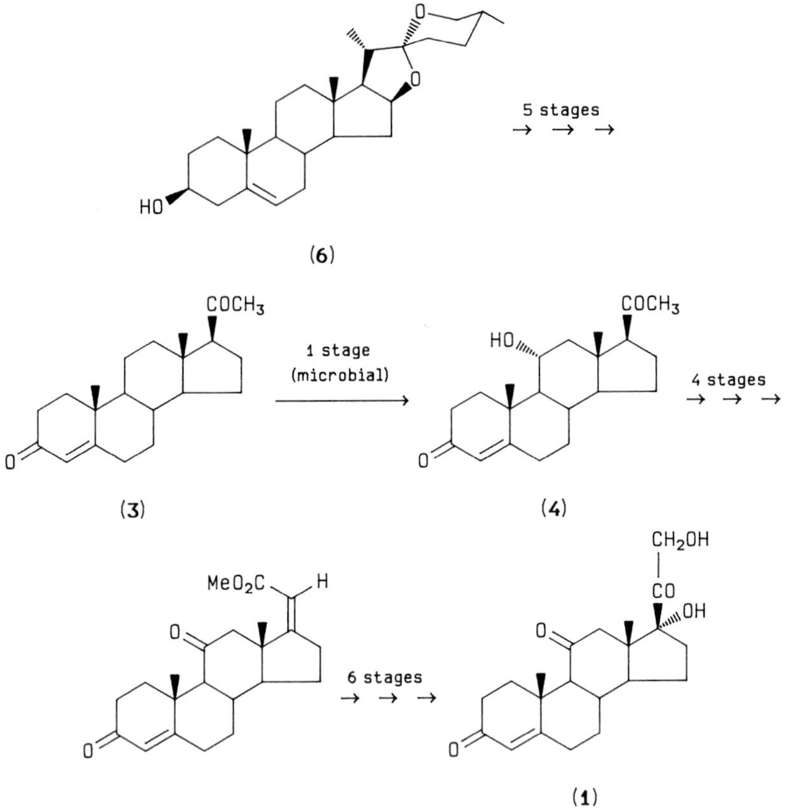

(6)

5 stages
→ → →

(3)

1 stage
(microbial)
─────────→

(4)

4 stages
→ → →

MeO₂C

6 stages
→ → →

(1)

Scheme 2

juice that is expressed from the leaves in the course of commercial fibre production and, as a secondary product, is relatively inexpensive. Hecogenin has a
ketonic oxygen at C-12, and a route for its transposition to C-11 had already been

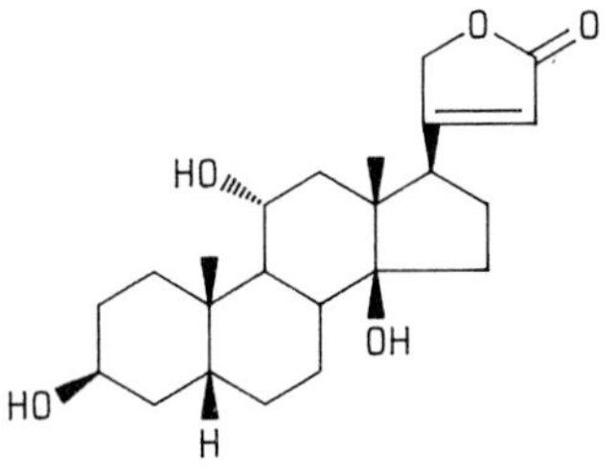

(7) Sarmentogenin

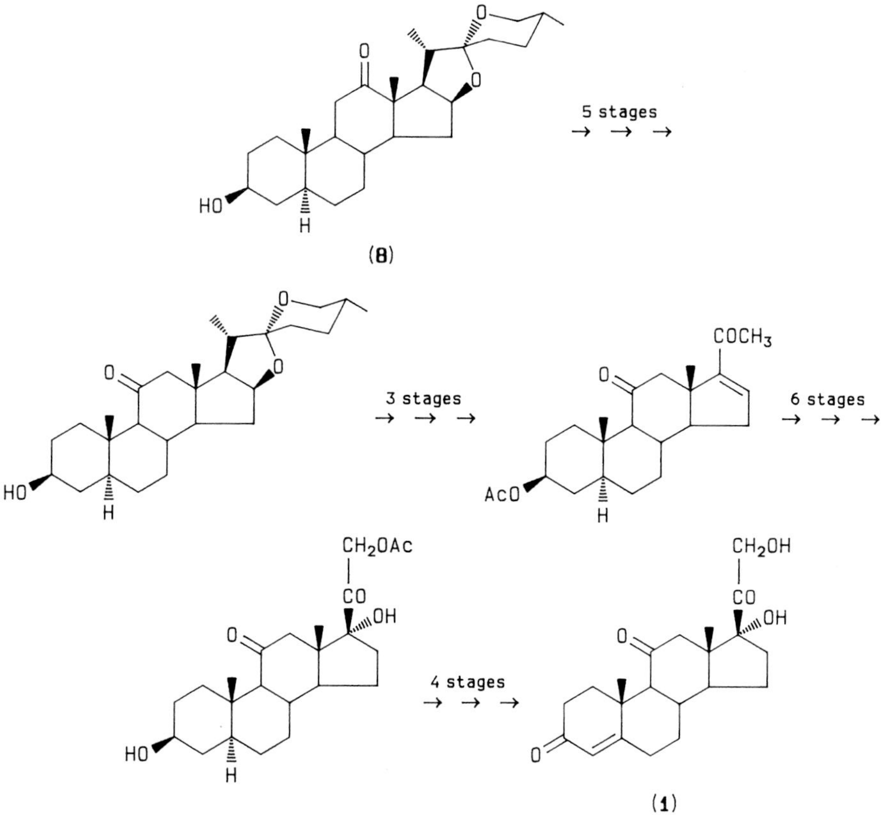

Scheme 3

devised. Further work at Glaxo Laboratories Ltd. resulted in viable methods for the extraction and purification of hecogenin and its conversion into cortisone in a 18-stage process (Scheme 3) (3).

Almost as early as the search for alternative methods of synthesis of cortisone, but initially much less successful, was the search for other compounds with similar biological activity. Cortisol (9) was the only one whose activity stood up to proper inspection. This, too, can be isolated from the adrenal glands of cattle, though in notably lower yield than cortisone. However, in man it predominates over cortisone. The two compounds show biological effects that are virtually identical because they are readily interconverted *in vivo;* the biological effects are generally attributable to cortisol rather than cortisone (4).

The first success in the search for surrogate compounds came when Fried and Sabo of Squibb (5) were investigating a route for converting the inactive 11α-

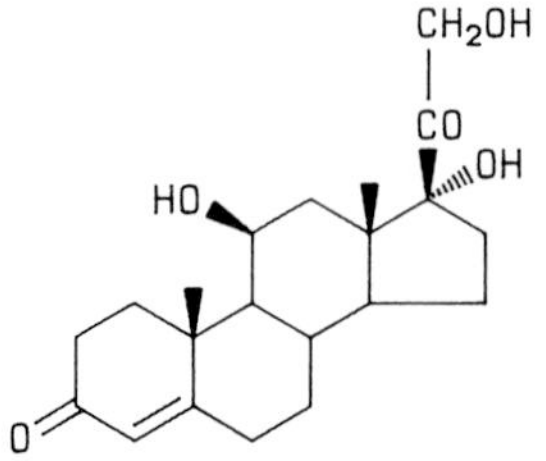

(9) Cortisol

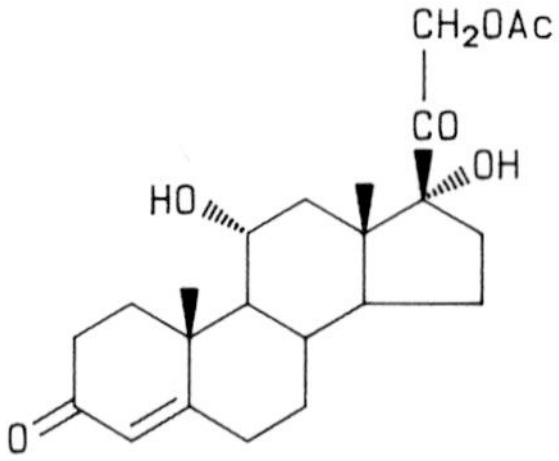

(10)

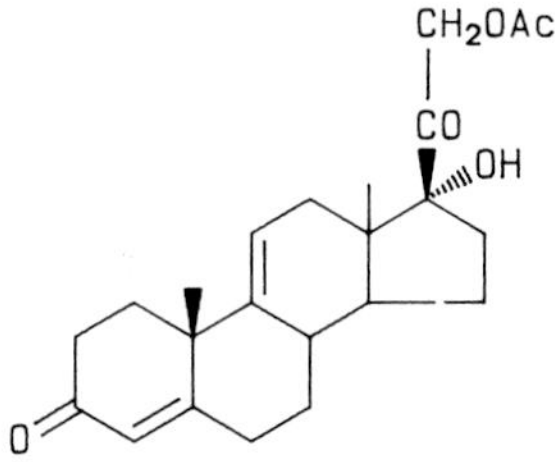

(11)

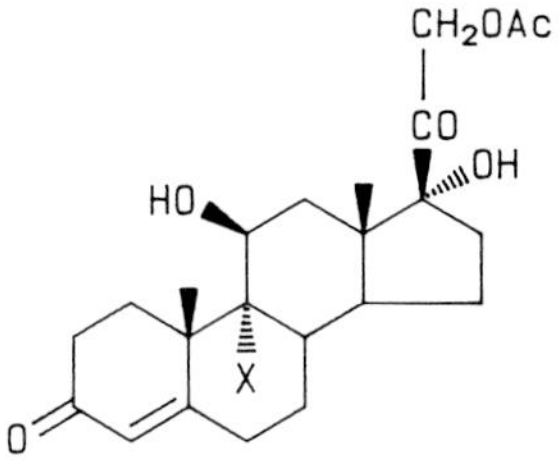

(12) X = Br
(13) X = F

hydroxy isomer (10) of cortisol 21-acetate into cortisol and wisely chose to check intermediates for activity. Addition of hypobromous acid to the 9(11)-dehydro-compound (11) gave 9α-bromocortisol 21-acetate (12), which was found to have about one-third of the activity of cortisone acetate in the liver glycogen assay.*
The other halogens were therefore tried in place of bromine and the activity was found to increase with decreasing atomic weight of the halogen.

9α-Fluorocortisol 21-acetate (13) has 11 times the activity of cortisone acetate but the substitution also has the effect of increasing to an even greater extent the unwanted mineralocorticoid activity, which causes retention of sodium and water in the body. The compound is therefore used only for the relatively rare cases in which this property is useful, for example, in Addison's disease.

The second success came from the Schering Corporation with the finding that the 1-dehydro derivatives of cortisone (14; prednisone) and of cortisol (15; prednisolone) were four times as active as the parents in their anti-rheumatic activity (6). Furthermore, they did not cause a proportionate increase in sodium retention and they were therefore rapidly brought into clinical use.

With these successes, there were renewed efforts to find yet other compounds with the required activity (4, 7). Notable among the successful substitutions were

---

*Cortisone and congeners promote breakdown of protein and increase deposition of the resulting carbohydrate (glycogen) in the liver.

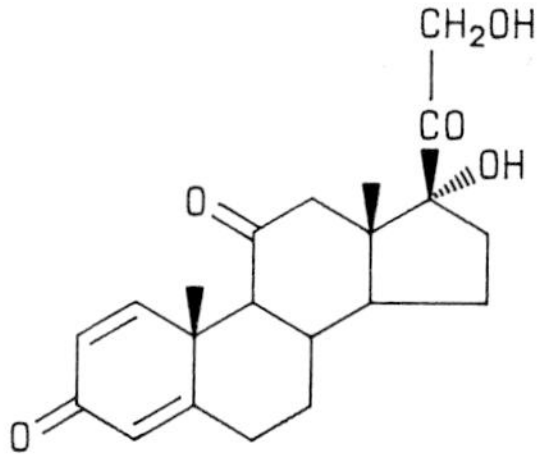

(**14**) Prednisone

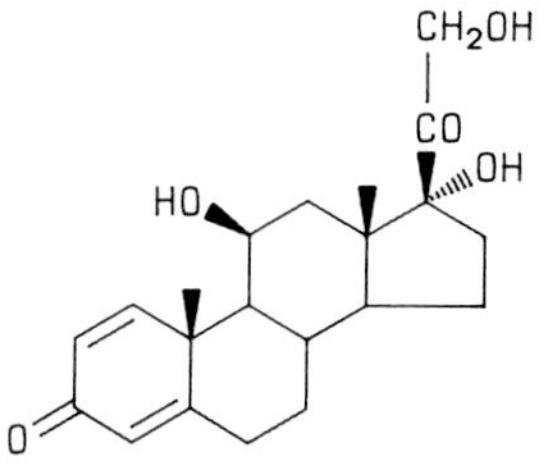

(**15**) Prednisolone

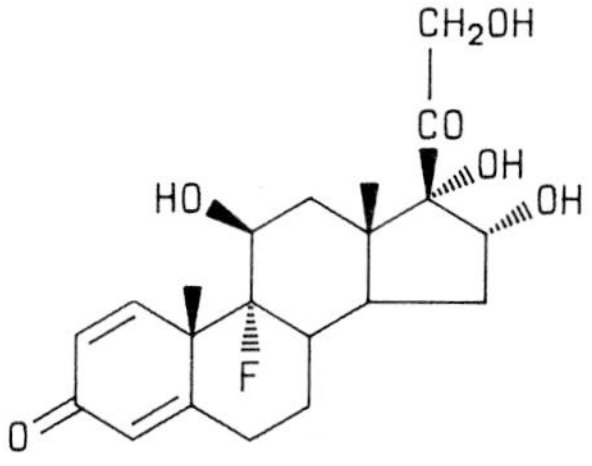

(**16**) Triamcinolone

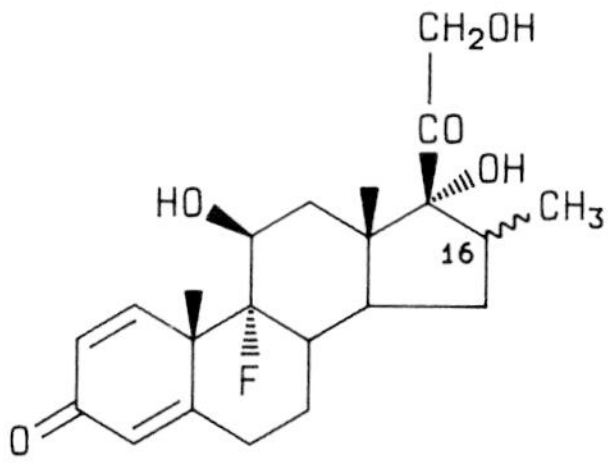

(**17**) 16α: Dexamethasone
(**18**) 16β: Betamethasone

the incorporation of a 16α-hydroxyl group, a 6α-fluorine atom and a 6α-, 16α- or 16β-methyl group. These too enhanced activity and, together with a 9α-fluorine atom, gave compounds such as triamcinolone (**16**), dexamethasone (**17**) and betamethasone (**18**) of greatly increased potency. Furthermore, the groups at C-16 overcame the tendency of the 9α-fluoro substituent to cause sodium and water retention, and the new compounds were added to the growing list of clinically available corticosteroids.

II.   MECHANISM OF ACTION

The mechanisms by which the adrenocorticoids produce a variety of biological effects has been and continues to be a fruitful area for investigation (8). One of the first important steps in the elucidation of the mechanism of action was the discovery that glucocorticoids* could regulate the activity of specific enzymes such as tyrosine aminotransferase and tryptophan oxygenase, attributable to enzyme induction by the steroids. Next it was shown that this enzyme induction was inhibited by blockade of protein or RNA synthesis.

The resultant theory that messenger RNA (mRNA) was involved was substan-

*Steroids, such as cortisol, that increase deposition of glycogen in the liver.

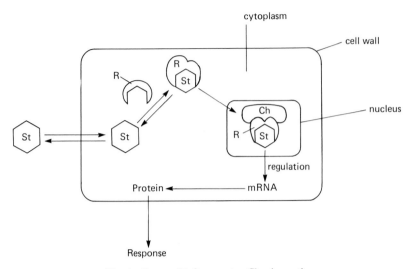

Fig. 1   St, steroid; R, receptor; Ch, chromatin.

tiated by a demonstration of glucocorticoid-induced build up of mRNA when protein synthesis was inhibited. The mechanism of the induction of mRNA production became clear with the finding that glucocorticoids bind to intracytoplasmic receptors and that the resultant complexes then migrate to the nucleus and bind to the chromatin or DNA, supporting the idea that the transcriptional level is involved (Fig. 1). Many of the proteins whose production is so regulated by glucocorticoids have now been identified, together with their role in hormonal action.

The glucocorticoids have been shown to inhibit the complex inflammatory and immunosuppressive responses in many ways, influencing the functions of various cell types and their movement and distribution. Some of these effects may be mediated by the products of the arachidonic acid cascade (prostaglandins, thromboxanes, endoperoxides and leukotrienes) and some steroids act by controlling the levels of arachidonic acid. Thus it is known that phospholipase A_2 activity, required for the formation of arachidonic acid, is controlled by a peptide (macrocortin) whose synthesis is in turn dependent on glucocorticoid action (9).

The synthetic glucocorticoid analogues with increased activity and selectivity of action usually show high affinity for the intracellular glucocorticoid receptors and their improved action can be partly attributed to this. However, effects on transport (for example, by altered binding to plasma components) are also of importance. Further, the introduced substituents and double bonds often slow metabolism to inactive steroids (metabolic inactivation may occur by reduction of ring A, 6β-hydroxylation, or oxidation or reduction of the dihydroxyacetone side-chain).

III. CLINICAL UTILITY

The original indication for treatment with cortisone and the subsequently synthesised analogues was rheumatoid arthritis, and this continues to be an important field of use, despite the side effects attendant upon chronic (long-term) therapy. However, it was soon discovered that the compounds had antiallergic activity and, given systemically, alleviated the symptoms of asthma. They were equally useful in hay-fever and in various conditions of the skin, such as eczema and psoriasis, but here the secondary effects of systemic corticosteroid therapy (deposition of fat, loss of calcium from the bones, suppression of the adrenal glands, suppression of the immune system) were too severe to warrant their general use, especially in children. One way of minimising side effects involves application of the steroid locally to the inflamed tissue, so allowing smaller systemic concentrations of the hormone, the skin being the easiest target.

Topical application of cortisol for treatment of skin conditions was first reported in 1952, and the newer analogues were tried as they appeared. They were, however, of somewhat indifferent efficacy. The situation improved with the introduction of triamcinolone acetonide (**19**) and, subsequently, of fluocinolone acetonide (**20**), in both of which topical activity was much enhanced. This latter compound, for example, as a 0.025% cream or ointment, was very effective in clearing the eruptions of eczema and, in many instances, of psoriasis. It did not, it is true, cure the underlying cause of the conditions, but the remission of symptoms, following the use of the steroid, was sufficiently long-lived to be clinically useful.

(**19**) X = H, Triamcinolone acetonide
(**20**) X = F, Fluocinolone acetonide

IV. THE VASOCONSTRICTOR ASSAY OF MCKENZIE AND STOUGHTON

McKenzie and Stoughton, in attempting to quantitate the effect of occlusion (i.e., sealing the area of skin over which the compound has been applied under an impermeable material such as polythene) on percutaneous absorption of steroids, made use of the clinical observation that such treatment led to pallor of the lesion and the surrounding skin. They postulated that the vasoconstriction that causes this is, in part, responsible for anti-inflammatory action. In experiments with dexamethasone (**17**), triamcinolone acetonide (**19**) and fluocinolone acetonide (**20**) on human subjects, they found that occlusion reduced 100-fold the concentration of the compounds that would cause vasoconstriction, as measured by pallor of the treated skin. Furthermore, by this criterion, dexamethasone was 100 times less active than either of the other two.

McKenzie used the same method to compare 20 steroids and found that whereas 21-acetates were about 10 times more "active" than the corresponding free alcohols, 21-phosphates were less active. Particularly striking was the thousandfold increase in activity in going from triamcinolone to its acetonide, although they were equiactive on intradermal injection; it appeared that the difference in activity on topical application is a reflection of the effect of the acetonide grouping upon absorption. Ideally, the steroid should pass through the horny layer of the stratum corneum to achieve an effective concentration in the epidermis but should not pass readily into the dermis and thence the systemic circulation.

McKenzie's study showed, significantly, that the most powerful vasoconstriction was shown by those substances that had been shown, clinically, to be the most effective topical anti-inflammatory agents (*10*).

V. EARLY WORK AT GLAXO

In examining McKenzie's results, it appeared that an important factor in determining the vasoconstrictor effect was the lipophilicity of the compound; the more lipophilic the compound, the more activity was enhanced. We set about, therefore, the preparation of lipophilic derivatives of the active steroids. We concentrated on derivatives of betamethasone, 9α-fluoro-16β-methylprednisolone (**18**) [whose synthesis (Scheme 4) had been developed at Glaxo] (*11*), not merely because it was readily available to us, but because it has very high activity systemically. Further, it could be borne in mind that skin contains various enzymes capable of metabolising steroids and that substituents, such as those in betamethasone, that minimise this process, may also be of value in topical steroids. In the event, the choice proved to be a wise one, since betamethasone derivatives usually had the highest activity of all the steroids that we tested (*12*).

In our studies we used McKenzie's method because it used the most appropriate animal, man, in a way sufficiently untraumatic to ensure ready volunteers from the staff! Graded dilutions of the test compound in ethanol were applied to a randomized pattern of circular areas on the flexor surface of the forearm, along

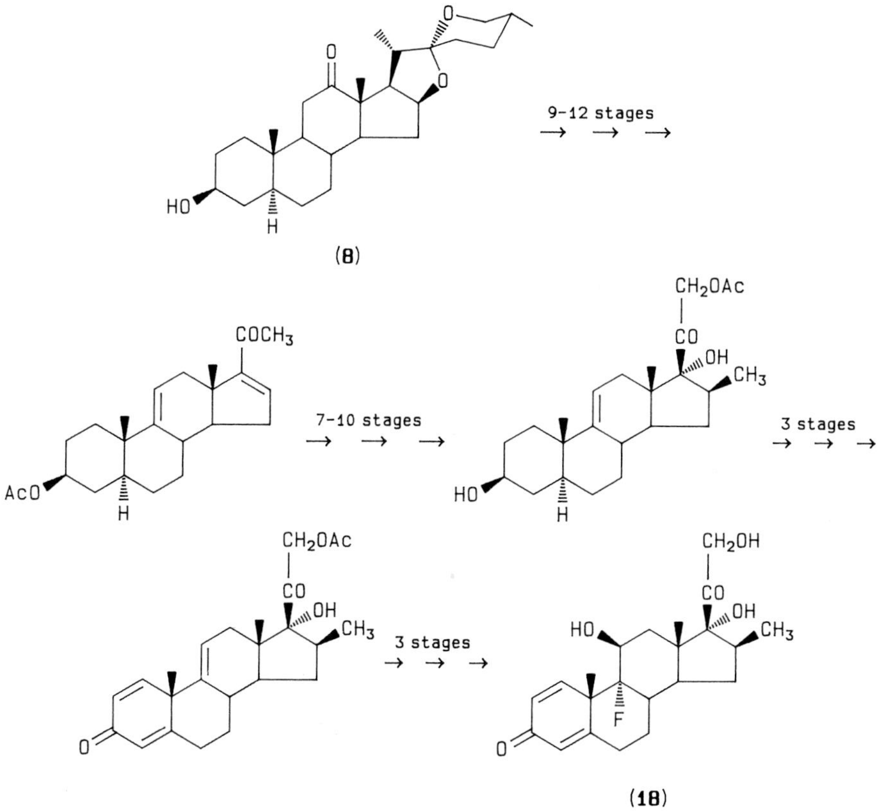

Scheme 4

with similar dilutions of fluocinolone acetonide, which was used as standard. The arm was then occluded with polythene and after 15 hours the polythene was removed, and the skin was allowed to settle for 1 hour and then "read". The minimum concentration of test compound that would cause vasoconstriction, as indicated by pallor of the skin, was compared with the concentration of fluocinolone acetonide that would do so. Fluocinolone acetonide was arbitrarily assigned a score of 100, and higher scores indicate more active compounds. In examining a series of compounds with related structures, it was usually possible to discern a pattern of structure–activity relationship.

Our first attempts at making more lipophilic derivatives of betamethasone involved the preparation of esters of the unhindered primary 21-hydroxyl group with acids of increasing molecular weight. This could be done, for example, by treatment of betamethasone with the appropriate acid chloride or acid anhydride. It was found that the aliphatic 21-esters showed increasing activity with increasing molecular weight peaking with the isobutyrate (McKenzie score 90) (cf. betamethasone, McKenzie score 0.8).

Encouraged by these results, we set about the masking of both the 17- and 21-hydroxy groups so as to increase the lipophilicity further. Among the first groups tried were the alkyl 17,21-orthoesters, and very soon we found the high activities that we were seeking.

Methyl or ethyl betamethasone 17,21-orthoesters had activities that increased from the orthoformate to the orthobutyrate (McKenzie score 400) and then began to decrease. In a small clinical trial, the methyl orthovalerate (21) (McKenzie score 150) was tested in psoriasis, and was found to be very effective. Some preliminary work was done towards developing this derivative, but its pharmaceutical properties proved unsuitable; in particular, it was not sufficiently stable in the media that would be used.

(21) Betamethasone 17,21-methyl   (22) Betamethasone 17-valerate
orthovalerate

However, the 17-monoesters of betamethasone (e.g., 22) obtained by very gentle treatment of orthoesters with an organic or a mineral acid, proved to be at least as active as the cyclic derivatives, which may, indeed, have been converted into the 17-esters on the skin.

For straight-chain 17-esters, biological activity increased from acetate to valerate (McKenzie score 360) and then dropped fairly sharply. Branched-chain esters were also investigated; activity appeared to peak at the isobutyrate (McKenzie score 470). It is interesting that, over a wide range of acids, 17-monoesters were more active than were the 21-esters, possibly because of their greater resistance to chemical or enzymatic hydrolysis.

17-Monoesters of a number of other active steroids were synthesised; they included derivatives of cortisone, hydrocortisone, prednisone, prednisolone and dexamethasone. However, they usually proved to be less active than the corresponding esters of betamethasone.

Betamethasone 17-valerate [22, Betnovate (Glaxo)] was selected for further trial and subsequently for development. Its activity in the McKenzie test (score 360) was among the highest that we could achieve at that time, and in a pilot clinical trial it appeared superior to fluocinolone acetonide. Although, in common with other 17-monoesters, it is readily converted by base to the corresponding 21-monoester, and thence into betamethasone, it is stable enough in ointments and creams to allow an adequate shelf-life.

Betamethasone 17-valerate was tested clinically, as a 0.12% preparation, in eczema and psoriasis against fluocinolone acetonide (0.025%) and some other steroid preparations. In 14 out of 20 trials, it was considered superior to the other steroid; in the remainder, it was at least as effective. No side effects were observed with any of the steroids (*13*).

The 17-monoesters of betamethasone may be prepared by treatment of betamethasone with a trialkyl orthoester, in presence of toluene-*p*-sulphonic acid as catalyst, to give the alkyl betamethasone orthoester, followed by gentle treatment with acid (Scheme 5). An interesting alternative method involves treatment of the corresponding 21-monoester with a strong base under anhydrous conditions, particularly with lithium dimethyl copper. This last reaction presumably proceeds via a cyclic derivative, as indeed does the converse transformation, brought about by aqueous alkali (Scheme 5).

Betnovate was marketed in 1963, as cream and ointment, and with or without an anti-infective. It has proved a valuable aid in the clinic in cases of eczema, psoriasis and other dermatoses. Side effects, arising from absorption through the skin and manifestations of systemic activity, have been minimal under proper dosage conditions.

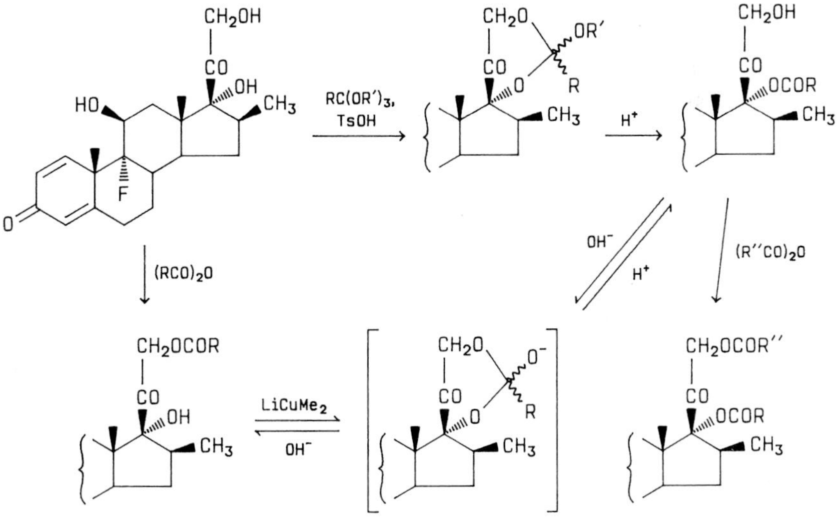

Scheme 5

We next looked at 17,21-diesters of betamethasone and some related steroids. They are readily prepared by conventional acylation methods from 17-mono-esters; the esterifying acids may be the same or different (Scheme 5). Again high activity was found and here it appeared that the total number of carbon atoms in the two ester functions was important, activity becoming optimal at around six carbon atoms. Thus, both betamethasone 17,21-dipropionate (**23**) (McKenzie score 1660) and the corresponding 9α-chloro compound [**24**, beclomethasone dipropionate, Propaderm) (Allen & Hanburys)] (McKenzie score 500) have proved clinically useful—the first being marketed by Schering-Plough, the second by Allen & Hanburys.

(**23**) X = F, Betamethasone 17,21-dipropionate
(**24**) X = Cl, Beclomethasone 17,21-dipropionate

VI. USE OF TOPICALLY ACTIVE STEROIDS IN ASTHMA

Although steroids have been used systemically in asthma since the early days of the discovery of their activity, their use was limited by the side effects that have already been discussed. With the discovery of compounds that were very potent anti-inflammatory agents on the skin, the question arose of whether they would be equally effective, topically, on the airways of the lung. Beclometha-sone dipropionate (**24**) was tried as an aerosol that could be inhaled and was found to be very effective in controlling asthmatic symptoms in the majority of patients. In proper dosage (not more than 300–400 μg/day) it showed no sys-temic effects, and the only side effect noted (in about 8% of patients) was a mild fungal infection of the throat. Under the proprietary name Becotide (Allen & Hanburys), the preparation has been outstandingly successful, and as a nasal spray its use was later extended to treatment of hay-fever and allied allergic complaints affecting the nose.

Under the proprietary name Bextasol (Glaxo) betamethasone 17-valerate (**22**) was subsequently marketed in aerosol form for a similar range of conditions.

VII. 17-ESTERS OF 21-DEOXYSTEROIDS AND OF 21-HALO-21-DEOXYSTEROIDS

Although removal of the 21-hydroxy group from, for example, cortisone or hydrocortisone, gives inactive compounds, simultaneous introduction of the 9,11-fluorohydrin group can restore the activity to a reasonable level; this is exemplified in fluorometholone (**25**). It was, therefore, of some interest to prepare 17-esters of such compounds and to test them for topical activity.

(**25**) Fluorometholone

Clearly, the orthoester method of acylation of a 17-hydroxy group is not applicable to 21-deoxysteroids. Instead, we prepared them by use of vigorous acylation methods (acid anhydride with perchloric acid as catalyst) on the 21-deoxysteroid; in most instances a relatively small amount of the 11,17-diacyloxy compound was formed at the same time, but this could be removed by crystallisation (Scheme 6).

A second method (Scheme 6) for the preparation of the esters involves the conversion of a 17-monoester of a 17,21-dihydroxy-20-ketone into its 21-mesylate and then treating this with sodium iodide in boiling pyridine. Alternatively, a 17α-acyloxy-21-bromo-20-ketone, on heating with pyridine, triethylamine, dimethyl sulphoxide or, more conventionally, sodium bisulphite, was reduced to the 21-unsubstituted compound. This behaviour is in marked contrast to that of the free 17α-hydroxy-21-bromo-20-ketones, which react with pyridine and other amines by conventional nucleophilic displacement at carbon. The presence of the acyloxy-group at C-17 certainly inhibits nucleophilic displacement at C-21 (see below) and so presumably allows the alternative debromination reaction to occur.

The 21-deoxybetamethasone 17-esters were active in the McKenzie test, though the range of acids that gave very potent compounds was rather small. However, the 17-propionate (**26**) was considerably more active (McKenzie score 1075) than most of the betamethasone 17-esters and 17,21-diesters. It was,

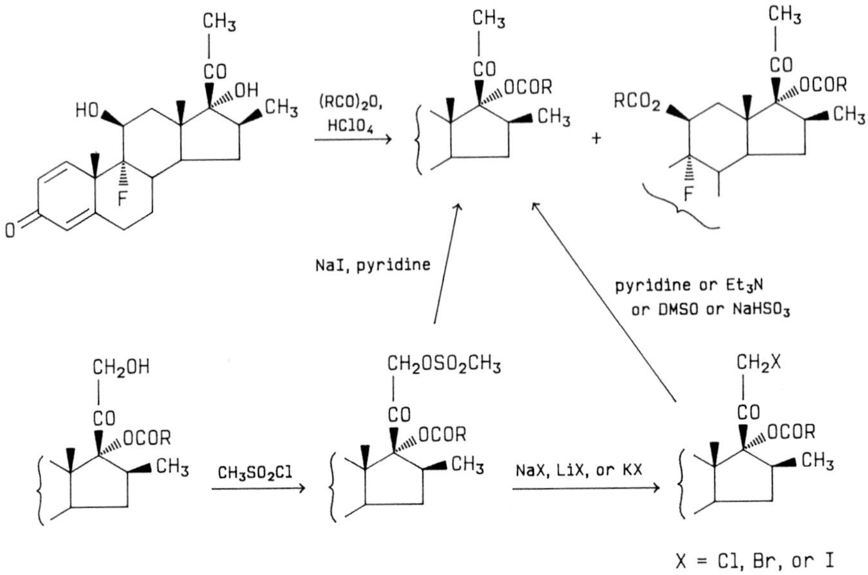

Scheme 6

however, overtaken by the 21-halo compounds that are discussed in the next paragraphs.

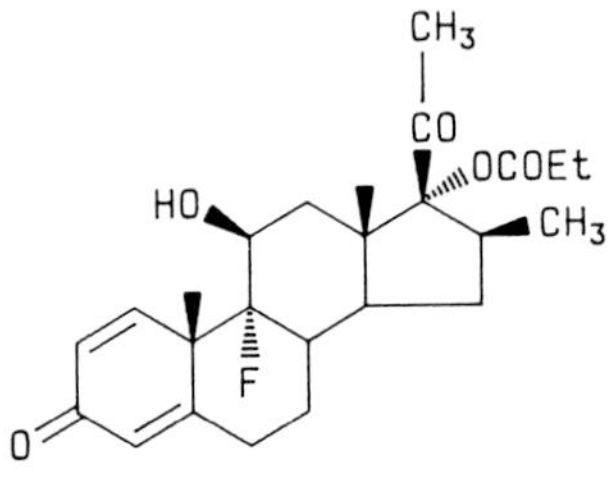

(**26**) 21-Deoxybetamethasone 17-propionate

In view of the fact that one could dispense with an oxygen function at C-21, we next tried the effect of a halogen atom at that position. Although 21-fluoro-17α-hydroxy-20-ketones had been shown to have systemic anti-inflammatory activity in animal tests, 21-chloro analogues were devoid of activity (7). We were therefore interested to try the effect of acylating the 17-hydroxy group in the presence of various 21-halogens.

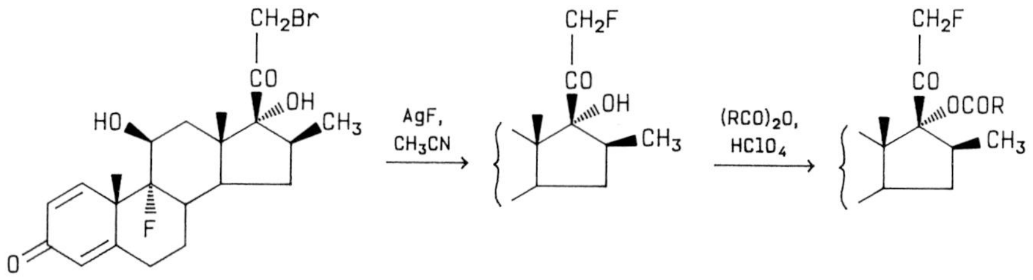

Scheme 7

The compounds were best prepared from the appropriate 17α-acyloxy-21-hydroxy-20-ketone by mesylating at C-21 and then reacting the mesylate with lithium chloride, lithium bromide or potassium iodide in acetone or ethyl methyl ketone, sometimes mixed with dimethylformamide (Scheme 6). Reaction with potassium iodide was very slow indeed, taking several days to complete, and the 21-iodo compounds were better prepared via the 21-bromo compounds, which reacted with potassium iodide rather faster than did the 21-mesylate.

21-Fluoro-17α-acyloxy-20-ketones were prepared from 21-bromo-17α-hydroxy-20-ketones, first by reaction with silver fluoride in acetonitrile to give the 21-fluoro-17α-hydroxy-20-ketone, which was then acylated by use of an acid anhydride and a strong acid catalyst (Scheme 7).

In the McKenzie test, the 21-halo compounds achieved the highest scores yet. Best were the 21-fluoro and 21-chloro compounds and, again, optimum activity was found with relatively short ester moieties. 21-Chloro-9α-fluoro-11β-hydroxy-16β-methyl-17α-propionyloxypregna-1,4-diene-3,20-dione (**27**, clobetasol propionate) (McKenzie score 1850) was selected for further trial and was found to be very potent (*14*). Under the proprietary name Dermovate (Glaxo), it was marketed in 1973. However, the systemic activity is increased along with the topical activity, and it is relatively easy to absorb enough of the material for these systemic effects to show themselves. It is particularly important, therefore, that the recommended dose is not exceeded.

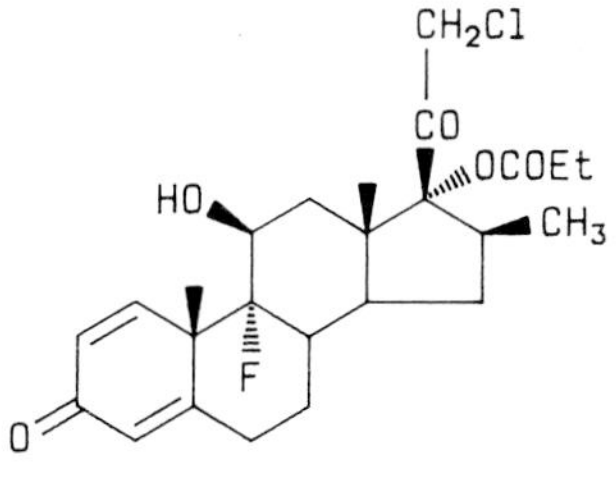

(**27**) Clobetasol 17-propionate

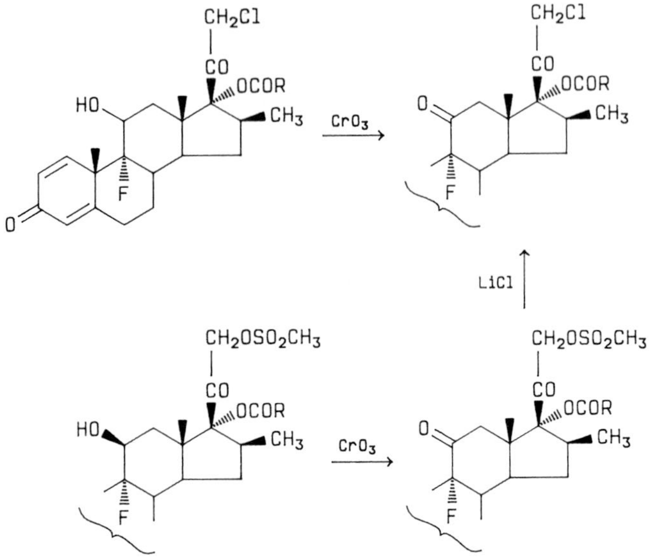

Scheme 8

VIII. EFFECT OF OXIDISING THE 11β-HYDROXY GROUP TO A KETONE GROUP

Selected active 11β-hydroxy compounds have been oxidised to the 11-ketones. In general they were less active than the 11β-hydroxy-compounds, and were not pursued. It is probable that they had to be reduced, *in vivo,* to the 11β-ols before displaying activity. However in the 9,21-dihalo compounds the McKenzie scores, though a great deal lower than those for the 11β-hydroxy compounds, were of an order that made them interesting *per se.*

The 11-ketones may be prepared either by chromic acid oxidation of the corresponding 11β-ols, or, alternatively, the oxidation may be done at an earlier stage (for example, oxidation of the 21-mesyloxy-17α-acyloxy-20-ketone) and the product then converted into the 21-halo compound by nucleophilic displacement in the usual way (Scheme 8).

One of the more active compounds was the 21-chloro-17-butyrate (**28,** clobetasone butyrate) (McKenzie score 263). This compound became of special interest when its topical activity was compared with the unwanted systemic activity.* Thus the therapeutic ratio of these effects was ~0.01 for betametha-

---

*Systemic activity is measured by the degree of thymus involution in the mouse.

$$CH_2Cl$$
$$|$$
$$CO$$

(28) Clobetasone 17-butyrate

sone, about 2 for most of the selected esters described above and about 30 for clobetasone butyrate (**28**). It was therefore developed as a safe compound for use in mild dermatoses. In addition to its lesser systemic activity, it appeared to have a somewhat smaller effect in thinning of the skin, a common side effect of long continued treatment with topical corticosteroids (*15*). The compound was therefore marketed under the proprietary name Eumovate (Glaxo) as a 0.05% cream and ointment.

IX. NEWER STEROIDS IN RESEARCH

In all early researches no active compounds were found that did not have at least a two-carbon side-chain at the 17-position, bearing a 20-carbonyl function. However, we have found a range of compounds, namely, derivatives of 17α-hydroxy-17β-carboxyandrostanes, with a one-carbon side-chain that are active in the McKenzie test.

Thus in the set of compounds derived from betamethasone both the 17α-hydroxyl and the 17β-carboxyl need to be esterified to obtain good activity. Highest activity (McKenzie score 400–800) is associated with the 17-propionate series, the carboxylic acid being esterified with methyl, chloromethyl and fluoromethyl groups. Hydrolysis of either ester group would result in inactive compounds which may allow the selection of systemically deactivated compounds.

These compounds can be prepared from 17,21-dihydroxy-20-ketones as shown in Scheme 9. Of the routes shown, the most selective in the presence of an 11β-hydroxyl group is that utilising intramolecular 17-acylation, via mixed anhydrides, of the 17β-carboxylic acid.

Activity was also found in a series of analogous 17-carbothioates. These compounds, bearing 16-methyl groups, could be prepared from 17α-acyloxy-17β-carboxylic acids. Steric hindrance at the 20-carbon made it necessary to use an intramolecular transformation to the carbothioic acid, as shown in Scheme 10. Such methods were not satisfactory in the presence of a 17α-hydroxy group, but in this case carboxyl activation with carbonyl diimidazole and reaction with

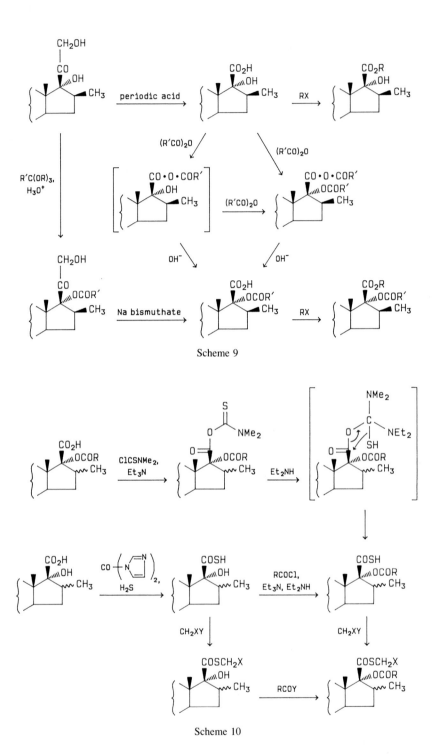

Scheme 9

Scheme 10

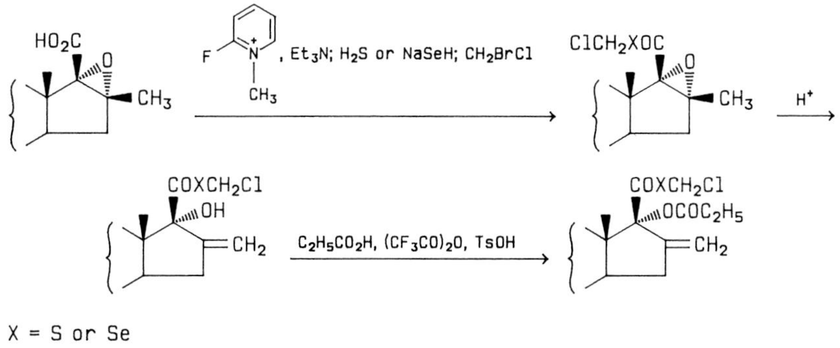

X = S or Se

Scheme 11

hydrogen sulphide was very useful, especially for the preparation of halomethyl carbothioates where the halomethylthiol is not available.

For the 16-methylene analogues the best route proceeded from the $16\alpha,17\alpha$-epoxy-17β-carboxylic acids through Mukaiyama-type activation of the carboxylic acid with a 2-haloazaaromatic compound, as shown in Scheme 11, the epoxide being subsequently rearranged with acid to provide the 16-methylene-17α-ol. This procedure also worked to produce carboselenic acids, which gave esters that were active but were regarded as unlikely to be acceptable as drugs.

From these new areas, it is likely that new compounds can be progressed to the market. These compounds should display a greater freedom from side effects than those currently in use.

REFERENCES

1. L. F. Fieser and M. Fieser, "Steroids," p. 650. Reinhold, New York, 1959.
2. P. C. Spensley, *Chem. Ind. (London)*, 426 (1952); R. K. Callow, J. W. Cornforth, and P. C. Spensley, *Chem. Ind. (London)*, 699 (1951).
3. B. A. Hems, *Chem. Ind. (London)*, 442 (1959).
4. I. E. Bush, *Pharmacol. Rev.* **14**, 317 (1962).
5. J. Fried and E. F. Sabo, *J. Am. Chem. Soc.* **75**, 2273 (1953).
6. H. L. Herzog, A. Nobile, S. Tolksdorf, W. Charney, E. B. Hershberg, and P. L. Perlman, *Science* **121**, 176 (1955).
7. E. W. Boland, *Am. J. Med.* **31**, 581 (1961); T. L. Popper and A. S. Watnick, *in* "Antiinflammatory Agents, Chemistry and Pharmacology" (R. A. Scherrer and M. W. Whitehouse, eds.), Vol. 1, p. 245. Academic Press, New York, 1974; I. Ringler, *in* "Methods in Hormone Research" (R. I. Dorfman, ed.), Vol. 3, p. 227. Academic Press, New York, 1964; L. H. Sarett, A. A. Patchett, and S. Steelman, *in* "Progress in Drug Research" (E. Jucker, ed.), Vol. 5, p. 11. Birkhauser, Basel, 1963.
8. J. D. Baxter and G. G. Rousseau, "Glucocorticoid Hormone Action." Springer-Verlag, Berlin, 1979.

9. R. J. Flower and G. J. Blackwell, *Nature (London)* **278,** 456 (1979).
10. A. W. McKenzie, *Arch. Dermatol.* **86,** 611 (1962); A. W. McKenzie and R. B. Stoughton, *Arch. Dermatol.* **86,** 608 (1962).
11. J. Attenburrow, J. E. Connett, W. Graham, J. F. Oughton, A. C. Ritchie, and P. A. Wilkinson, *J. Chem. Soc.,* 4547 (1961); T. R. Carrington, S. Eardley, J. Elks, G. F. H. Green, G. I. Gregory, A. G. Long, and J. C. P. Sly, *J. Chem. Soc.,* 4560 (1961); G. I. Gregory, J. S. Hunt, P. J. May, F. A. Nice, and G. H. Phillipps, *J. Chem. Soc.,* 2201 (1966).
12. G. H. Phillipps, *in* "Mechanisms of Topical Corticosteroid Activity" (L. Wilson and R. Marks, eds.), Churchill, London, 1976).
13. D. I. Williams, D. S. Wilkinson, J. Overton, J. A. Milne, W. B. McKenna, A. Lyell, and R. Church, *Lancet* **1,** 1177 (1964).
14. C. G. Sparkes and L. Wilson, *Br. J. Dermatol.* **90,** 197 (1974); P. Woodbridge, *Practitioner* **121,** 732 (1974).
15. D. D. Munro and L. Wilson, *Br. Med. J.* **iii,** 626 (1975).

CHAPTER 10

Steroid Contraceptives

F. J. ZEELEN
Organon Scientific Development Group
Oss, The Netherlands

I. INTRODUCTION

Some 65 million women, all over the world, use steroid contraceptives to control their fertility. This has proven to be a very reliable method. It is surpassed in overall safety only by the use of intra-uterine devices, but the latter method has a slightly higher failure rate.

In this chapter the steroids contained in these preparations are described together with the key steps of their syntheses, and this is followed by a discussion of the different dosage schemes. The long-acting preparations, most of which are in the development stage, illustrate a novel and interesting area of medicinal chemistry which will become important in the future.

A. HISTORY

The principle of hormonal contraception has been known since 1919, when Haberlandt implanted ovaries from pregnant rabbits under the skin of normal fertile rabbits and found that these animals became infertile. This shows that hormones released by the ovaries can prevent pregnancy. After the isolation and structure elucidation of the estrogens estrone (**1**) (1932) and estradiol (**2**) (1935) and of the progestagen progesterone (**3**) (1934), it could be proven that these hormones can inhibit ovulation in experimental animals.

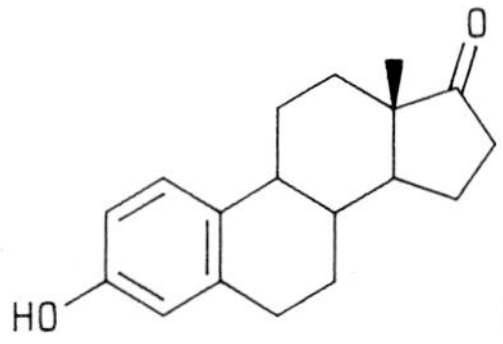

(**1**) 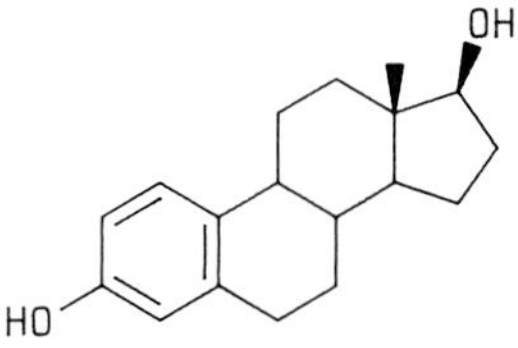   (**2**) 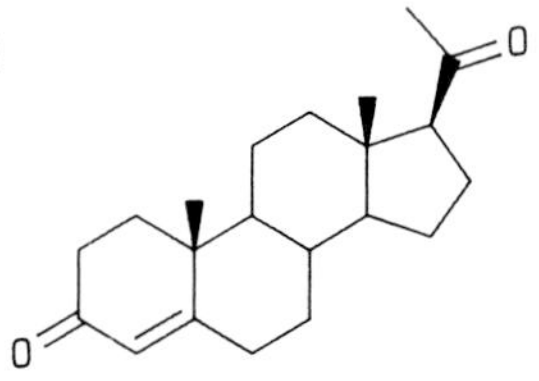   (**3**)

In 1944 Bickenbach and Paulikovics showed in a pilot experiment (1 patient!) that a daily injection of 20 mg of progesterone could inhibit ovulation. Due to the low solubility of progesterone it is impossible to prepare concentrated solutions suitable for injection. Injections of crystalline suspensions of progesterone are painful, and this method of administration is not attractive for a contraceptive preparation. The oral activity of progesterone is extremely low; in one study 300 mg of progesterone had to be given daily to induce some progestational effect (*1*). In order to make it a useful approach potent, orally active steroids had to be found.

B. ETHISTERONE (**4**)

Inhoffen *et al.* prepared the 17α-ethynyl derivative (**4**) of the male hormone testosterone (**5**) (*2*). The androgenic activity of the new derivative is very low, but surprisingly it shows progestational activity. On injection its potency is about one-third that of progesterone, but in contrast with progesterone it is also active by the oral route.

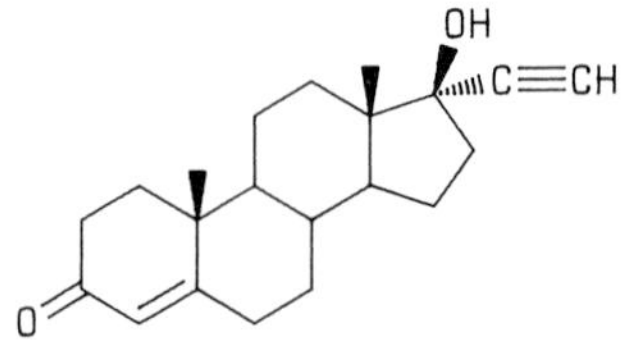

(**4**) 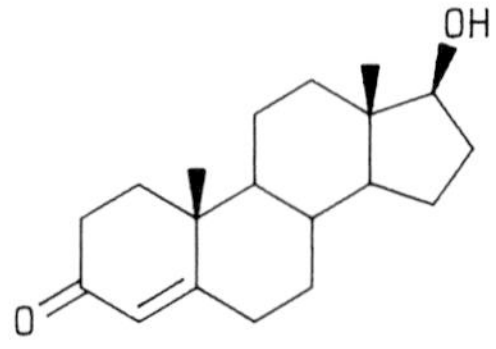   (**5**)

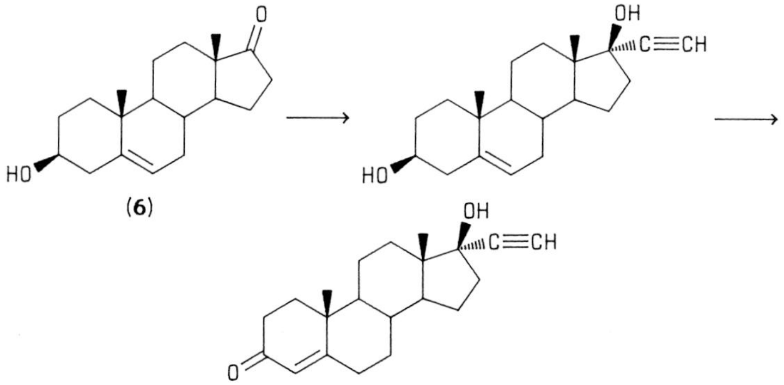

Scheme 1

A key step in the synthesis of ethisterone is the stereoselective addition of an ethynyl group to the 17-ketosteroid, 3β-hydroxyandrost-5-en-17-one (6). Oppenauer oxidation then completes its synthesis (Scheme 1).

Ethisterone (4) became the first oral progestagen introduced into clinical practice. However, its oral activity is still low and many analogues have been synthesized in the effort to find more potent compounds.

C. THE FIRST 19-NORSTEROIDS

Norethisterone (norethindrone) (7), which lacks the 19-methyl group of ethisterone, and the isomeric norethynodrel (8) proved about five times as potent, which made these compounds suitable candidates for clinical investigations. The first studies gave variable results which could be correlated with the presence of a potent estrogenic impurity (mestranol) (9) in the first batches of both compounds 7 and 8 in amounts as high as 3% (*1*).

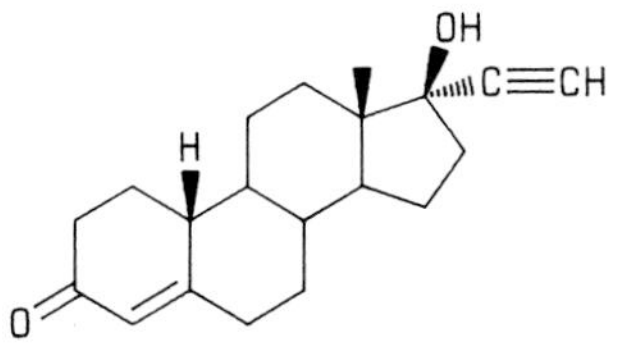

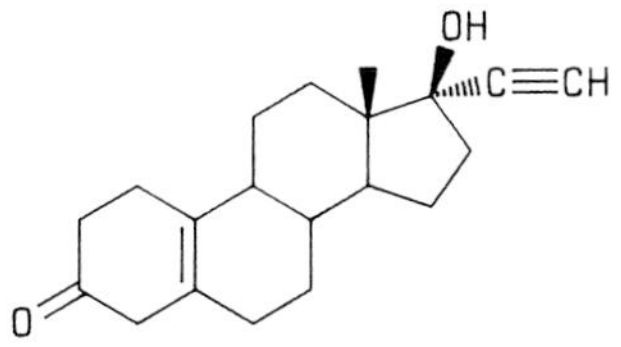

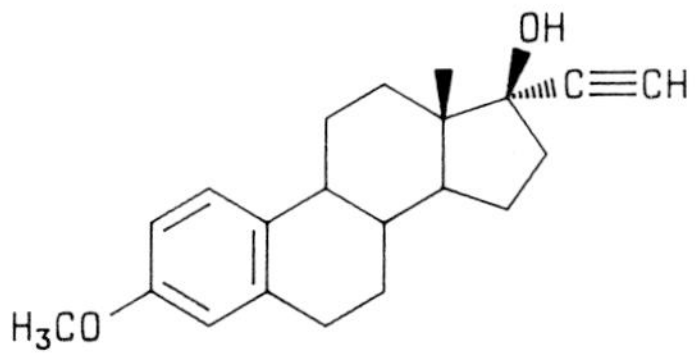

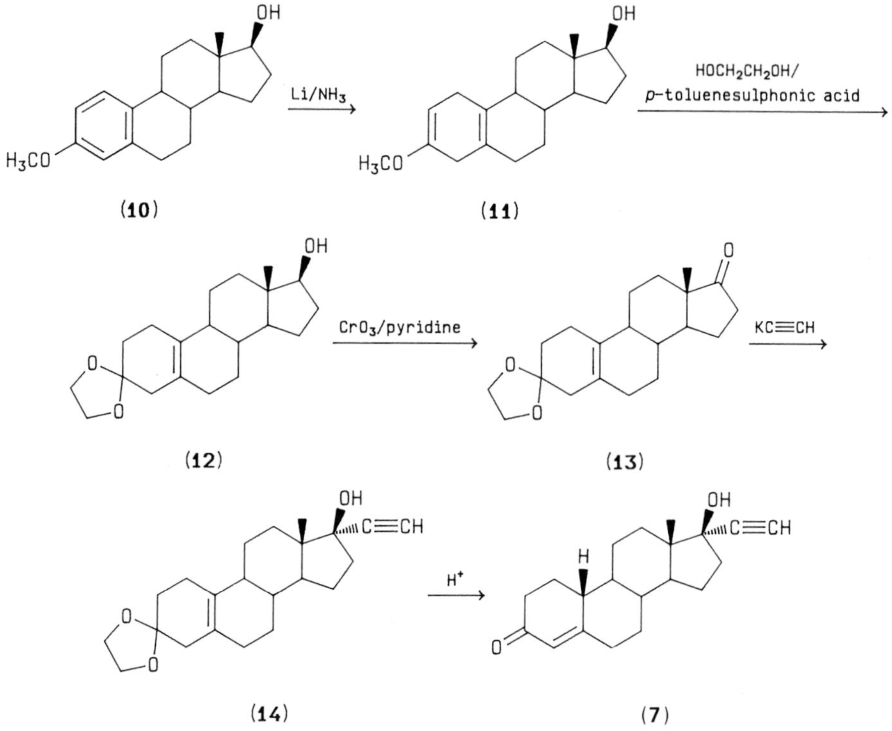

Scheme 2

To understand why this impurity could be present we have to know the synthetic route to these 19-norsteroids (Scheme 2). A key step in the synthesis is the Birch reduction of the estradiol ether (**10**) leading to the unstable enol ether (**11**). In the synthesis of norethisterone this enol ether was not purified but converted directly to the ketal (**12**) and oxidized to the 17-ketone (**13**). This was then converted into the 17α-ethynyl-17β-hydroxy derivative (**14**) followed by removal of the protecting group to give the desired product (*3*). Unreacted estra-1,3,5(10)-triene-3,17-diol 3-methylether (**10**) may be carried through the procedure to produce the potent estrogen impurity mestranol (Scheme 3).

However, it was proved in early experiments that the presence of a *small* amount of estrogen is important as it helps to prevent break-through bleeding. In the first large-scale contraceptive trial, 830 women took a tablet containing 10 mg of norethynodrel plus 0.15 mg of mestranol daily from day 5 through day 24 of the menstrual cycle. This successful trial marks the birth of steroid contraception (*4*) and it paved the way for the combined preparations (estrogen and progestagen). Extensive clinical development work was to follow since it was evident from the first trial that the doses of the estrogen and progestogen were too high. For contraception norethynodrel (**8**) is now usually given in doses of 2.5

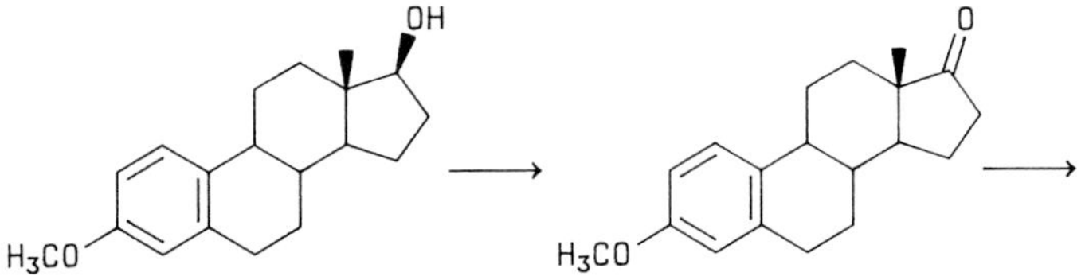

(10)

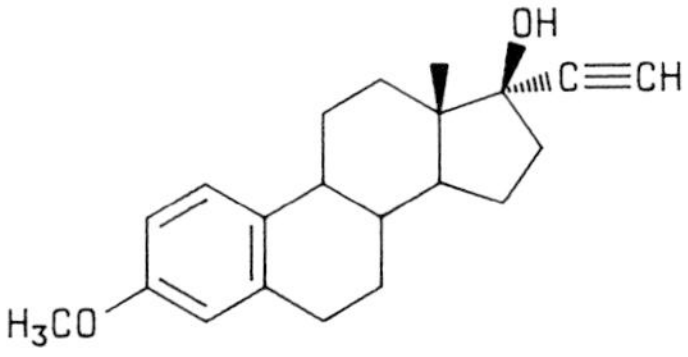

(9)

Scheme 3

mg combined with 0.1 mg of mestranol (9), or 5 mg of norethynodrel is given combined with 0.075 mg of mestranol.

II.   THE FIRST GENERATION OF STEROIDS

A.   THE PROGESTAGENS

Norethisterone (7) and norethynodrel (8) were mentioned in the introduction. After oral administration both steroids are about equipotent. However the affinity

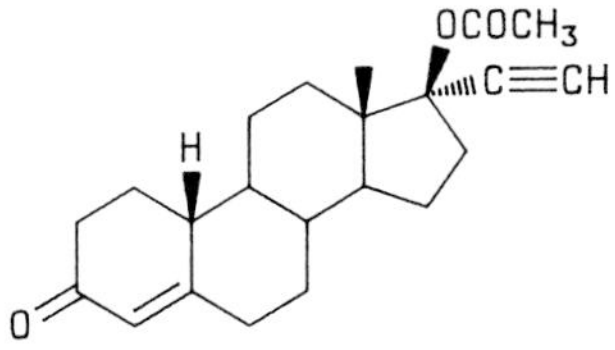

(15)

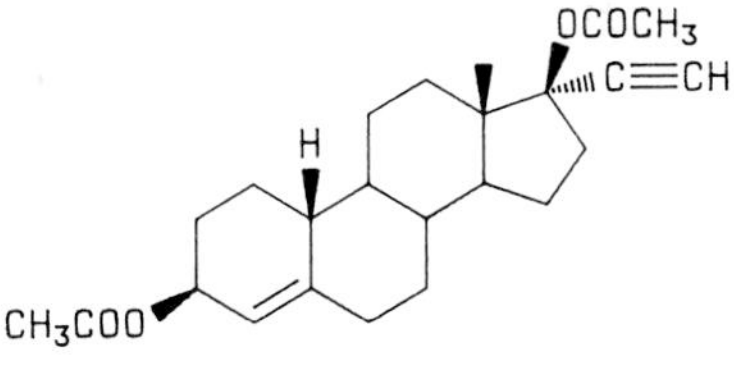

(16)

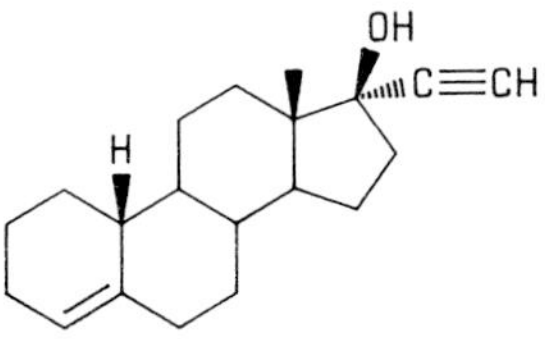

(17)

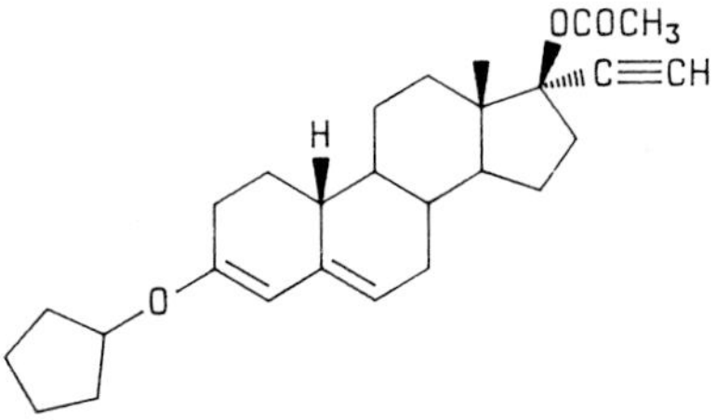

(18)

of norethynodrel for the progesterone receptor is only one-quarter that of norethisterone. This suggests that norethynodrel is a pro-drug, converted in the body
to the more potent drug norethisterone. This was proven by metabolism studies.
Other pro-drugs of norethisterone which were developed are norethisterone acetate (15), ethynodiol diacetate (16), lynestrenol (17) and quingestanol acetate
(18). These compounds have a comparable potency.

B.   THE ESTROGENS

   Mestranol (9), the estrogen which was used in the first trials, also proved to be
a pro-drug. It is oxidized efficiently in the liver to ethinylestradiol (19). This
estrogen has become the major estrogen used in contraceptive preparations.

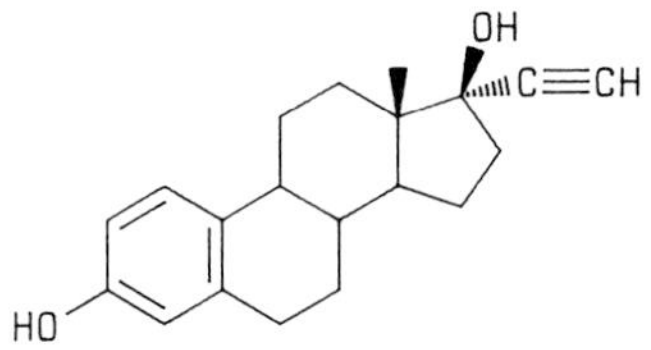

(19)

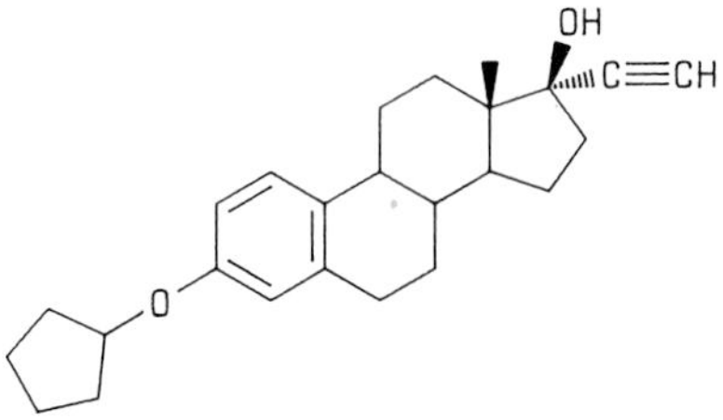

(20)

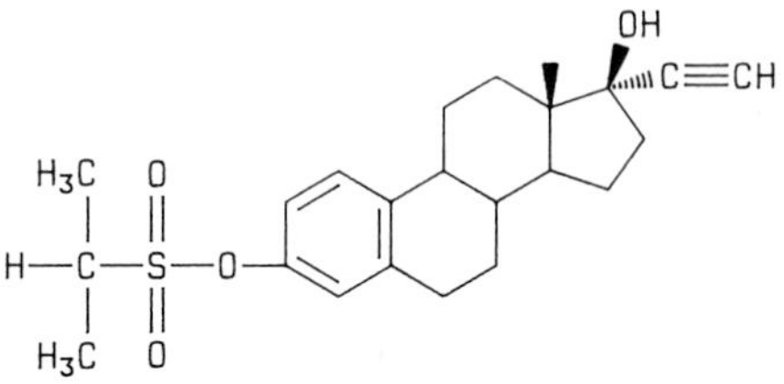

(21)

   Lipophilic pro-drugs of ethinylestradiol (19) were developed as long acting
estrogens. Lipophilic compounds may accumulate in fat tissues or be administered via injection in an oil to form a depot from which the lipophilic substance is
gradually released. The most important examples are quinestrol (20) and ethinylestradiol sulfonate (21).

III.   SYNTHESIS

A.   PARTIAL SYNTHESIS

   The key steps in the production of the 19-norsteroids are the conversion of
readily available androsta-1,4-diene-3,17-dione (22) into estrone (23) either by

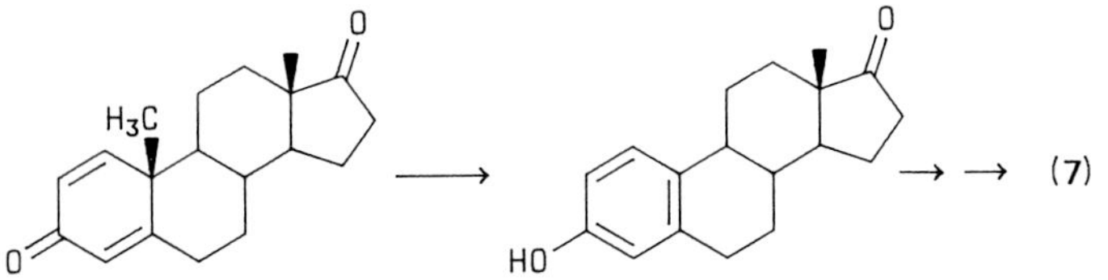

(22) → (23) → → (7)

Scheme 4

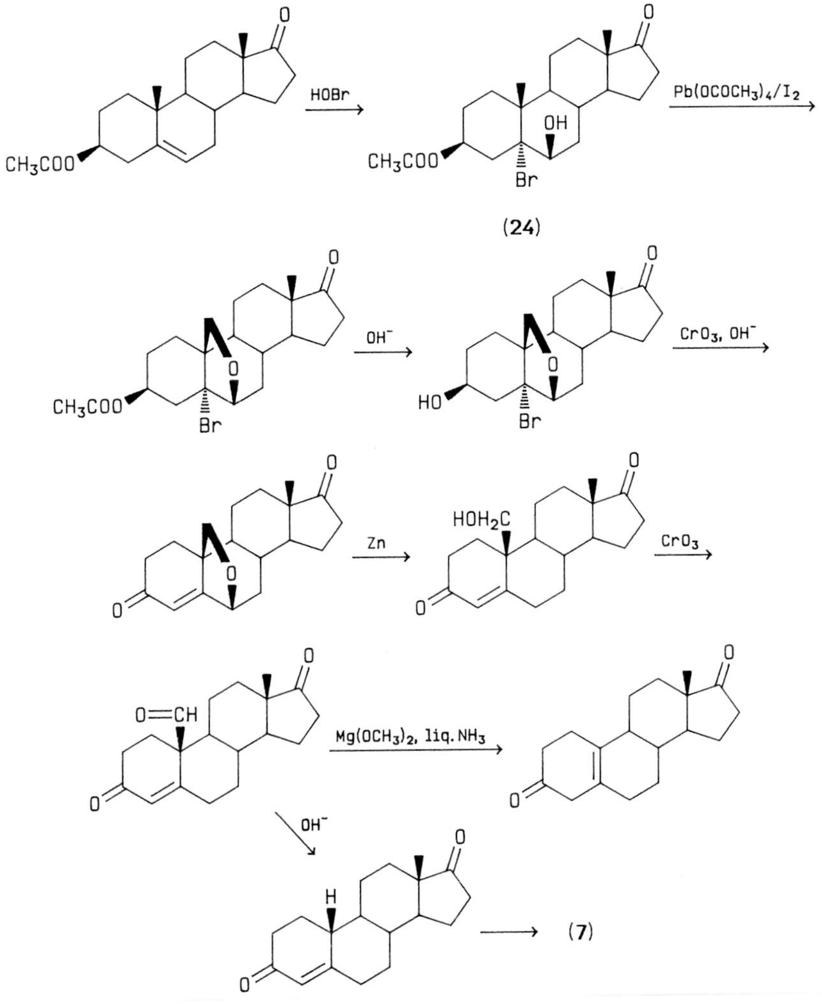

Scheme 5

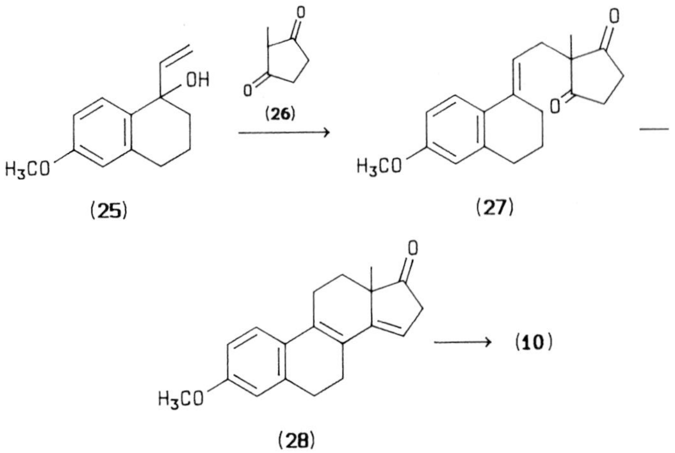

Scheme 6

pyrolysis in the presence of a hydrogen donor (5) or by reductive aromatization (6) (Scheme 4), and the Birch reduction which has been discussed in Section I.

An improved route (Scheme 5) is based on the functionalization of the 19-methyl group through intramolecular oxidation of the 6β-hydroxysteroid (24) using lead tetraacetate and iodine (7).

B. TOTAL SYNTHESIS

Notwithstanding the stereochemical complexity of these steroid molecules, some total syntheses were developed (8). Key steps in an approach pioneered by

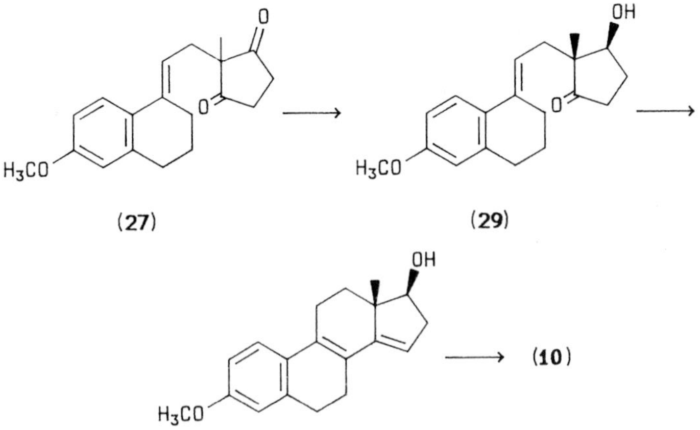

Scheme 7

Ananchenko and Torgov (9) are the coupling of 1-ethenyl-6-methoxy-1,2,3,4-tetrahydronaphthalen-1-ol (**25**) with 2-methylcyclopentane-1,3-dione (**26**) followed by ring closure to give the steroid (**28**) (Scheme 6).

A disadvantage of this approach is that racemates are formed. The first solution to this problem came when it was found that the dione (**27**) could be reduced stereoselectively by the yeast *Saccharomyces uvarum* to a ketol (**29**) possessing the configuration of the natural steroids (Scheme 7) (*10*).

Newer syntheses have been developed but the major part of the production of contraceptive steroids is still based on these, by now classical, approaches. It is interesting to note that the world production of steroids used for contraception is about 15 tons/year.

IV. THE SECOND GENERATION OF PROGESTAGENS: NORGESTREL

Norgestrel (**30**) is a more potent analogue of norethisterone and has been prepared by total synthesis from 2-ethylcyclopenta-1,3-dione (*11*). It originally reached the market as a racemate but, since all contraceptive activity resides in the enantiomer with the configuration of the natural steroids, the racemate is being gradually replaced by the (−) isomer.*

(**30**) (−)-Norgestrel
(levonorgestrel)

(**30**) (+)-Norgestrel
(dextronorgestrel)

V. INTERMEZZO

Drug development follows a regular pattern. Whenever a successful pioneering discovery is made a number of pharmaceutical companies try to enter that field. At that moment, however, knowledge of the mechanism of action is usually limited and relevant screening and follow-up tests are still under development. As the only compass for the chemist is the lead compound, various simple

---

*In old literature one sometimes finds the name "*d*-norgestrel" for levonorgestrel. This strange nomenclature stemmed from the first determination of the absolute configuration of the natural steroid series, which was based on the correlation of natural 3β-hydroxy-4-ene steroids with *d*-glyceraldehyde. For that reason some authors named all steroids with the natural configuration *d*-steroids.

derivatives and pro-drugs are made in this first phase. This has the advantage that a number of research groups get involved in the study of the field and build up the necessary know-how and experience.

In the next phase, when a relevant quantitative screening test is available, the chemists can start searching for more potent compounds. This decreases the amounts of compounds which have to be taken by the patient but does not automatically result in better drugs.

When clinical experience has advanced to the stage where action and side effects of the drug are known to such a degree that relevant animal models, (mimicking desirable and undesirable effects) are developed, the chemist can start to search for better compounds.

Since the steroid contraceptives show very few unwanted side effects, studies in large user populations proved necessary to find the uncommon side effects. Systematic studies, whereby a thousand or more women were followed over a number of years, were only started in the period 1968–1970.

Meanwhile, chemists were in a difficult position. Many interesting progestational and estrogenic steroids were synthesized but no test systems were available to select compounds of interest for further development.

We know now that steroid contraceptives show a number of desirable side effects. For example, they decrease iron deficiency anaemia, benign breast disease, pelvic inflammatory disease, functional ovarian cysts, menstrual disorders and premenstrual tension. Undesirable side effects are an increased risk of cardiovascular problems (venous thromboembolism, thrombotic stroke, hemorrhagic stroke and acute myocardial infarction) and of some liver diseases (cholelithiasis and hepatocellular adenoma). These side effects are all rare: we also have to realise that most studies were done with patients using the older, higher dose preparations. However in patients who already have an increased risk for cardiovascular problems, for example those with bad smoking habits, the effects may cumulate.

To translate these results into an indicator for the selection of novel steroids one has to use a working hypothesis to explain the origin of these rare side effects with the aim of developing a practical test model. The 11-substituted steroid desogestrel (**31**) is the first example of a steroid of the third generation. It was not only selected for development on the basis of its potency but also in view of its lack of androgenicity. Androgenicity may, via its influence on the high density lipoprotein-cholesterol complex in the blood, be associated with an increased risk for ischemic heart disease.

VI. THE THIRD GENERATION OF PROGESTAGENS: DESOGESTREL

Many analogues have been synthesized to study the effect of substitution on the potency and selectivity of action of lynestrenol (**17**). The most promising line of investigation followed 11β-substitution. A quantitative analysis of the struc-ture–activity relationships showed that two effects are important (*12*).

1. Bulky 11β-substituents induce, through 1,3-diaxial interaction with the 18-methyl group, a change in the shape of the steroid skeleton leading to better binding to the progesterone receptor and decreased binding to serum proteins. This enhances the potency of the compound.

2. By contrast, long substituents interfere with receptor binding and so de-crease potency.

Results with the other 11-substituents which induce a similar change in the shape of the steroid molecule are in line with these data. One example is the high potency found for a series of 11-methylene derivatives (originally prepared as intermediates for the synthesis of some 11β-substituted steroids).

(**31**)

The potent 11-substituted analogues were studied for their selectivity of action and this led to the selection of desogestrel (**31**) for further development. Its potency and selectivity of action were confirmed in clinical studies, and it reached the market in 1981.

Key steps in the synthesis of desogestrel (**31**) are the intramolecular oxidation of the 18-methyl group in the steroid (**32**), using lead tetraacetate and iodine to furnish the lactone (**33**), conversion of the lactone by Grignard reaction and Wolff–Kishner reduction to a 18-ethylsteroid (**34**), and Wittig reaction of the 11-ketone (**35**) to give the 11-methylene derivative (**36**). After removal of the protecting ketal groups to give the dione (**37**), selective thioacetalization, eth-ynylation and selective reduction yield desogestrel (**31**) (Scheme 8) (*13*).

VII.   MECHANISM OF ACTION
AND DOSAGE FORMS

The first half of the normal 28-day menstrual cycle is dominated by the ripening follicle and is therefore called the *follicular phase*. A critical role is played by the follicular stimulating hormone (FSH) produced by the hypophysis. FSH stimulates the growth of the ripening follicle and induces the formation of receptors for luteinising hormone (LH) in the theca cells and the granulose layer around this follicle. Circulating LH can then interact with these LH receptors and

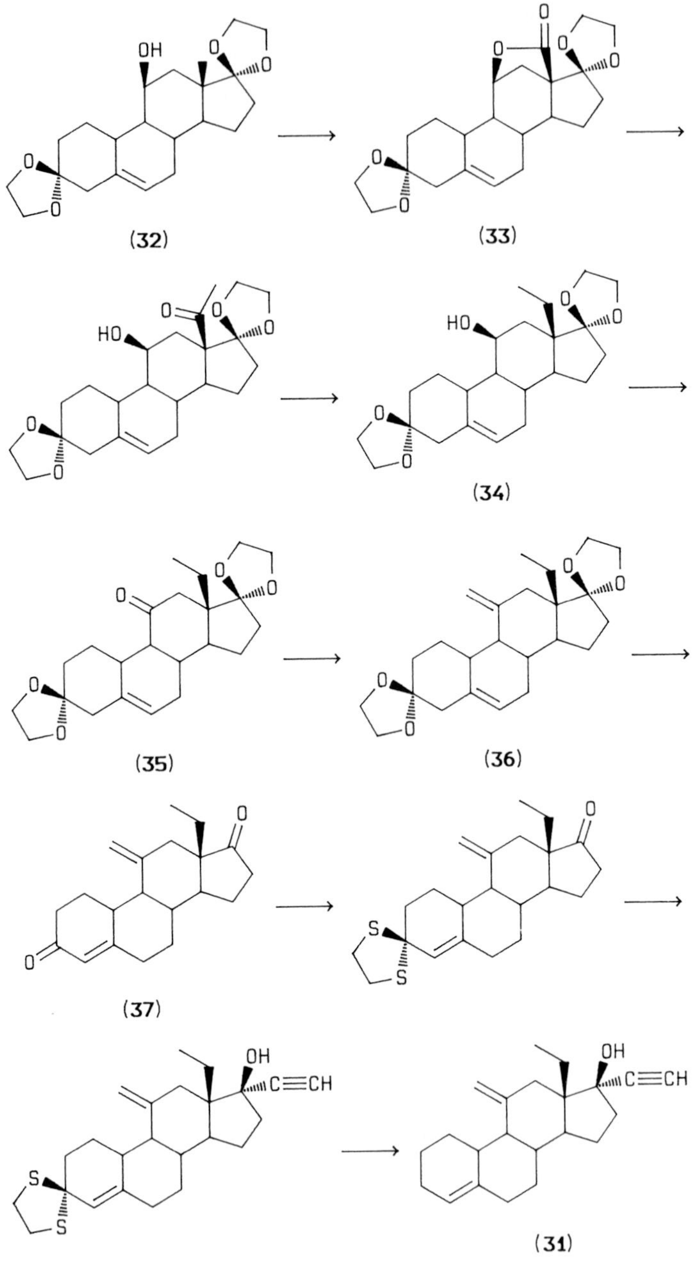

Scheme 8

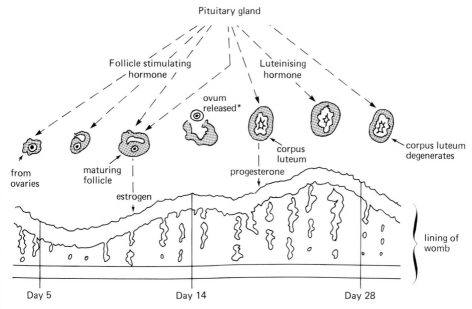

Fig. 1   The menstrual cycle. Asterisk indicates where the ovum is released, and it passes along the Fallopian tube into the uterus. If fertilized the ovum divides and becomes implanted in the lining of the uterus. A placenta forms and produces the hormone chorionic gonadotrophin. This hormone prevents the degeneration of the corpus luteum and stimulates secretion of estrogen and progesterone.

induce the production of estradiol. Estradiol stimulates regeneration and proliferation of the uterine endometrium and promotes the development of estradiol and progesterone receptors (Fig. 1).

The hormonal system is regulated by feedback mechanisms. In the case of FSH there is a negative inhibitory feedback relationship with estradiol, while in the case of LH there is a negative inhibitory feedback at low levels of estradiol and a positive stimulatory feedback at high levels of estradiol.

If all goes well the estrogen levels gradually reach a peak, which is sufficiently high to trigger the preovulatory gonadotropin release. Serum concentrations of LH and to lesser extent FSH increase rapidly which, provided a follicle is in the appropriate stage of maturity, leads to rupture of this follicle and expulsion of the ovum (*ovulation*). The remaining granulosa cells increase in size and form the corpus luteum. This marks the start of the *luteal phase*.

If the ovum is fertilized it is further transported, while dividing, in about 3 days through the Fallopian tube to the uterus where it takes another three days to prepare for nidation. To make this possible, the development of the uterus towards this event has to be synchronous. During these 6 days the development of the fertilized ovum can be hindered by excessive levels of estrogens.

An important factor in the luteal phase is the rise in progesterone levels in the blood which induces a change in the uterine endometrium to the secretory state essential for possible implantation of the fertilized ovum.

Another effect of progesterone is a transformation of the cervical mucus to a viscous state, so hindering the passage of spermatozoa.

In the absence of implantation the corpus luteum degenerates after approximately 10 days. The progesterone and estradiol production decrease rapidly, initiating shedding of the uterine endometrium (menstruation), which marks the start of the new cycle.

The administration of the combination of an estrogen and a progestagen for 20–22 days results in a number of effects. First it blocks ovulation; secondly it interferes with phasic development of the uterine endometrium which decreases the chance for successful implantation; and thirdly the cervical mucus may become so viscous that it hinders sperm penetration. The fall of estrogen and progestagen levels at the end of treatment stimulates the shedding of the endometrium leading to regular bleeding. This is important since it proves to the user that the contraceptive is effective.

A.   THE COMBINED PREPARATIONS

The high efficacy of the combined preparations rests on the above mentioned multiple activities. The dosages of the steroids used in the modern combined preparations are much lower than those used in the first investigations. The daily dose of ethinylestradiol (19) varies between 0.02 and 0.05 mg. Mestranol (9) is about half as potent as ethinylestradiol and its dose varies between 0.05 and 0.10 mg/day.

The progestagens of the first generation are used in the following dose range.

Progestagen	Dosage (mg/day)
Norethisterone (7)	0.5–2
Norethynodrel (8)	2.5–5
Norethisterone acetate (15)	0.6–4
Ethynodiol diacetate (16)	0.5–2
Lynestrenol (17)	0.75–2.5

The more potent second generation progestagen levonorgestrel [(−)-(30)] is used in the range 0.125–0.25 mg/day. The dose of the more selective third generation progestagen desogestrel (31) is 0.15 mg/day.

The reliability of the newer combinations has been proven in extensive clinical investigations.

B. THE PHASIC PREPARATIONS

In order to lower the amounts of steroids which have to be administered, attempts have been made to translate the present knowledge of contraceptive mechanism into new formulations.

Since the estrogen is of major importance in the follicular phase a sequential regimen was tried. In a first trial (*14*) 0.1 mg of ethinylestradiol (**19**) was given daily from day 5 to day 15 of the cycle followed by daily administration of the combination of 0.1 mg of ethinylestradiol (**19**) and 25 mg of the progestagen dimethisterone (**38**) from day 16 to day 20. This approach was not very successful. Efficacy was lower than desired, and a number of side effects were found.

(**38**)

A variation is the "*once-a-week pill*" developed in East Germany (*15*) where during the first 3 weeks of the cycle 1 mg of ethinylestradiol sulfonate (**21**) is administered followed in the fourth week by 2 × 5 mg of norethisterone acetate (**15**).

Clinical experiments have also been carried out with a "*once-a-month pill*". An oil-filled capsule containing 2.0 mg of the long-acting estrogen quinestrol (**20**) and 2.5 mg of the progestagen quingestanol acetate (**18**) was given every 4 weeks. The pill was poorly accepted by the users and the contraceptive efficacy was low (*16*).

In a second generation of sequential preparations the dosage regimen consisted of 10 days of estrogen treatment followed by 11 days of treatment with estrogen plus progestagen. Better results are achieved with the "*normophasic*" schedule. In this case the progestagen treatment starts before the ovulation phase. Even a "*triphasic*" sequence has reached the market.

C. THE MINIPILL

In an attempt to develop preparations which would only have peripheral effects progestagens were given continuously in a low dose. With these preparations it was found that a fair contraceptive effect could be achieved. However the efficacy is much lower when one or two tablets are missed. Since these preparations are given on a continuous basis they lack the induced monthly drop in estrogen and progestagen levels which is important to achieve a regular bleeding pattern. Irregular menstruation occurs in 30–60% of users so that these preparations have never become popular. The complete mechanism of action has not been unravelled in detail. It is evident that the original goal has not been achieved completely since these preparations induce anovulatory cycles in 15–40% of women. Examples of these preparations are norethisterone (7), 0.35 mg/day; ethynodiol diacetate (16), 0.35 mg/day; lynestrenol (17), 0.50 mg/day and levonorgestrel [(−)-(30)], 0.03 mg/day.

D. LONG-ACTING DOSAGE FORMS

During the last decade the development of long-acting contraceptive dosage forms has been an important research topic. This type of contraception is important for women who need contraception but for whom the daily oral intake is unsuitable. Very long-acting dosage forms may also be important in countries with an underdeveloped medical infrastructure.

The only possibility to achieve a duration of action of a week or longer is through slow release from a depot. A number of approaches are possible but only a few have reached an advanced stage.

a. Microcrystalline Suspensions

For poorly soluble compounds like most steroids, aqueous microcrystalline suspensions may serve as a suitable depot. The dissolution rate and solubility of a compound in water correlate with its hydrophobicity and, to a lesser extent, its melting point. The greater the hydrophobicity and the higher the melting point the lower will be the solubility of a compound in water and the slower will be its rate of dissolution. Thus esterification with a hydrophobic acid can decrease the dissolution rate of a drug.

(39)

(40)

An example of such a contraceptive preparation is the combination of 25 mg of the progestagen medroxyprogesterone acetate (**39**) and 5 mg of the estrogen estradiol cypionate (**40**) suspended in 1 ml of an aqueous vehicle. When injected at 28-day intervals it proved an effective and acceptable contraceptive (*17*).

An important and often used preparation consists of a microcrystalline suspension of medroxyprogesterone acetate alone. Best results in this minipill type approach were obtained with 150 mg injected intramuscularly every 3 months (*18*).

b. Oil Depots

Another possibility for controlling the release of hydrophobic steroids is to use an oil depot. The steroid is extracted gradually from the oil; again the duration of action may be regulated by esterification. Very potent compounds must be used.

A useful compound is the heptanoate ester of norethisterone (**41**). Injection of 200 mg of this ester dissolved in 1 ml of a 1:1 mixture of castor oil and benzyl benzoate once every 60 days proved an acceptable contraceptive treatment. Similarly, injection of 200 mg of the norprogesterone derivative **42** dissolved in 1 ml of arachis oil containing 2% of benzyl alcohol inhibited ovulation for 5–10 months (*19*).

(41)   (42)

c. Biodegradable Microspheres and Capsules

In this approach the depot is formed by incorporation of the steroid in a biodegradable polymer. Erosion of the polymer releases the steroid, although diffusion out of the polymer also may be of importance. The rate of release depends on the stability of the polymer, the size of the microsphere or capsule, and the physical properties of the steroid.

A pilot study with norethisterone (**7**) in injectable microspheres (60–240 μm) of polylactic acid (**43**), indicated that a 6-month duration of action may be achieved. A similar pilot study has been reported using levonorgestrel [(−)-(**30**)] in a subdermal capsule made of poly-ε-hydroxycaproic acid (**44**) (*20*).

$$HO[COCH(CH_3)O]_nH \qquad HO[CO(CH_2)_5O]_nH$$

(43)   (44)

TABLE I
Some Steroids[a]

Desogestrel (**31**)
    54024-22-5   (17α)-13-Ethyl-11-methylene-18,19-dinorpregn-4-en-20-yn-17-ol
Dimethisterone (**38**)
    79-64-1 (anhydrous)   (6α,17β)-17-Hydroxy-6-methyl-17-(1-propynyl)-androst-4-en-3-one
    41354-30-7 (monohydrate)
Estradiol (**2**)
    50-28-2   (17β)-Estra-1,3,5(10)-triene-3,17-diol
Estradiol cypionate (**40**)
    313-06-4   (17β)-Estra-1,3,5(10)-triene-3,17-diol 17-cyclopentanepropanoate
Estrone (**1**)
    53-16-7   3-Hydroxyestra-1,3,5(10)-trien-17-one
Ethinylestradiol (**19**)
    57-63-6   (17α)-19-Norpregna-1,3,5(10)-trien-20-yne-3,17-diol
Ethinylestradiol sulfonate (**21**)
    28913-23-7   (17α)-19-Norpregna-1,3,5(10)-trien-20-yne-3,17-diol 3-(2-propanesulfonate)
Ethisterone (**4**)
    434-03-7   (17α)-17-Hydroxypregn-4-en-20-yn-3-one
Ethynodiol diacetate (**16**)
    297-76-7   (3β,17α)-19-Norpregn-4-en-20-yne-3,17-diol diacetate
Levonorgestrel [(−)-(**30**)]
    797-63-7   (17α)-13-Ethyl-17-hydroxy-18,19-dinorpregn-4-en-20-yn-3-one
Lynestrenol (**17**)
    52-76-6   (17α)-19-Norpregn-4-en-20-yn-17-ol
Medroxyprogesterone acetate (**39**)
    71-58-9   (6α)-17-(Acetyloxy)-6-methylpregn-4-ene-3,20-dione
Mestranol (**9**)
    72-33-3   (17α)-3-Methoxy-19-norpregna-1,3,5(10)-trien-20-yn-17-ol
Norethisterone (**7**)
    68-22-4   (17α)-17-Hydroxy-19-norpregn-4-en-20-yn-3-one
Norethisterone acetate (**15**)
    51-98-9   (17α)-17-(Acetyloxy)-19-norpregn-4-en-20-yn-3-one
Norethisterone heptanoate (**41**)
    3836-23-5   (17α)-17-[(1-Oxoheptyl)oxy]-19-norpregn-4-en-20-yn-3-one
Norethynodrel (**8**)
    68-23-5   (17α)-17-Hydroxy-19-norpregn-5(10)-en-20-yn-3-one
Norgestrel (**30**)
    6533-00-2   (17α)-(±)-13-Ethyl-17-hydroxy-18,19-dinorpregn-4-en-20-yn-3-one
Org-2154 (**42**)
    67490-00-0   (16α)-16-Ethyl-21-[(1-oxodecyl)oxy]-19-norpregn-4-ene-3,20-dione
Progesterone (**3**)
    57-83-0   Pregn-4-ene-3,20-dione
Quinestrol (**20**)
    152-43-2   (17α)-3-Cyclopentyloxy-19-norpregna-1,3,5(10)-trien-20-yn-17-ol
Quingestanol acetate (**18**)
    3000-39-3   (17α)-3-Cyclopentyloxy-19-norpregna-3,5-dien-20-yn-17-ol 17-acetate
Testosterone (**5**)
    58-22-0   (17β)-17-Hydroxyandrost-4-en-3-one

[a] This table lists the steroids mentioned with the CAS number and the scientific name as used by *Chemical Abstracts*. Further references can be found through *Chemical Abstracts*. The names and CAS numbers of the compounds discussed in this chapter are summarised in this table.

Removal of the biodegradable microspheres is impossible, while removal of a biodegradable capsule is only possible as long as the capsule is intact. Here little can be done should side effects be experienced or in the case that the user desires to stop with the contraceptive. For that reason the duration of action should not be too long, for example not more than 3–6 months.

d. Non-biodegradable Subdermal Implants and Vaginal Rings

An experiment with implants of 200 mg of levonorgestrel [(−)-(**30**)] packed in 20.4 cm of polydimethylsiloxane tubing showed contraceptive action for more than 5 years (*21*). The rate of release, in this case 0.030 mg per day, is controlled by the diffusion rate through the silicon rubber tubing. The non-biodegradable implants have to be removed by microsurgery at the end of use. This limits the possible implantation sites and creates a cosmetic problem.

In a related approach norethisterone (**7**) was incorporated into a poly-dimethylsiloxane core surrounded by a thin diffusion layer of that same silicon rubber and formed into a ring suitable for vaginal application. In a pilot study these devices were tested over a 90-day period. With devices releasing 0.050 mg a day of norethisterone an unacceptable high pregnancy rate was found. Raising the daily released dose to 0.2 mg a day increased the ovulation inhibiting potency but also induced an irregular bleeding pattern. Results obtained in a study with a similar type ring, releasing 0.02 mg per day of levonorgestrel [(−)-(**30**)], indicated a stronger ovarian effect than observed with the 0.05 mg/day norethisterone device whereas the number of days with bleeding and spotting was less than seen with the 0.2 mg/day norethisterone device (*22*).

Another contraceptive vaginal ring consists of a polydimethylsiloxane core with a thin layer of levonorgestrel [(−)-(**30**)] and estradiol (**2**) (ratio 2:1), which in turn is covered with an overcoat of polydimethylsiloxane tubing. Contraceptive efficacy and control of the menstrual cycle were good (*23*).

REFERENCES

1. J. Rock, R. C. Garcia, and G. Pincus, *Recent Prog. Horm. Res.* **13**, 323 (1957).
2. H. H. Inhoffen, W. Logemann, W. Hohlweg, and A. Serini, *Berichte* **71**, 1024 (1938).
3. H. J. Ringold, G. Rozenkranz, and F. Sondheimer, *J. Am. Chem. Soc.* **78**, 2477 (1956).
4. G. Pincus, C. R. Garcia, J. Rock, M. Paniagua, A. Pendleton, F. Laraque, R. Nicolas, R. Borno, and V. Pean, *Science* **130**, 81 (1959).
5. H. H. Inhoffen, *Angew. Chem.* **A59**, 207 (1947).
6. H. L. Drijden, G. M. Webber, and J. J. Wieczorek, *J. Am. Chem. Soc.* **86**, 742 (1964).
7. K. Heusler, J. Kalvoda, Ch. Meystre, H. Ueberwasser, P. Wieland, G. Anner, and A. Wettstein, *Experientia* **18**, 464 (1962); C. M. Siegmann and M. S. de Winter, *Recl. Trav. Chim. Pays-Bas* **89**, 442 (1970).

208   F. J. Zeelen

8. R. T. Blickenstaff, A. C. Ghosh, and G. C. Wolff, "Total Synthesis of Steroids." Academic Press, New York, 1974.
9. S. A. Ananchenko and I. V. Torgov, *Tetrahedron Lett.*, 1553 (1963).
10. P. Bellet, G. Nominé, and G. Matthieu, *C. R. Ser. C* **263**, 88 (1966); H. Gibian, H. Kieslich, H. J. Koch, H. Kosmol, C. Rufer, E. Schröder, and R. Vössing, *Tetrahedron Lett.*, 2321 (1966).
11. H. Smith, G. A. Hughes, C. H. Douglas, D. Hartley, B. J. McLoughlin, J. B. Siddal, G. R. Wendt, G. C. Buzby, D. R. Herbst, K. W. Ledig, J. W. McMenamin, D. W. Pattison, J. Suida, J. Tokolics, R. A. Edgren, A. B. A. Jansen, B. Gadsby, D. H. R. Watson, and P. C. P. Philips, *Experientia* **19**, 394 (1963).
12. A. J. v. d. Broek, A. I. A. Broess, M. J. v. d. Heuvel, H. P. de Jongh, J. Leemhius, K. H. Schönemann, J. Smits, J. de Visser, N. P. van Vliet, and F. J. Zeelen, *Steroids* **30**, 481 (1977).
13. A. J. v. d. Broek, C. v. Bokhoven, P. M. J. Hobbelen, and J. Leenhuis, *Recl. Trav. Chim. Pays-Bas* **94**, 35 (1974).
14. G. K. Aydar and R. B. Greenblatt, *J. Med. Assoc. State Ala.* **31**, 53 (1961).
15. K. H. Chemnitius, C. Clausen, W. Stölzner, and A. Naumann, *Zentralbl. Pharm.* **116**, 537 (1977).
16. D. R. Mishell and N. D. Freid, *Contraception* **8**, 37 (1973); S. Tejuja, S. D. Choudhury, N. C. Saxena, U. Malhotra, and G. Bhinder, *Contraception* **10**, 375 (1974).
17. K. Fotherby, G. Benagiano, H. K. Toppozada, A. Abel-Rahmann, F. Navaroli, B. Arce, R. Ramos-Cordero, C. Gual, B. M. Landgren, and E. Johanisson, *Contraception* **25**, 261 (1981).
18. T. Siriwongse, W. Snidvongs, P. Tantayaporn, and S. Leepipatpaiboon, *Contraception* **26**, 487 (1982).
19. E. M. Coutinho, J. C. de Souza, J. C. Barboza, and V. Dourada Silva, *Contraception* **25**, 551 (1982); H. K. Toppozada, S. Koetsawang, V. E. Aimakhu, T. Khan, A. Pretnar, T. K. Chatterjee, M. P. Molitor-Peffer, R. Apelo, R. Lichtenberg, P. C. Crosignano, J. C. de Souza, C. Gomez-Rogers, A. A. Haspels, R. H. Ciray, P. Diethelm, G. Benagiano, and J. Annus, *Contraception* **25**, 1 (1982).
20. L. R. Beck, V. Z. Pope, C. E. Flowers, D. R. Cowsar, T. R. Rice, D. H. Lewis, R. L. Dunn, A. B. Moore, and R. M. Gilley, *Biol. of Reprod.* **28**, 186 (1982); S. J. Ory, C. B. Hammond, S. G. Yangsy, R. Wayne Hendren, and C. G. Pitt, *Am. J. Obstet. Gynecol.* **145**, 600 (1983).
21. S. Diaz, M. Pavez, P. Miranda, D. N. Robertson, J. Sivin, and H. B. Croxatto, *Contraception* **25**, 447 (1982); B. M. Landgren, M. A. Oriowo, and E. Diczfalusy, *Contraception* **24**, 29 (1981).
22. B. M. Landgren, E. Johannisson, B. Masironi, and E. Diczfalusy, *Contraception* **26**, 567 (1982).
23. I. Sivin, D. R. Mishell, Jr., A. Victor, S. Diaz, F. Alvarez-Sanchez, N. C. Nielson, O. Akinla, T. Pyorala, E. Coutinho, A. Faundes, S. Roy, P. F. Brenner, T. Ahren, M. Pavez, V. Brache, O. F. Giwa-Osagie, M. O. Fasan, B. Zausner-Guelman, E. Darze, J. C. Gama da Silva, J. Diaz, T. M. Jackanicz, J. Stern, and H. A. Nash, *Contraception* **24**, 341 (1981).

CHAPTER 11

Injectable Cephalosporin Antibiotics: Cephalothin to Ceftazidime

C. E. NEWALL

Department of Microbiological Chemistry
Glaxo Group Research Ltd.
Greenford, England

I. INTRODUCTION

Fleming's observations in 1929, which led to the isolation and development of penicillin in the mid-1940s, were the beginning of an era of antibacterial drug discovery which continues to this day (*1*). At the time of their introduction, penicillin G (**1**) and penicillin V (**2**), the first of the commercially available β-lactam antibiotics, revolutionised antibacterial chemotherapy by providing effective treatment of life threatening infections caused by some bacteria, including the very common *Staphylococcus aureus* (see Table I). However, the activity of these early compounds was largely restricted to Gram-positive* bacteria, such as staphylococci and streptococci. It also soon became apparent that bacterial resistance caused by penicillinases, which destroyed the antibiotics, was becoming a problem, particularly in hospitals. Extensive studies of the chemistry of the penicillins were rewarded by the development of efficient methods for the isolation of 6-aminopenicillanic acid (6-APA). The availability of this key intermediate led to the development by workers at Beecham during the early 1960s of the

---

*Bacteria are termed Gram-positive or Gram-negative according to the uptake of dye stain in a test devised by a Danish physician H. J. Gram. Gram-positive bacteria have a peptidoglycan outer cell wall; Gram-negative bacteria possess a peptidoglycan cell wall (Fig. 1) and a second barrier, a lipopolysaccharide cell membrane (Fig. 1, Chap. 1).

TABLE I
Some Clinically Important Bacteria

Organism	Gram type	May cause or be associated with
Staphylococcus aureus	+	Skin and soft tissue infections, septicaemia, endo-carditis, accounts for ~25% of all hospital infections
Streptococci	+	Several types—commonly cause sore throats, upper respiratory tract infections and pneumonia
Escherichia coli	−	Urinary tract and wound infections, common in the gastro-intestinal tract and often causes problems after surgery, accounts for ~25% of all hospital infections
Proteus species	−	Urinary tract infections
Salmonella species	−	Food poisoning and typhoid fever
Shigella species	−	Dysentery
Enterobacter species	−	Urinary tract and respiratory tract infections, septi-
Klebsiella species	−	caemia
Pseudomonas aeruginosa	−	An 'opportunist' pathogen, can cause very severe infections in burn victims and other compromised patients, i.e., cancer patients, commonly causes chest infections in patients with cystic fibrosis
Haemophilus influenzae	−	Chest and ear infections, occasionally meningitis in young children
Bacteroides fragilis	−	Septicaemia following gastro-intestinal surgery

penicillinase-resistant narrow-spectrum antibiotics methicillin (**3**), cloxacillin (**4**) and the broader spectrum oral penicillin, ampicillin (**5**).

The antibacterial action of penicillins and other, more recently discovered, classes of β-lactam antibiotics derives from their ability to interfere with the synthesis and maintenance of the bacterial cell wall. Unlike mammalian cells,

(**1**) R = PhCH$_2$— Penicillin G   (**2**) R = PhOCH$_2$— Penicillin V

(**3**) R = (OMe / OMe) Methicillin   (**4**) R = (Cl, Me) Cloxacillin

(5) R = Ph—CH— (D) Ampicillin   (6) R = Ph—CH— (D) Piperacillin

                      |
                      NH₂

        NH
        |
        CO
        |
        N   O
        |
        N   O
        |
        Et

which are adapted to life in the controlled environment of the body, single-celled organisms like bacteria must be able to survive in conditions of varying pH, temperature and osmolarity. With the exception of certain species such as *Chlamydia* which live as parasites within mammalian cells, bacteria have evolved a fairly flexible, yet physically strong cell wall. This is composed of the polymer peptidoglycan, which is constructed from sub-units of an *N*-acetylmuramyl pen-

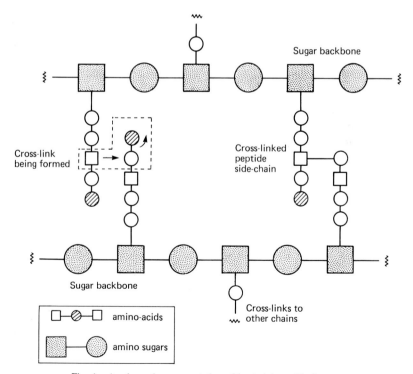

Fig. 1   A schematic representation of bacterial peptidoglycan.

tapeptide, linked and cross-linked to form a net-like 'bag' (Fig. 1) capable of withstanding the osmotic forces caused by differing concentrations of salts within the cell and in the surrounding medium. In order to grow and divide, bacteria must continually modify their cell wall, breaking and reforming cross-links and inserting new *N*-acetylmuramyl pentapeptide units. Whilst doing this they are vulnerable to the action of β-lactam antibiotics, which inhibit enzymes ['penicillin binding proteins' (PBPs)] responsible for carrying out these modifications.

Interest in the development of penicillins has continued worldwide and some newer injectable compounds, such as piperacillin (**6**), exhibit good broad-spectrum activity against a wide range of Gram-positive and Gram-negative bacteria. However, the broad-spectrum penicillins have a major disadvantage in that they are rapidly destroyed by β-lactamase enzymes produced by many strains of bacteria; indeed production of these enzymes is probably the most important cause of bacterial resistance to penicillins. This problem has been addressed in part by the discovery and development of β-lactamase inhibitors, such as clavulanic acid (**7**), discussed in more detail in Chap. 12.

(**7**) Clavulanic acid

Since the 1930s the metabolites from fungi and other similar organisms have been very extensively investigated in the search for new bioactive molecules. In 1945 Brotzu isolated a strain of *Cephalosporium acremonium*, which produced several antibiotics, from a sewage outfall in Cagliari, Sardinia. The organism was sent to the Sir William Dunn School of Pathology in Oxford, where Abraham's group isolated three structurally different types of antibiotic; one of these was a penicillin [penicillin N (**8**)] possessing a different 6-substituent, and the

(**8**) Penicillin N

(**9**) Cephalosporin C

(**10**) Cephalosporin P₁

others, cephalosporin C (**9**) and cephalosporins P1–P5 [e.g., P1 (**10**)], were novel (*2*).

The most interesting of these was cephalosporin C, which exhibited weak broad-spectrum activity. This compound was clearly structurally related to the penicillins, in particular to penicillin N which had the same aminoadipoyl side-chain. Although cephalosporin C was much less active against sensitive strains of staphylococci than penicillin G it was unaffected by penicillinases produced by resistant strains and retained its activity against these bacteria. This observation was regarded as so significant that several companies, including Eli Lilly and Glaxo, decided to develop this new class of antibiotic which issued from Abraham's group at Oxford. Fermentation studies were soon underway to improve the production of cephalosporin C at the expense of the less desirable penicillin N and cephalosporin P. At the same time chemical studies aimed at the preparation of analogues with greatly improved antibacterial activity were begun.

Unlike the penicillin molecule, which can be readily modified only by changing the 6-acylamino substituent, cephalosporin C had two convenient points of attack, at the 7-position in a manner analogous to modification of the penicillin 6-position and at the 3-position where the acetoxymethyl group held out much promise for new chemistry. An early priority was to provide a key intermediate for the synthesis of compounds with new 7-acylamino substituents by removing the aminoadipoyl side-chain, hence the discovery of a method of removing this side-chain was a crucial step forward. Many methods of achieving this have now been described: one of the most commonly used involves the conversion of the 7-amide function of an N-protected diester of cephalosporin C into an imino chloride with phosphorus pentachloride/pyridine. Subsequent treatment with an appropriate alcohol affords an imino ether, which may readily be hydrolysed with aqueous acid to give the ester of 7-amino cephalosporanic acid [7-ACA (**11**)] in high yield (Scheme 1) (*3*).

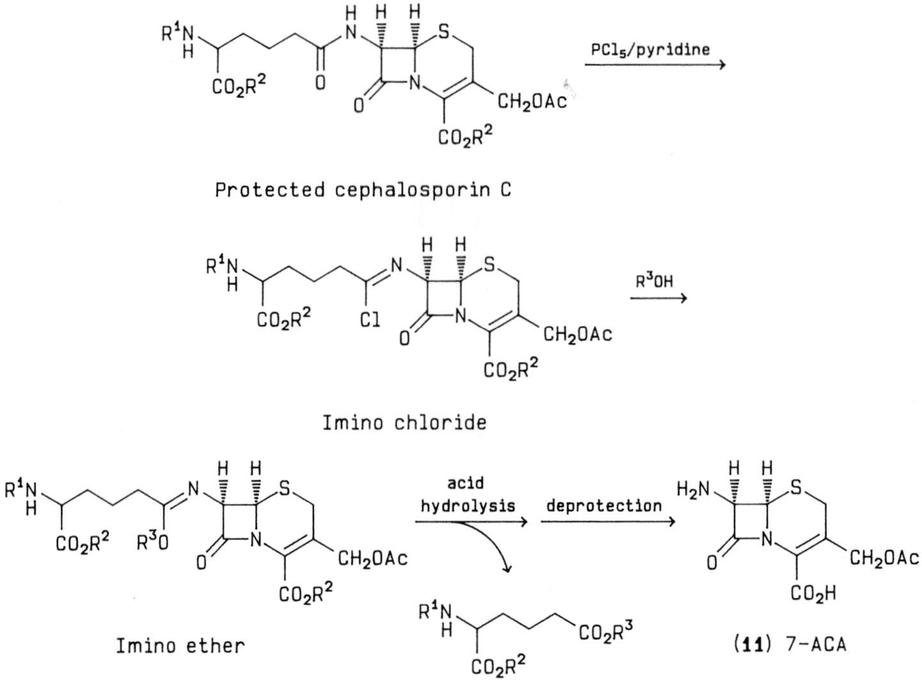
PCl5/pyridine
Protected cephalosporin C
R3OH
Imino chloride
acid hydrolysis
deprotection
Imino ether
(11) 7-ACA

Scheme 1 Generalized scheme for the preparation of 7-ACA.

II. PREPARATION OF MODIFIED FIRST-GENERATION CEPHALOSPORINS

The scene was now set for the chemical modification of 7-ACA which, like 6-APA, has little activity in its own right. Early studies concentrated on acylation of the 7-amino group and led to cephalothin (**12**), the first cephalosporin to be used in the clinic. Cephalothin had good activity against many common pathogens, notably *Staph. aureus* and *Escherichia coli,* and was stable to staphylococcal penicillinase. However, it carried the 3-acetoxymethyl substituent of cephalosporin C, which is relatively unstable to mammalian esterases, and was partially converted into the less active 3-hydroxymethyl derivative (**13**) *in vivo.* Thus, some of the activity of a dose of cephalothin may be lost within a short time of administration, reducing the clinical effect.

This particular problem of metabolic instability could clearly be addressed by modifying the 3-substituent, and it was soon found that displacement of the acetoxy group by pyridine gave a compound, cephaloridine (**14**), with similar antibacterial properties which was stable to mammalian esterases. Cephaloridine

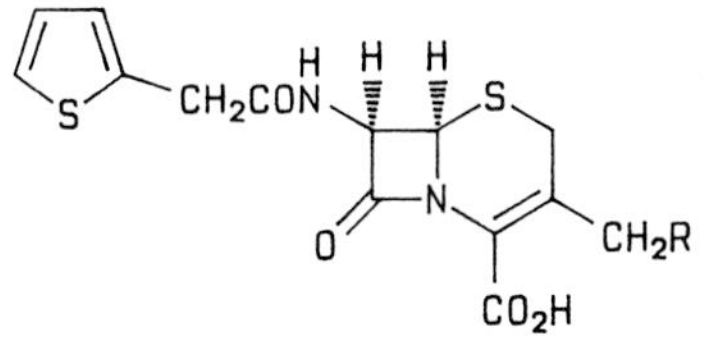

(12) R = OAc Cephalothin
(13) R = OH

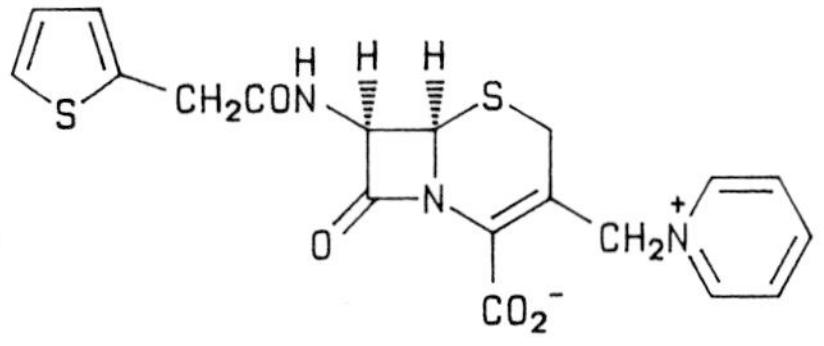

(14) Cephaloridine

was first made available in the mid-1960s and remains in current clinical use. It has very occasionally been associated with some nephrotoxicity (kidney toxicity) in patients with renal disease, particularly if high doses are used, but otherwise it is well tolerated and is generally very effective against sensitive bacteria.

Cephalothin and cephaloridine must both be given by injection as neither compound is absorbed from the gastro-intestinal tract, and much effort was put into a search for oral cephalosporins. In the late 1960s the first of these, cephalexin (15), was developed independently by groups at Eli Lilly and Glaxo. Cephalexin is a 3-methyl cephalosporin and may be prepared either from cephalosporin C or by rearrangement of a penicillin sulphoxide (Scheme 2) (4). It has broad-spectrum activity and is very effective in the treatment of less severe infections, particularly in non-hospitalised patients.

Although cephaloridine is unaffected by Gram-positive penicillinases and remains the most effective cephalosporin for the treatment of infections caused by Gram-positive bacteria, it was soon found that some Gram-negative bacteria were able to produce β-lactamases which were capable of destroying it. Furthermore, it was realised that the β-lactamases capable of deactivating cephaloridine

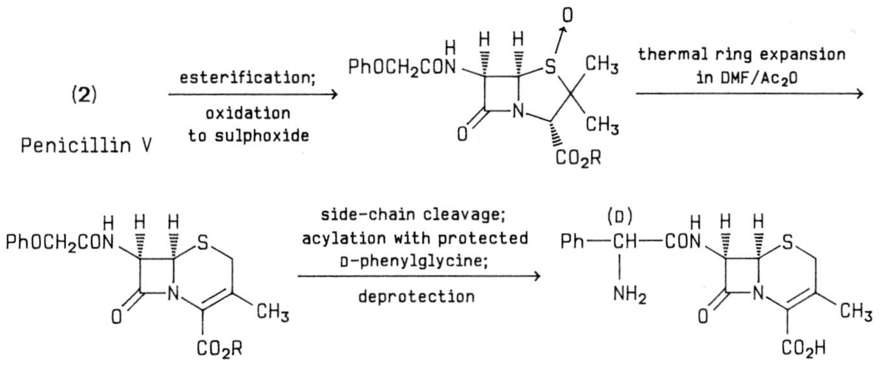

(15) Cephalexin

Scheme 2   Preparation of cephalexin (15) from penicillin V (2).

and other first-generation injectable cephalosporins were widespread in the community and that bacterial resistance caused by these enzymes was becoming a problem, particularly in hospitals where the frequent use of antibiotics applied ecological pressures which favoured their emergence. The search for β-lactamase stable cephalosporins began.

III.   PREPARATION OF SECOND-GENERATION CEPHALOSPORINS

Two solutions to the above mentioned problem were possible; one was to administer lactamase inhibitors such as clavulanic acid with compounds like cephalothin and cephaloridine. However, a more satisfactory solution was to make compounds which were stable to β-lactamases, and a great deal of effort was put into this approach. One strategy was to prepare compounds in which the β-lactam ring was sterically crowded in order to hinder the approach of the nucleophilic group of the β-lactamase to the β-lactam ring. However, most attempts to do this resulted in compounds virtually devoid of antibacterial activity; this is not surprising as the activity of these molecules derives from the ability of the β-lactam ring to interact (probably by acylation) with the enzymes responsible for synthesising and maintaining the bacterial cell wall. However, two types of active and β-lactamase stable compounds were found.

The first type was the 7α-methoxycephalosporins (cephamycins) derived from cephamycin C (16), which had been isolated from *Streptomyces clavuligerus* by workers at Merck. Replacement of the aminoadipoyl side-chain of cephamycin C by the thienylacetyl group carried by cephaloridine provided cefoxitin (17), which proved to be stable to both β-lactamases and mammalian esterases. This compound has a broader spectrum of activity than the first-generation cephalosporins, mainly because of its stability to lactamases; however, it is painful on injection and is often given with a local anaesthetic.

(16) R = (with H_2N–CHCH$_2$CH$_2$CH$_2$— and HO$_2$C)   Cephamycin C

(17) R = (thienyl)—CH$_2$—   Cefoxitin

(18) Cefuroxime

The second group of compounds which combined stability to β-lactamases with good antibacterial activity were the oximinocephalosporins. The first of these was Glaxo's cefuroxime (**18**) (*5*). Cefuroxime exhibits a high level of resistance to clinically important β-lactamases and is not hydrolysed by mammalian esterases. It is safe and well tolerated by humans, even at high doses, and has been used very successfully for a number of years.

Despite their improved level and spectrum of activity the second-generation compounds like cefuroxime and cefoxitin still do not provide complete antibacterial cover as they have little or no useful activity against many of the more intractable bacteria which in the late 1970s were beginning to cause concern, especially in critically ill patients suffering from serious underlying diseases. Thus patients with renal and respiratory tract diseases, with cystic fibrosis, severe wounds, burns and immunosuppressed cancer and organ transplant patients are at risk from infection by opportunistic pathogens such as *Pseudomonas aeruginosa*. This and many other bacteria occur very commonly, often as part of the normal body flora, and usually only become pathogenic when the body's natural resistance mechanisms are depressed in some way. This can occur in patients in shock, namely, in severe burn and accident victims, as a result of preexisting disease or as a result of immunosuppressive chemotherapy. Once established, an infection by one of these pathogens may prove to be rapidly fatal, for example if it results in septicaemia or meningitis, or it may lead to a chronic and weakening infection which may be very difficult to eradicate. Until recently the only antibiotics generally effective for the treatment of these serious infections, particularly those caused by *Pseudomonas,* were the aminoglycosides, such as gentamicin (**19**). These have a mechanism of action different from the penicillins and cephalosporins, being inhibitors of bacterial protein synthesis rather than of cell wall biosynthesis. The aminoglycosides kill bacteria very rapidly. However, they can cause adverse reactions, and blood concentrations have to be carefully monitored to avoid levels which might lead to ototoxic (ear) or nephrotoxic

(**19**) Gentamicin A   (**20**) Cefoperazone

(kidney) effects. Furthermore, resistance to the aminoglycosides can occur and, because of the toxicity of these compounds, cannot be overcome simply by increasing the dose. There was clearly a need for a new generation of very potent β-lactam antibiotics intended primarily for hospital use, and many of the major pharmaceutical companies began research programmes aimed at finding compounds with the desirable combination of properties.

IV.   PREPARATION OF THIRD-GENERATION CEPHALOSPORINS

Several penicillins, for example piperacillin (6), were found to have very good activity against many bacteria, including some strains of *Pseudomonas;* however, β-lactamase producing strains remained resistant. Cephalosporins with a similar ureido 7-substituent, such as cefoperazone (20), have also been found to possess good broad-spectrum activity but are relatively unstable to the lactamases produced by some Gram-negative bacteria.

The first public evidence that cephalosporins with the desired properties could be prepared came with the disclosure of cefotaxime (21) by Roussel-Uclaf. This compound possesses the methoximino group characteristic of cefuroxime and the 3-acetoxymethyl group of cephalothin but carries a new aryl substituent in the side-chain. Cefotaxime was somewhat less active against *Staph. aureus* than other cephalosporins but was more active against many Gram-negative bacteria. It had some activity against *Ps. aeruginosa*. It was unstable to mammalian esterases, being converted, like cephalothin, into the corresponding 3-hydroxymethyl derivative in the body; however, this was claimed to be less of a disadvantage in the case of cefotaxime since the desacetyl metabolite (22) also possessed considerable antibacterial activity, although less than that of the parent compound. It soon became clear that several other companies were also actively involved in research in this area. With the exception of the research at Glaxo the main interest seemed to be focussed on methoximes (cf. cefuroxime), although the patents generally disclosed a wide variety of more complex alkoximino groups.

Most of these new cephalosporins (23–26) differed only in the nature of the 3-substituent; some of these [e.g., the tetrazolylthiomethyl group carried by cefmenoxime (24)] were derived from earlier cephalosporins but others, notably the triazinedione carried by ceftriaxone (26), were novel. These compounds exhibited broadly similar patterns of antimicrobial activity, with only moderate activity against staphylococci, excellent activity against most Gram-negative bacteria and some activity against *Pseudomonas*. All were generally stable to β-lactamases, although some variation in their relative stabilities has been reported. With the exception of cefotaxime (21), all appear to be metabolically stable.

(**21**) R = —CH$_2$OAc   Cefotaxime

(**22**) R = —CH$_2$OH   Desacetyl cefotaxime

(**23**) R = —H   Ceftizoxime

(**24**) R = —CH$_2$S—   Cefmenoxime

(**25**) R = —CH$_2$S—   Cefodizime

(**26**) R = —CH$_2$S—   Ceftriaxone

None of the compounds is orally absorbed, and they are all given by injection or intravenous infusion. Their routes and rates of elimination from the body tend to be different, and these factors are likely to influence their suitability for use in different disease states. Most of the antibiotic is normally eliminated from the body via the urine but with some of the compounds a significant proportion of the dose is eliminated in the bile and faeces, increasing the possibility of gastro-intestinal side effects, such as diarrhoea, by disturbing the normal bacterial flora of the lower intestine. Of course, biliary excretion can be advantageous in some cases, for example when the patient has an infection involving the gall bladder or bile duct. Generally speaking a long elimination half-life is desirable as compounds like ceftriaxone (**26**), which are slowly excreted, need to be given less often. However, care needs to be taken with patients whose ability to eliminate drugs is undeveloped (e.g., babies) or impaired (e.g., the elderly and patients with renal failure).

Although all the methoximes (**21, 23–26**) have some activity against *Ps. aeruginosa* and would be suitable for the treatment of infections caused by relatively sensitive strains of this organism, none of them approach the activity of

(27) Cefsulodin

(28) Ceftazidime

gentamicin or the *Pseudomonas*-specific cephalosporin cefsulodin (**27**). However, the Glaxo antibiotic ceftazidime (**28**) has excellent activity against *Pseudomonas*, being very active against gentamicin-sensitive strains and much more active than aminoglycosides against most gentamicin-resistant strains. Ceftazidime's activity against most other Gram-negative bacteria is similar to that of the methoximes but there is some loss of activity against *Staph. aureus*. It is very effective against Gram-negative bacteria, including *Ps. aeruginosa, in vivo* and is more active against staphylococci in experimental infections than might be expected from its minimum inhibitory concentrations (MICs) against these bacteria *in vitro*. Ceftazidime's relatively long elimination half-life, low blood-serum binding, good tissue penetration and rapid bactericidal action probably provide an explanation for its effectiveness against staphylococci *in vivo*.

Many methods have been developed for the synthesis of these new compounds. In most cases the 7-acylamino substituent is fully elaborated prior to attachment to the cephalosporin nucleus. Thus, oximation of ethyl acetoacetate affords the 2-hydroximino ester (**29**), which may be chlorinated in the 4-position with sulphuryl chloride. Reaction of the resulting 4-chloro ester with thiourea in aqueous ethanol for about an hour at room temperature affords the syn isomer of the 2-aminothiazolyloximino ester (**30**) in a yield of about 60% (*6*). Tritylation of the amino group proceeds smoothly with trityl chloride in the presence of pyridine and the resulting N-protected ester may then be O-alkylated, for example with dimethyl sulphate, and saponified to give the N-tritylated 2-methoximino side-chain acid (**32**) (Scheme 3). Alternatively, ethyl 2-hydroximino-3-oxobutyrate (**29**) may be successively O-alkylated and brominated to give the 4-bromo-2-methoxyimino ester (**33**), cyclisation of which with thiourea affords the corresponding 2-amino side-chain ester (**34**). In all these reactions care must be taken to minimise the formation of the anti isomers of the oximes, which tend to be produced when the desired syn isomers are exposed to acid, particularly in anhydrous media.

The side-chain acid (**35**) for ceftazidime may readily be prepared from the N-protected oxime ester (**31**) by reaction with *t*-butyl bromoisobutyrate in dimethyl

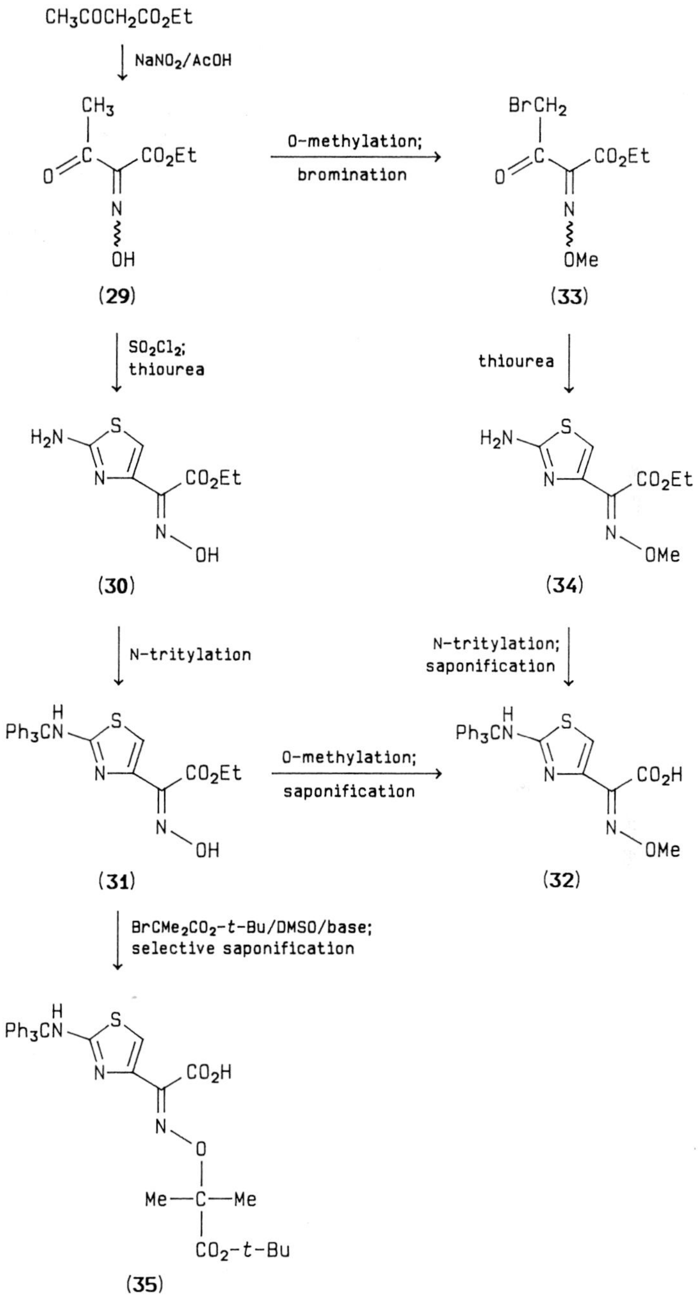

CH₃COCH₂CO₂Et

↓ NaNO₂/AcOH

(29)

O-methylation;
bromination
⟶

(33)

SO₂Cl₂;
thiourea ↓

thiourea ↓

(30)

(34)

N-tritylation ↓

N-tritylation;
saponification ↓

(31)

O-methylation;
saponification
⟶

(32)

BrCMe₂CO₂-t-Bu/DMSO/base;
selective saponification ↓

(35)

Scheme 3   Preparation of the side-chain acids for ceftazidime, cefmenoxime, etc.

sulphoxide in the presence of sodium carbonate followed by selective saponification of the less sterically hindered ethyl ester group.

Although the synthesis of the side-chain will normally be completed before it is attached to the cephalosporin nucleus, apart from minor adjustments to the functionality, this need not always be the case. Thus, workers at Takeda devised a synthesis of radiolabelled cefmenoxime which involved the formation of the thiazole ring as almost the last step (Scheme 4) (7). They reacted the 7-aminocephalosporin acid (36) with 4-chloro-3-oxobutyryl chloride (prepared by the addition of chlorine to diketene) to give the 7-(4-chloro-3-oxobutyramido) compound, which was reacted with sodium nitrite and acetic acid to give the oxime (37). Careful O-methylation with dimethyl sulphate followed by esterification with diphenyl diazomethane provided the methoximino ester (38). This was reacted with ^{14}C-labelled thiourea and de-esterified with trifluoroacetic acid/anisole to give ^{14}C-radiolabelled cefmenoxime (24).

Once the side-chain acid has been prepared in a suitably protected form it may be coupled with the appropriate derivative of 7-ACA. The coupling methods normally used for the attachment of side-chains to penicillins and cephalosporins are similar to those used in peptide synthesis and involve the formation of an activated derivative of the carboxylic acid group. Thus, a pre-formed acid halide,

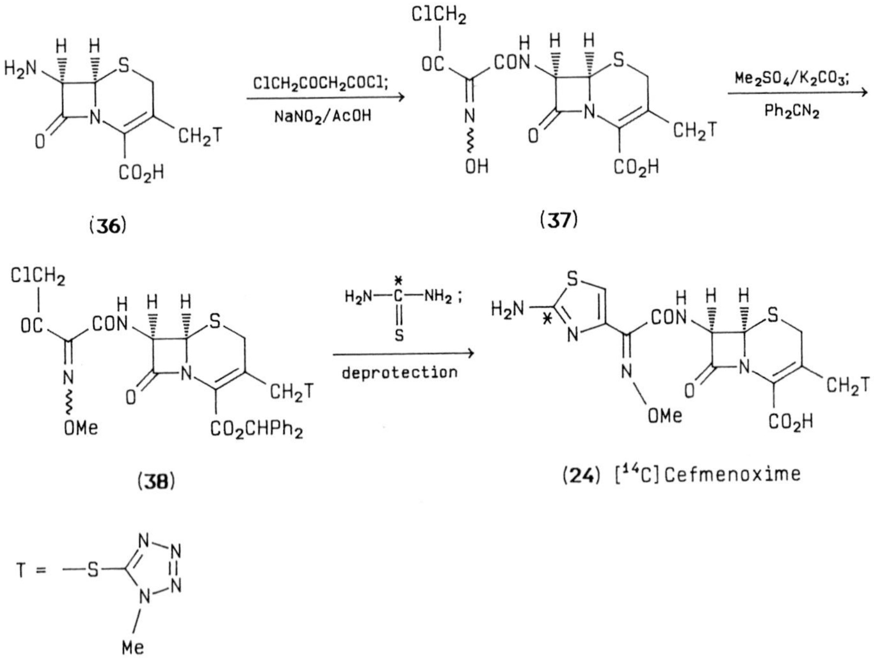

Scheme 4   Synthesis of radiolabelled cefmenoxime.

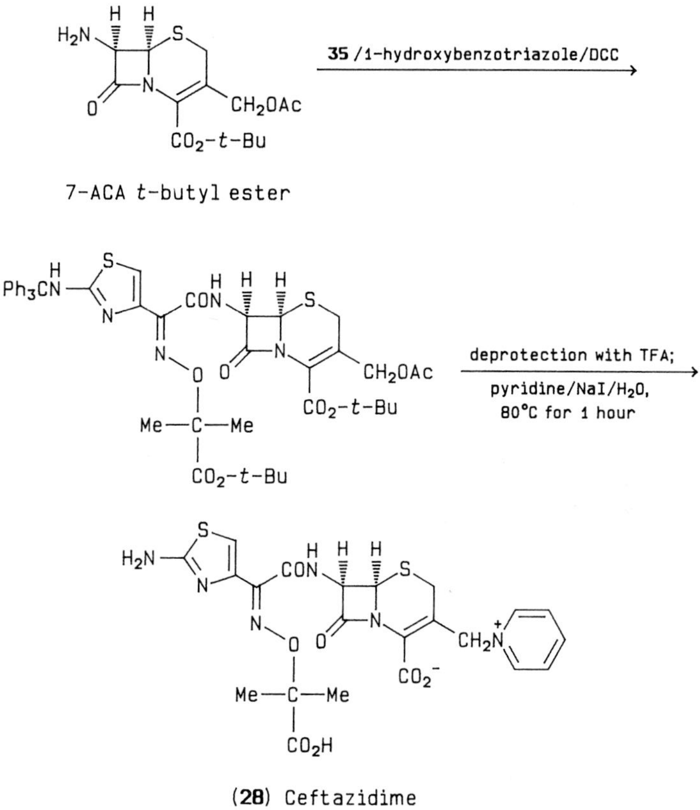

7-ACA *t*-butyl ester

35 /1-hydroxybenzotriazole/DCC

deprotection with TFA;
pyridine/NaI/H$_2$O,
80°C for 1 hour

(**28**) Ceftazidime

Scheme 5   Preparation of ceftazidime from 7-ACA.

activated ester or anhydride may be used, or the activated species may be formed *in situ* by the use of a coupling reagent such as dicyclohexyl carbodiimide (DCC). The latter reagent is now commonly used in conjunction with 1-hydroxybenzotriazole, forming a very reactive benzotriazolyl ester of the side-chain acid *in situ;* this usually reacts with the 7-ACA derivative to give the coupled cephalosporin in high yield and with minimum formation of by-products.

After the side-chain has been attached the synthesis may be complete, apart from removal of any protecting groups. However, some more fundamental adjustment of functionality may be required. An example of this is the displacement of an acetoxy group from the 3-substituent by pyridine, as in the final stages of a synthesis of ceftazidime (**28**) illustrated in Scheme 5.

A number of sulphur and other nitrogen nucleophiles may also be used in similar 'last-step' displacement reactions. However, an alternative strategy, proceeding via the appropriate 3-substituted 7-aminocephalosporin, is usually preferable as it provides a more convergent synthesis. Thus, in the case of ceftriaxone (26), the 3-mercapto-2-methyl-1,2,4-triazine dione (39) (from which the 3-substituent is derived) may be prepared in two steps by the reaction of methylhydrazine with potassium thiocyanate, followed by cyclisation with dimethyl oxalate. Condensation with 7-ACA provides the 3-substituted-7-aminocephalosporanic acid, which may be condensed with the N-protected side-chain acyl chloride to give, ultimately, ceftriaxone (26) (8).

The application of this strategy to the synthesis of ceftazidime required a good way of preparing 7-amino-3-pyridiniummethylcephalosporanic acid (40), an intermediate not previously used in synthesis. One method of preparing this compound is to remove the side-chain from cephaloridine (14) by a standard procedure involving phosphorus pentachloride. The 7-aminobetaine (40) is conveniently isolated from the reaction as a pure, highly crystalline dihydrochloride salt (Scheme 7). Alternatively, the acetoxy group of an N-protected form of cephalosporin C may be displaced by pyridine and the side-chain then removed with PCl$_5$ to give the same intermediate. Coupling with the protected side-chain acid (35) followed by removal of the t-butyl and trityl protecting groups gives ceftazidime.

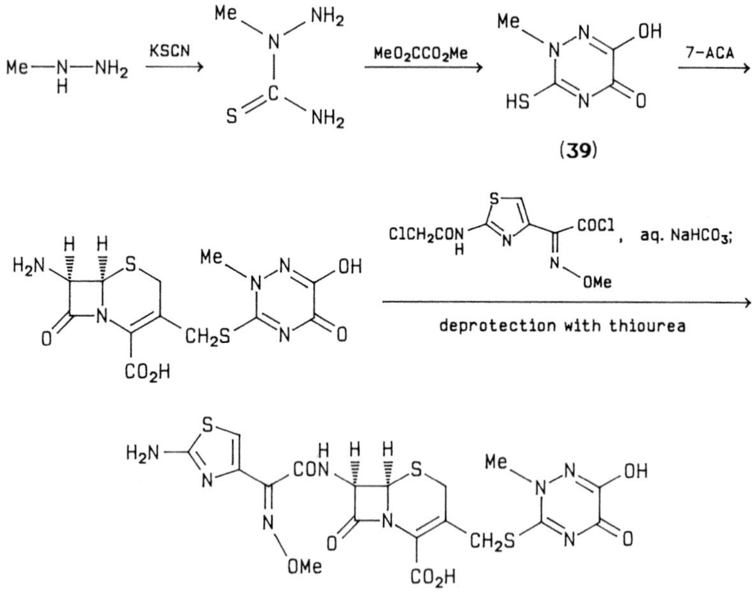

Scheme 6   Preparation of ceftriaxone from 7-ACA.

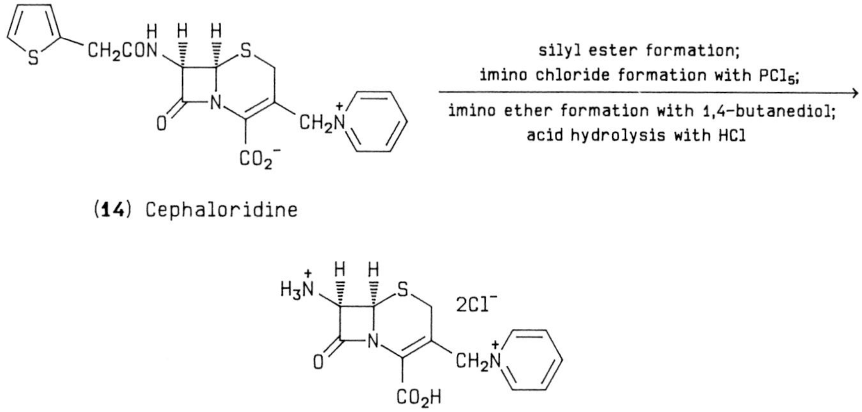

(**14**) Cephaloridine

(**40**)

Scheme 7   Preparation of 7-amino-3-pyridiniummethylcephalosporanate from cephaloridine.

V. CONCLUSION

Some of these third-generation broad-spectrum cephalosporin antibiotics are now on the market and several more are at an advanced stage of clinical trial. Their impact on clinical practice is likely to be significant and they will probably extend the use of cephalosporins into areas where other agents, such as the aminoglycosides, have been the antibiotics of choice. Ceftazidime, in particular, with its exceptional activity against *Pseudomonas,* seems set to challenge the supremacy of the aminoglycosides in the treatment of severe infections caused by Gram-negative bacteria (9).

Notwithstanding the very good activity of these compounds, bacterial strains resistant to them will eventually emerge. Indeed, many of these almost certainly exist already but have not yet been identified in the clinic. They will tend to move into the ecological niches created by the eradication of today's sensitive strains and are likely to come to our notice within the next few years. We must try to anticipate their appearance, and work on new generations of 'mega-cephalosporins' has already begun.

REFERENCES

1. S. M. Roberts, *Chem. Ind. (London),* 162 (1984).
2. E. P. Abraham, and P. B. Loder, *in* ''Cephalosporins and Penicillins, Chemistry and Biology'' (E. H. Flynn, ed.), pp. 1–26. Academic Press, New York, 1972.
3. L. D. Hatfield, W. H. W. Lunn, B. G. Jackson, L. R. Peters, L. C. Blaszczak, J. W. Fisher, J. P.

Gardner, and J. M. Dunigan, *in* "Recent Advances in the Chemistry of β-Lactam Antibiotics" (G. I. Gregory, ed.), pp. 109–124. Special Publication No. 38, The Royal Society of Chemistry, London, 1981.

4. R. D. G. Cooper and D. O. Spry, *in* "Cephalosporins and Penicillins, Chemistry and Biology," (E. H. Flynn, ed.), pp. 183–254, Academic Press, New York, 1972.

5. P. C. Cherry, M. C. Cook, M. W. Foxton, M. Gregson, G. I. Gregory, and G. B. Webb, *in* "Recent Advances in the Chemistry of β-Lactam Antibiotics" (J. Elks, ed.), pp. 145–152. Special Publication No. 28, The Chemical Society, London, 1977.

6. R. Bucourt, R. Heymes, A. Lutz, L. Pénasse, and J. Perronnet, *Tetrahedron* **34,** 2233 (1978).

7. M. Ochiai, A. Morimoto, and T. Mujawaki, *J. Antibiot.* **34,** 186 (1981).

8. R. Reiner, U. Weiss, U. Brombacker, P. Lanz, M. Montavon, A. Furlenmeier, A. Angehrn, and P. J. Probst, *J. Antibiot.* **33,** 783 (1980).

9. P. Acred, D. M. Ryan, M. A. Sowa, and C. M. Watts, *J. Antimicrob. Chemother.* **8,** Suppl. B, 247 (1981); P. W. Muggleton, *ibid,* 1; P. B. Harper, *ibid,* 5.

CHAPTER 12

Clavulanic Acid and Related Compounds: Inhibitors of β-Lactamase Enzymes

A. G. BROWN

Beecham Pharmaceuticals Research Division
Chemotherapeutic Centre
Betchworth, England

I. INTRODUCTION

It is now well over 50 years since the discovery of penicillin by Fleming. In that time, and particularly in the last 25 years, a wide variety of β-lactam antibiotics have been obtained (i) as microbial metabolites, (ii) as semi-synthetic antibacterials prepared by the chemical modification of naturally occurring β-lactams, and (iii) by total synthesis. Today the most widely used β-lactam antibiotics are derivatives of the penicillin (**1**) and cephalosporin (**2**) families, but new entities such as clavulanic acid (**3**) and thienamycin (**4**) are about to gain widespread therapeutic application (*1*). In this chapter the discovery, development and chemotherapeutic application of one of these newer β-lactams, namely clavulanic acid (**3**), is related. In addition, the discovery and potential of the olivanic acids and thienamycin is described.

During their early studies on the purification and evaluation of penicillin, Abraham and Chain recognised that bacteria could produce an enzyme capable of destroying the antibiotic (*2*). They called this enzyme penicillinase, though nowadays it is more generally referred to as β-lactamase. β-Lactamases destroy penicillins and cephalosporins by hydrolysing the β-lactam ring to yield a penicilloic acid derivative (**5**) in the case of penicillins or a variety of products (e.g.,

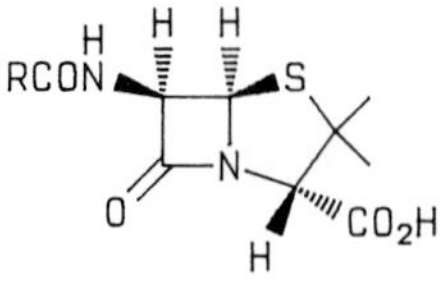

(1)

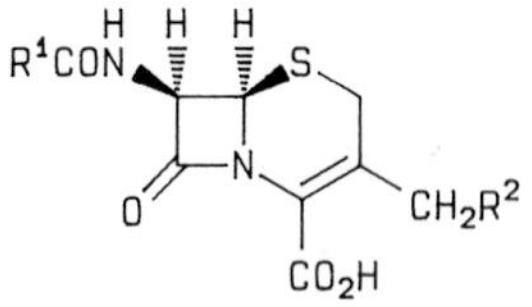

(2)

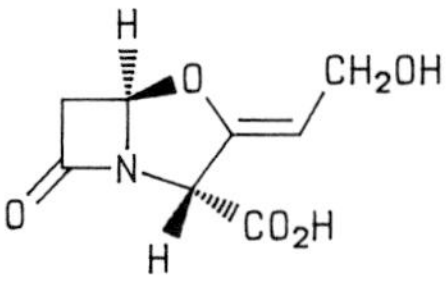

(3) Clavulanic acid

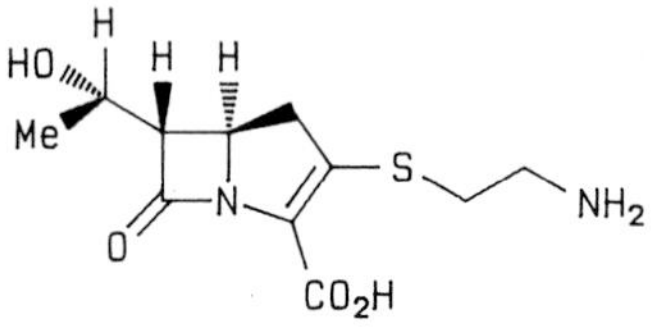

(4) Thienamycin

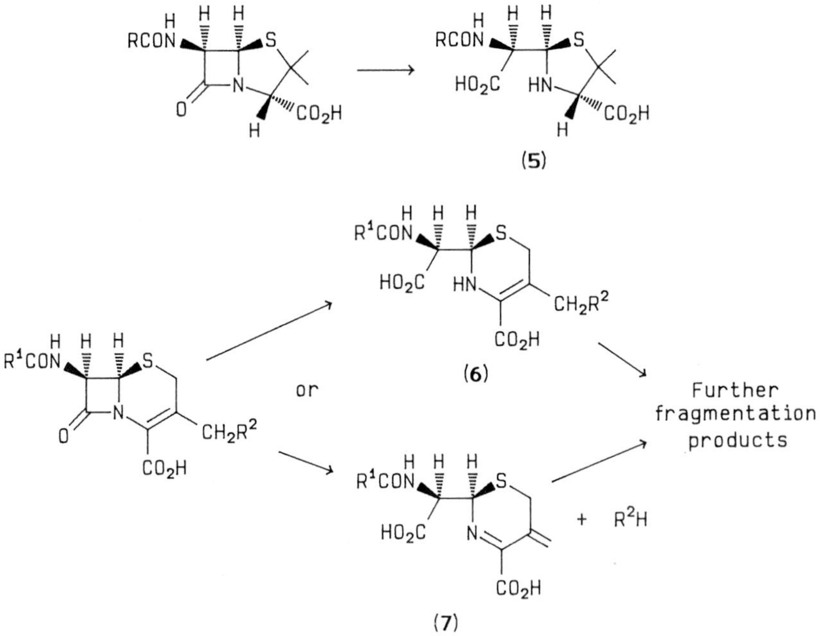

(5)

(6)

or

Further
fragmentation
products

(7)

Scheme 1   General reaction scheme for the hydrolysis of penicillins and cephalosporins by β-lactamase.

6 and **7**) with cephalosporins depending upon the nature of the R^2 substituent (Scheme 1).

The ability of bacteria to produce a variety of β-lactamases has proved over the years to be the major mechanism by which resistance develops to antibiotic therapy with penicillins and cephalosporins. Indeed initial attempts in the late 1950s and early 1960s to overcome resistance due to β-lactamase production (particularly by staphylococci) led to the successful development of penicillins with a high degree of stability towards this enzyme, namely, penicillins such as compounds **8–11** and the semi-synthetic cephalosporins [e.g., cefuroxime (**12**) (see Chap. 11)].

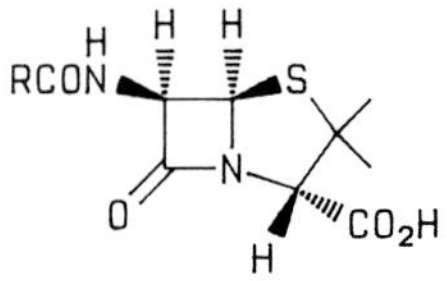

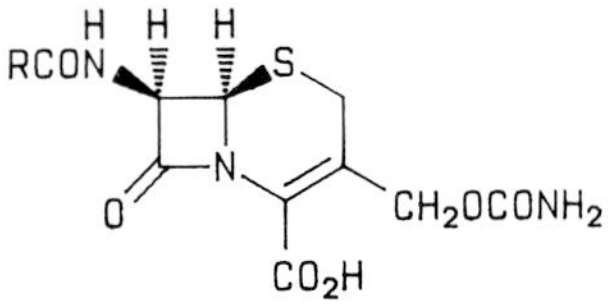

(12) Cefuroxime

(8) Methicillin R =

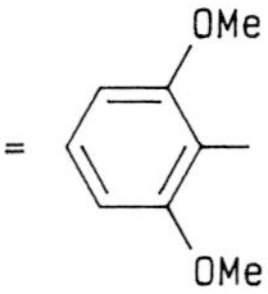

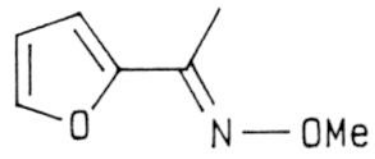

(9) Cloxacillin
X = H, Y = Cl R =

(10) Flucloxacillin
X = F, Y = Cl

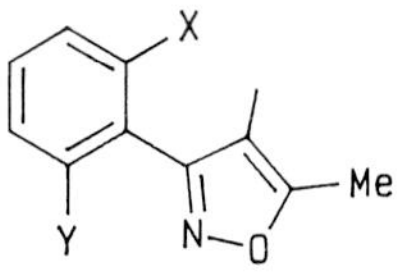

(11) Nafcillin R =

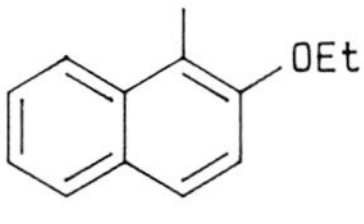

Since their discovery a large amount of work has been published on the production, biochemistry and chemistry of β-lactamases (*3*). Those produced by Gram-positive and Gram-negative bacteria can be classified and divided according to whether they are plasmid-mediated or chromosomally mediated,* and on the basis of their substrate (e.g., penicillin or cephalosporin) and inhibition profiles (*4*) (Table I).

*Chromosomally mediated β-lactamases are carried on the chromosomes (DNA) of the bacterium; thus they will always be present in varying amounts in the species producing them. Plasmids are small pieces of circular bacterial DNA which may be passed from one bacterial strain or species to another; this represents an important source of transmissable bacterial resistance.

TABLE I

Classification of β-Lactamases and Inhibition by Clavulanic Acid (CA)[a]

Mediation	β-Lactamase type	Class	Examples	Inhibited by CA
Chromosomal	Cephalosporinase	I	*Enterobacter cloacae* P99	−
			Citrobacter freudii Mantic	−
			Escherichia coli JT 410	−
			Bacteriodes fragilis	+
	Penicillinase	II	*Proteus mirabilis* C889	+
	Broad spectrum	IV	*Klebsiella pneumoniae* E 70	+
			Branhamella catarrhalis 1908	+
Plasmid	TEM	III	TEM-1, TEM-2; *E. coli* JT 4	+
			SHV-1	+
	OXA	V	OXA-1, OXA-2, OXA-3	+
	PSE		PSE-1, PSE-2, PSE-3, PSE-4	+
			Pseudomonas aeruginosa Dalgleish	+
Plasmid	Penicillinase	Gram-positive	*Staphylococcus aureus* Russell	+

[a] Adapted from Ref. *4.*

II. ISOLATION OF CLAVULANIC ACID

In the late 1960s, results from detailed studies on the production of β-lactamases and on the preparation and microbiological properties of new penicillins led Dr. George Rolinson at Beecham to consider the possibility of screening microorganisms for naturally occurring β-lactamase inhibitors using an assay based on β-lactamase inhibition. A microbiological screen (5), which became known within Beecham as the KAG assay, was set up and applied to culture filtrates obtained from a variety of fungi and actinomycetes. The screen is based on the traditional hole-in-plate antibacterial assay system. Agar containing a fixed amount of penicillin G is inoculated with the β-lactamase-producing strain *Klebsiella aerogenes* A and incubated. If no β-lactamase inhibitor is present the *K. aerogenes* A grows as an opaque lawn, because the penicillin G is destroyed. If, however, a solution containing an inhibitor is placed in a well cut in the plate, diffusion occurs into the agar, and now on incubation and as a result of inactivation of the β-lactamase, a clear zone of inhibition results around the well (see Fig. 1). Application of this KAG assay to isolates (~1000 actinomycetes and fungi) obtained from soil samples collected from varied habitats resulted in the identification of a number producing potent β-lactamase inhibitory activity; these cultures were subsequently found to be strains of *Streptomyces olivaceus* and were isolated from various soils procured from South Africa, Israel, New Zealand and Spain, brought in by itinerant company scientists (including the Research Director!) and marketing representatives. While the production, isolation and characterisation of the metabolites responsible for the β-lactamase inhibition of these *S. olivaceus* strains was being investigated, other *Streptomyces* species, known for their cephamycin (see Chap. 11) production, were also examined for β-lactamase inhibitory activity. Thus, when *S. clavuligerus* was grown, it was found to produce a metabolite with pronounced activity as a β-lactamase inhibitor, as measured by the KAG assay (Fig. 1). Initially this β-lactamase inhibitor was known as MM (or BRL) 14151 but was later called clavulanic acid (5, 6).

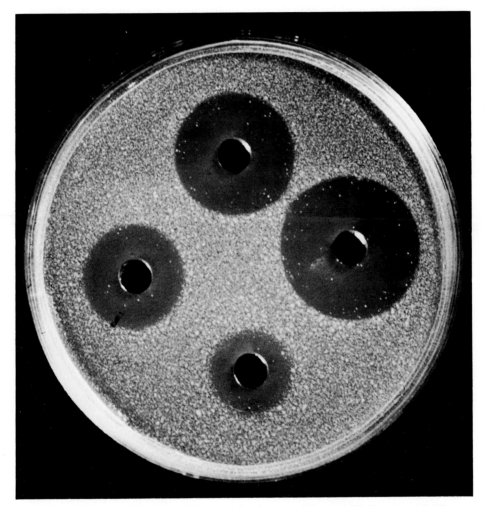

Fig. 1   Plate test for β-lactamase inhibitory activity. Agar containing penicillin G was seeded with *K. aerogenes;* wells contained clavulanic acid at 5.0, 2.5, 1.25 and 0.6 μg/ml. (From Ref. *9a*.)

Clavulanic acid (3) can be isolated as a crystalline alkali metal salt from culture filtrate by solvent extraction, for example, using *n*-butanol, or by ion-exchange chromatography. Its structure was established via ^{1}H and ^{13}C NMR and mass spectrometric studies on the methyl ester. An X-ray analysis of the *p*-nitrobenzyl ester confirmed the assigned structure, while a similar study on the *p*-bromobenzyl ester revealed the absolute configuration as (*R*) at C-2 and at C-5; these studies also confirmed the *Z* configuration of the exocyclic double bond. Thus clavulanic acid (3) was found to be (*Z*)-(2*R*,5*R*)-3-(β-hydroxyethylidene-7-oxo-4-oxa-1-azabicyclo[3.2.0]heptane-2-carboxylic acid. A trivial nomenclature similar to that used for penicillin and cephalosporin derivatives is usually preferred. By this procedure the parent ring system is called clavam and is numbered from oxygen as shown in structure **13**. This numbering system will be used henceforth.

(13) Clavam

Clavulanic acid was the first example of a "non-traditional" fused β-lactam to be isolated from a microorganism. In contrast to the traditional examples of penicillins and cephalosporins it contains an oxygen atom instead of a sulphur atom in the heterocyclic ring fused to the β-lactam ring, that is, it contains an oxazolidine ring instead of a thiazolidine or dihydrothiazine ring. It lacks an acylamino substituent at C-6 on the β-lactam ring and contains a β-hydroxyethylidene function at C-2. In addition to these structural features, clavulanic acid was novel in that it was also shown to be an extremely potent inhibitor of a wide range of β-lactamases.

It should be noted that following the Beecham discovery of clavulanic acid it became apparent that other groups (e.g., Glaxo and Japanese workers) had also detected clavulanic acid from *S. clavuligerus* and other *Streptomyces*. Since these first reports, other clavam derivatives, namely **14–18**, have been isolated

(14) R = CO$_2$H
(15) R = CH$_2$CH$_2$OH
(18) R = CH$_2$CHCO$_2$H
              |
             NH$_2$

(16) R = CH$_2$OH
(17) R = CH$_2$CHO

from *S. clavuligerus* and from other *Streptomyces* (7). Interestingly, three of these compounds, clavam-2-carboxylate (**14**), the hydroxyethyl clavam (**15**), and the alanyl clavam (**18**) have been shown to possess stereochemistry *opposite* to that of clavulanic acid at C-5.

III. BIOLOGICAL ACTIVITY OF CLAVULANIC ACID

Clavulanic acid is a potent inhibitor of a wide variety of β-lactamase types (Table I) as defined by an I_{50} value, that is, the concentration of clavulanic acid required to result in a 50% inhibition of the rate of hydrolysis of a standard penicillin or cephalosporin substrate. Such I_{50} values for an inhibitor are determined with and without preincubation of enzyme and inhibitor. Analysis of these results, as well as others from detailed kinetic studies, can indicate if an agent is a reversible or irreversible inhibitor and whether it is exerting competitive or non-competitive inhibition. Against the β-lactamases listed in Tables I and II clavulanic acid is a relatively poor inhibitor of class I types (sometimes called cephalosporinases) which are produced by a variety of genera such as *Enterobacter, Citrobacter, Proteus* (indole-positive species), *Serratia, Providentia,*

TABLE II
β-Lactamase Inhibition Spectrum for Clavulanic Acid;
Benzylpenicillin Substrate (1 mg/ml)[a]

Source of β-lactamase	I_{50} value[b] (µg/ml)
Escherichia coli JT4[c]	0.07
E. coli JT20[c]	0.3
Klebsiella aerogenes Ba95[c]	0.07
K. aerogenes E70	0.015
Proteus mirabilis C889	0.03
Serratia marcescens U39[c]	0.4
Pseudomonas aeruginosa 4482[c]	0.35
Ps. aeruginosa (Dalgleish)	0.007
Haemophilus influenzae 4482[c]	0.07
Staphylococcus aureus (Russell)	0.06
Bacillus cereus (mixture of types I and II)	17

[a] Adapted from Ref. *4.*

[b] Inhibitor incubated for 15 minutes with enzyme at pH 7.3 before addition of substrate.

[c] Contains resistance plasmid of TEM type.

Pseudomonas aeruginosa, and certain strains of *Escherichia coli, Shigella* and *Salmonella,* though it is very effective against those produced by *Bacteroides fragilis.** Class II (e.g., from *Proteus mirabilis*) and class IV (e.g., from *Klebsiella pneumoniae*) β-lactamases are readily inhibited by clavulanic acid as are the enzymes from the other classes, namely, III and V, which are plasmid mediated and which have been further subdivided into TEM, OXA, and PSE types. The β-lactamases of the TEM type are considered to be the main β-lactamases encountered in Gram-negative populations. The β-lactamase produced by the Gram-positive organism *Staphylococcus aureus* is very susceptible to clavulanic acid, as are those produced by most *Bacillus* sp.

(19) Amoxycillin R = HO—⟨⟩—CH—|NH₂

(20) Ampicillin R = ⟨⟩—CH—|NH₂

(21) Benzyl penicillin R = ⟨⟩—CH₂—

(22) Ticarcillin R = ⟨S⟩—CH—|CO₂H

When clavulanic acid is combined with a β-lactam such as amoxycillin (**19**) or ampicillin (**20**) which shows some instability towards β-lactamases, the resultant formulation has pronounced synergistic effects against a wide range of β-lactamase producing bacteria, such as strains of *S. aureus, K. pneumoniae (aerogenes), P. mirabilis, P. vulgaris, Branhamella catarrhalis, Bacteroides fragilis* and certain strains of *E. coli, Haemophilus influenzae, Neisseria gonorrhoeae, Shigella, Salmonella, Serratia* and *Pseudomonas** (namely those producing plasmid-mediated β-lactamases) (*8–9b*). The minimum inhibitory concentration (MIC) of amoxycillin (**19**) against β-lactamase producing strains of *S. aureus* and *E. coli* were 125 and >500 μg/ml. In the presence of 5 μg/ml clavulanic

*For more data on most of these bacteria, see Table I, Chap. 11.

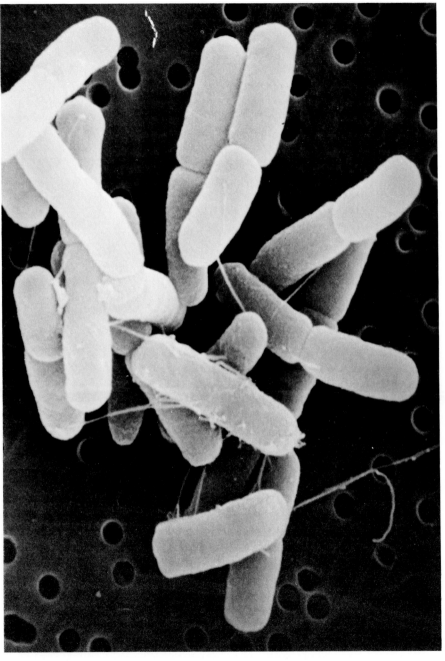

Fig. 2 Scanning electron micrograph showing the effect of amoxycillin (10 μg/ml) after 60 minutes at 37°C against a β-lactamase producing strain of *E. coli* JT39. (From Ref. *9b.*)

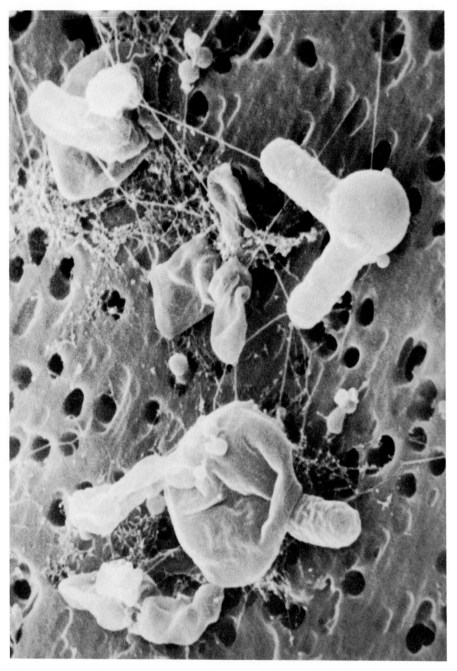

Fig. 3 Scanning electron micrograph showing bacteriolytic effects produced by amoxycillin (10 μg/ml) plus clavulanic acid (2.5 μg/ml) after 60 minutes at 37°C against a β-lactamase producing strain of *E. coli* JT39. (From Ref. *9b.*)

TABLE III
Effect of Clavulanic Acid (CA) on the Activity of Amoxicillin
against β-Lactamase Producing Organisms (MIC Values, μg/ml)[a]

Organism[b]	Amoxicillin + CA (μg/ml)			CA alone
	0	1.0	5.0	
Bacteroides fragilis (28)	33	0.48	0.14	13.1
Escherichia coli[c] (100)	>5000	94.5	13.2	24.8
Haemophilus influenzae[c] (15)	150	0.72	0.44	36.8
Klebsiella aerogenes (45)	315	1.75	0.89	33.2
Klebsiella aerogenes[c] (32)	>5000	126	20	33.6
Neisseria gonorrhoeae[c] (6)	>40	0.18	—	5.6
Proteus species (23)	433	11.6	4.2	62.9
Staphylococcus aureus (35)	106	0.72	0.17	17.1

[a] Adapted from Ref. 8.
[b] Numbers in parentheses indicate number of strains tested.
[c] Strains producing a plasmid-mediated β-lactamase.

acid, however, these MICs were reduced to 0.17 and 5 μg/ml, respectively (Table III; see also Figs. 2 and 3). Similarly striking synergistic effects are obtained with benzyl penicillin (21) and ticarcillin (22) plus clavulanic acid, as with first-generation cephalosporins such as cephalexin and cephaloridine. The newer cephalosporins such as cefuroxime (12), which have pronounced stability to β-lactamases, do not show synergistic effects with clavulanic acid. At the concentrations generally used to illustrate synergistic effects with various β-lactams, clavulanic acid itself shows a low level of antibacterial activity (MIC 25–125 μg/ml) against a variety of bacteria (Table III).

Clavulanic acid is well absorbed by a number of animal species (e.g., mouse, dog, squirrel monkey) when dosed by the subcutaneous, intramuscular and oral routes. Against experimental infections in mice caused by β-lactamase producing bacteria, clavulanic acid plus amoxycillin was very effective (Table IV). Extensive toxicological and metabolic studies on clavulanic acid allowed it to be cleared for detailed pharmacological investigations in man. Orally it is well absorbed in man, a dose of 125 mg resulting in a peak serum level of ~3.5 μg/ml 1 hour after administration, with a urinary recovery of 30–40%. Both amoxicillin and clavulanic acid are well absorbed when administered together by mouth to man, and the two compounds show similar serum profiles and half-lives.

Studies comparing the effects of clavulanic acid plus amoxycillin (Augmentin) on β-lactamase negative and β-lactamase producing cultures show that the action on the bacterial cell wall by the formulation involves the rapid formation of

TABLE IV

In Vivo Activity of Amoxycillin plus Clavulanic Acid (CA):
Mouse CD_{50} (mg/kg) ($\times 2$), Sub-cutaneous[a]

	Amoxycillin	
Organism	Alone	Plus CA (5 mg/kg)
Proteus mirabilis C889	>1000	14
Klebsiella aerogenes I 112	>1000	6.6
Klebsiella aerogenes Ba95[b]	>1000	25
Escherichia coli JT39[b]	>1000	7.7
Escherichia coli JT124[b]	>1000	17

[a] From Ref. *8*. Mice dosed 1 and 5 hours post infection.
[b] Strains producing a plasmid-mediated β-lactamase. CA alone was ineffective at 50 mg/kg.

sphereoplasts followed by cell lysis (Fig. 3). The same effects are seen with amoxycillin and β-lactamase negative cultures.

IV. CHEMISTRY OF CLAVULANIC ACID AND BIOLOGICAL ACTIVITY OF SOME DERIVATIVES

Clavulanic acid contains a number of functional groups which can be readily modified leading to a large variety of derivatives (*10*). The acid moiety is easily esterified using a diazoalkane or by alkylation of the corresponding alkali metal salt in a suitable solvent, or via an alcohol or thiol and a carbodiimide; the benzyl (**23**) and *p*-nitrobenzyl esters (**24**) are the most useful in that these ester functions can be conveniently removed via catalytic hydrogenolysis. Catalytic hydrogenation of methyl (**25**) or benzyl clavulanate (**23**) gave methyl or benzyl dihydroclavulanate (**26**) as a mixture of C-2 epimers. Hydrogenolysis of benzyl clavulanate in aqueous ethanol containing an equivalent amount of sodium hydrogen carbonate, at room temperature and atmospheric pressure with uptake of 1 mole of hydrogen, led to sodium clavulanate while clavulanic acid itself was easily obtained under similar conditions but using ethanol as solvent. Under more rigorous conditions of hydrogenolysis benzyl clavulanate (**23**) could be converted into the isoclavulanic acid derivative (**27**), which is the *E*-isomer of (**23**), and into a 9-deoxyclavulanic acid analogue (**28**). The allylic hydroxyl function can be acylated, etherified, sulphated, replaced by halogen (and hence azido leading to amino and acylamino functions), or by amino and sulphur nucleophiles and oxidised to an aldehyde. The allylic double bond can be isomerised photolytically as well as catalytically. An interesting product from the photolysis of

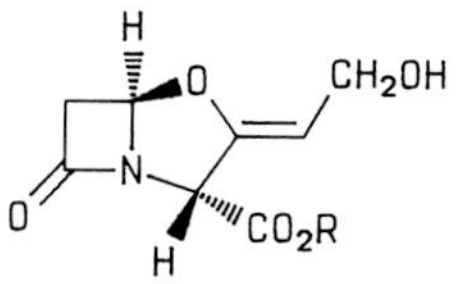

(23) R = CH₂C₆H₅
(24) R = CH₂C₆H₄-*p*-NO₂
(25) R = CH₃

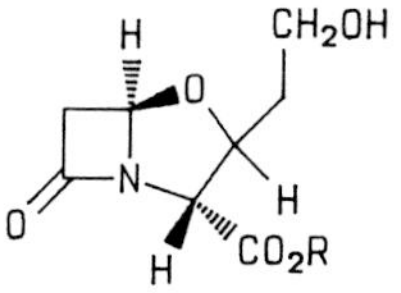

(26) R = Me or CH₂C₆H₅

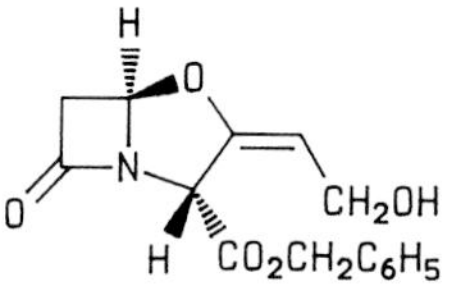

(27)

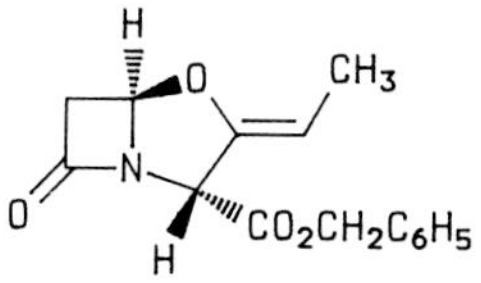

(28)

phenacyl clavulanate was the tetracyclic β-lactam oxatane (**29**). The alkene moiety in clavulanic acid can also be epoxidised and cleaved by ozonolysis. Certain derivatives undergo elimination reactions with the formation of a diene (a clavem), while alkylation can be carried out at C-3 and C-6. The β-lactam carbonyl group reacts with certain Wittig reagents (*11*) and the parent acid can be decarboxylated (*12*). The degradation of clavulanic acid or its esters under a variety of conditions produces a number of non-β-lactam species as well as rearrangement products (*13*). The pyrroles **30** and **31** can be obtained via azetidinone (**32**) on treatment of ester (**23**) with triethylamine and acetic acid, while hydrolysis (*14*) of clavulanic acid gave the amino ketone (**33**). The clavam

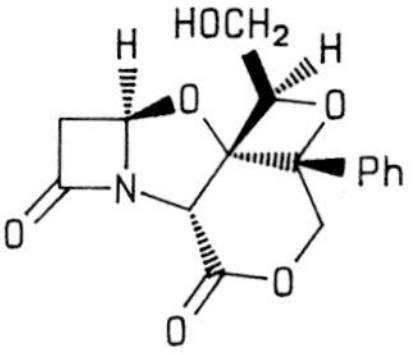

(29)

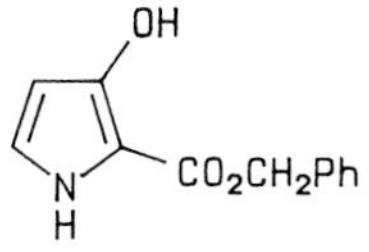

(30)

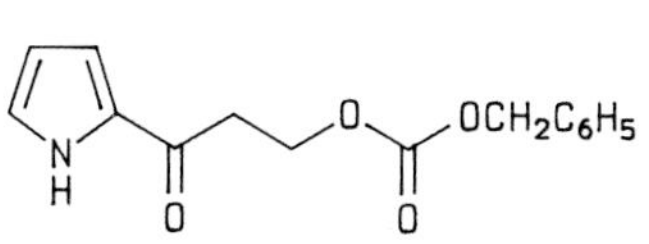

(31)

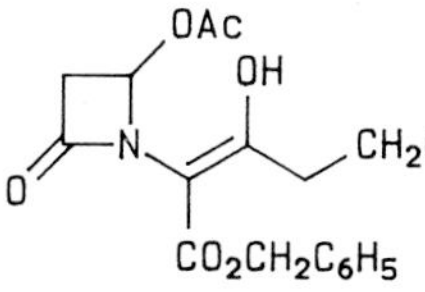

(32)

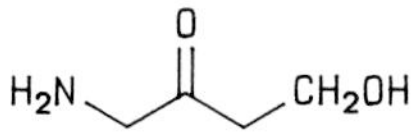

(33)

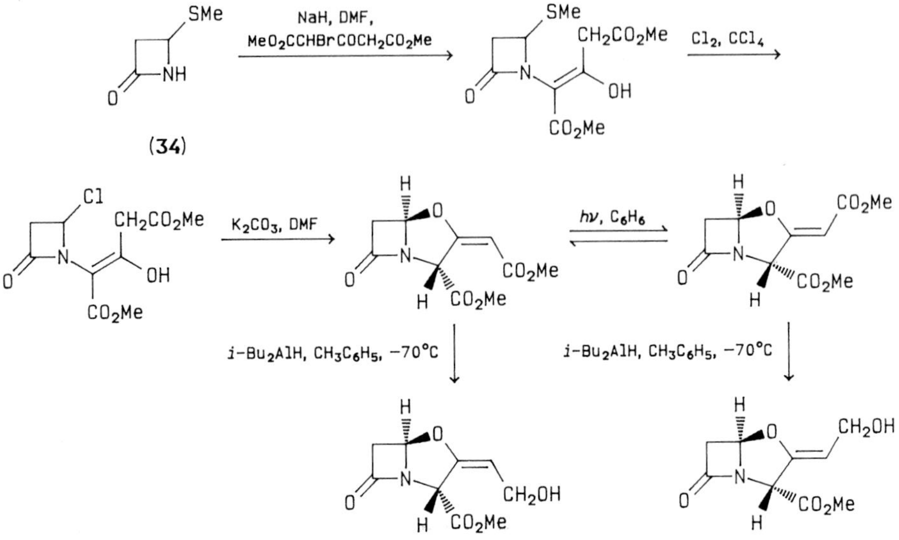

Scheme 2   Synthesis of (±)-methyl clavulanate.

nucleus has been a target for total synthesis, and the structure of clavulanic acid has been confirmed by the preparation of racemic methyl clavulanate (25) from the azetidinone (34) by the sequence of reactions shown in Scheme 2; (±)-methyl isoclavulanate (35) was also prepared as a consequence of this work (15).

The β-lactamase inhibitory (I_{50}) data for a number of representative clavam derivatives obtained from clavulanic acid are given in Table V. From these (16a) and other data one can identify a number of empirical structure–activity features.

1. Potent β-lactamase inhibitory activity appears to require a close structure analogy to clavulanic acid, only variation of the C-9 hydroxyl group being allowed; any modification resulting in removal of the double bond or destruction of the β-lactam moiety gives poor inhibitors, as does C-6 modification, C-5 inversion [i.e., (5R) stereochemistry is required], C-3 decarboxylation or C-3 amide formation.

2. Isoclavulanic acid (the E-isomer) derivatives are less active than the Z-isomers.

3. Clavem derivatives have limited interest.

4. In general terms β-lactamase inhibitory (and hence synergistic) activity is closely related to the size and hydrophilicity of the substituent replacing the hydroxy function, with small, hydrophilic groups yielding the most active compounds in any series.

TABLE V
β-Lactamase Inhibitory Properties of Some Derivatives of Clavulanic Acid[a]

CH$_2$R / CO$_2$H (clavulanic acid structure)

	Inhibitory activity, I$_{50}$ (µg/ml); β-lactamase from				
	Staphylococcus aureus Russell	Escherichia coli JT4 IIIa (RTEM)	Klebsiella aerogenes E 70 II	Proteus mirabilis C889 IV	Citrobacter freundii Mantio I
Clavulanic acid; R = OH	0.06	0.07	0.03	0.03	10
Deoxyclavulanic acid; R = H	0.12	0.09	0.05	—	5
Isoclavulanic acid	0.6	1.0	0.45	—	5
Acetate; R = OCOCH$_3$	0.04	—	>0.4	—	0.4
Carbamate; R = OCONHCH$_3$	1.5	2.5	2.5	—	0.45
Methyl ether; R = OMe	0.05	0.18	0.07	0.01	8.5
Benzyl ether; R = OCH$_2$Ph	0.005	0.1	0.04	0.02	4.4
Thioether; R = SMe	0.11	0.04	0.13	0.01	>>10[b]
Amine; R = N (CH$_2$Ph)$_2$	0.002	0.04	0.08	0.01	0.62

[a] Adapted from Ref. 16a.
[b] β-Lactamase from Enterobacter cloacae P99.

(**36**) 9-DCA   R = H
(**37**) 9-ADCA   R = NH$_2$

Detailed evaluation data on two typical derivatives are presented below to illustrate that extensive chemotherapeutic and toxicological comparisons of derivatives are necessary in order to select compounds with greater promise than their parent.

Sodium 9-deoxyclavulanic acid (**36**, 9-DCA) was found to have β-lactamase inhibitory properties similar to clavulanic acid (**3**) while 9-aminodeoxyclavulanic acid (**37**, 9-ADCA) had slightly improved activity against RTEM and *S. aureus* β-lactamases (*16b*). *In vitro* synergy data, however, indicated 9-DCA to be less effective than clavulanic acid, while 9-ADCA was better, at protecting amoxycillin. As 9-DCA gave poorer and 9-ADCA gave better mouse blood levels than clavulanic acid when dosed orally, 9-ADCA was found to give better results as a synergist with amoxycillin against experimental infections. Extensive toxicological studies in a variety of animal species, however, revealed 9-ADCA to be toxic. For example, in the rat an oral dose of 9-ADCA (100 mg/kg) resulted in changes in serum chemistry indicative of liver and kidney damage. In comparison clavulanic acid at 10 times this dose did not produce such effects.

V. MECHANISM OF ACTION OF CLAVULANIC ACID

The mode of action of clavulanic acid as a β-lactamase inhibitor has been examined in detail (*17*). The interaction with the β-lactamase TEM2 is illustrated in Fig. 4. An acyl–enzyme intermediate (formed by cleavage of the β-lactam ring by a hydroxy group of a serine residue and opening of the oxazolidine ring) is derived from the Michaelis complex; this intermediate now breaks down in three possible ways. It can (a) collapse to yield original enzyme plus degraded clavulanic acid, (b) form a transiently stable complex which ultimately hydrolyses to enzyme and degradation product(s) or (c) form irreversible complexes. A turnover of 115 clavulanic acid molecules occurs for every irreversible inactivation of enzyme. A similar mechanism is proposed for the inactivation of the chromosomally mediated β-lactamase from *K. aerogenes*. With *S. aureus* β-lactamase the interaction yields an acyl–enzyme intermediate which reacts fur-

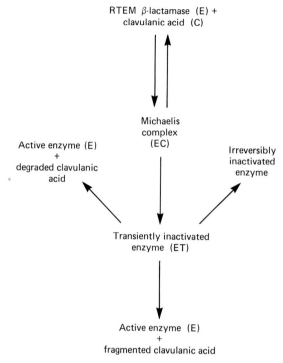

Fig. 4   Mechanism of inactivation of RTEM β-lactamase by clavulanic acid.

ther to give irreversibly inactivated enzyme, though hydrolysis of the intermediate can occur in the absence of an excess of clavulanic acid to give enzyme-degraded clavulanic acid.

With an idea of the mechanism of action of clavulanic acid, medicinal chemists set about the design, synthesis and microbiological evaluation of analogues such as penicillanic acid sulphone (**38,** sulbactam) (*18*), 6β-iodo- and 6β-bromopenicillanic acids (**39**) (*19*), 6α-chloropenicillanic acid sulphone (**40**) (*20*), 2β-chloromethylpenam sulphone (**41**) (*21*), alkyl sulphonamidopenicillanic acid sulphones (**42**) (*22*) and 6-acetylmethylenepenicillanic acid (**43**) (*23*). Of the β-lactamase inhibitors examined in detail the majority appear to be established like clavulanic acid as ''mechanism-based inactivators'' (or ''Trojan Horse inactivators''). In β-lactamase I (derived from a *B. cereus* organism) it is considered that serine-44 is the amino acid residue involved in acyl–enzyme intermediate formation when 6β-bromopenicillanic acid is the inhibitor. The location of the active site in the tertiary structure of the RTEM β-lactamase is under study via X-ray crystallography.

(38) R = H
(42) R = CF$_3$SO$_2$NH

(39) R = Br or I

(40)

(41)

(43)

VI.   THE OLIVANIC ACIDS
AND THIENAMYCINS

The KAG assay which led to the discovery of clavulanic acid also identified a series of *Streptomyces olivaceus* strains that produce antibiotic β-lactamase inhibitors. These compounds were isolated, purified and characterised (24) to give the olivanic acid (or carbapenem) family represented by the sulphate esters (44–46) and the closely related hydroxy compounds (47–50). At this time (early 1970s) Merck workers were characterising the thienamycins 4, 51 and 52 from *S. cattleya* and the epithienamycins (47–50) from *S. flavogriseus* (25). While the Beecham screen was based on β-lactamase inhibition, the Merck approach was geared to detecting inhibitors of peptidoglycan synthesis. To date about 40 carbapenems have been isolated from *Streptomyces* sp. Structurally the carbapenems differ from the penicillins in that they have a CH$_2$ unit instead of S and contain an endocyclic double bond; the substitutent at C-2 is usually a substituted alkyl or alkenylthio unit, while alkyl, hydroxyalkyl or alkylidene functions are present at C-6. The stereochemistry of the β-lactam ring protons can be cis or trans. The synthesis of derivatives of this ring system, especially close analogues of thienamycin and the olivanic acids, has received concentrated attention over the last 6 or 7 years. The strategies used have been reviewed (26). The β-lactamase inhibitory activities of representative carbapenems are given in Table VI (16a). It should be noted that the olivanics are potent β-lactamase inhibitors (up to 1000 times more active than clavulanic acid) and by contrast more effective against cephalosporinases (Class I type β-lactamases). Synergistic effects can be detected in combination with certain penicillins and cephalosporins, but evaluation is complicated by the pronounced antibacterial activity of the car-

TABLE VI

β-Lactamase Inhibitory Activity of Olivanic Acids (I_{50}, μg/ml)[a]

Olivanic acid	*Staphylococcus aureus* Russell	*Escherichia coli* JT 4	*Klebsiella aerogenes* E 70	*Enterobacter cloacae* P99
(44)	0.01	0.001	0.002	0.02
(45)	0.01	0.001	0.002	0.001
(46)	0.03	0.015	0.003	0.02
(47)	0.13	15	10	0.03
(48)	5	0.03	0.01	0.2
(49)	0.02	1.5	15	0.02
(50)	0.25	0.06	0.06	0.03
(3)	0.04	0.04	0.006	—

[a] Adapted from Ref. *16a*.

(44) MM4550   R = (structure with O^-, S^+, NHCOCH_3)

(45) MM13902   R = S (structure with NHCOCH_3)

(46) MM17880   R = S (structure with NHCOCH_3)

(47) MM22380 Epithienamycin A
R = S (structure with NHCOCH_3)

(48) MM22381 Epithienamycin C
R = S (structure with NHCOCH_3)

(49) MM22382 Epithienamycin B
R = S (structure with NHCOCH_3)

(50) MM22383 Epithienamycin D
R = S (structure with NHCOCH_3)

(51) R = (structure with NHCOCH_3)

(52) R = (structure with NHCOCH_3)

(53) MK 0787 R = (structure with N=CHNH_2)

bapenem inhibitor (*16, 27*). Thienamycin (**4**) and a chemically more stable *N*-formimidoyl derivative (**53**) are potent, broad-spectrum antibiotics (*28*).

A serious drawback with carbapenems, however, is their poor metabolic stability which generally leads to low urinary recovery. An enzyme, dehydropeptidase-I, from kidney has been shown to be responsible for the degradation of compounds such as thienamycin (**4**) and the olivanic acid (**45**) in man and other species (*29*). Merck workers have endeavoured to overcome this problem by the co-administration of an inhibitor of the dehydropeptidase enzyme (*30*).

VII. CONCLUSION

Currently a formulation (BRL 25000) of potassium clavulanate (125 mg) plus amoxycillin trihydrate (250 mg) called Augmentin* is marketed in a number of countries following satisfactory toxicological examination and detailed clinical trials (*9*). Augmentin is highly effective against urinary tract, skin and soft tissue, upper and lower respiratory tract and gonorrhoeal infections.

REFERENCES

1. R. B. Morin and M. Gorman, eds, "Chemistry and Biology of β-Lactam Antibiotics," Vols 1, 2, and 3. Academic Press, New York, 1982; G. N. Rolinson, *J. Antimicrob. Chemother.* **5**, 7 (1979).
2. E. P. Abraham and E. Chain, *Nature (London)* **146**, 837 (1940).
3. J. M. T. Hamilton-Miller and J. T. Smith, eds, "Beta-Lactamases." Academic Press, London, 1979.
4. C. Reading and T. Farmer, *in* "Antibiotics" (A. D. Russell and L. B. Quensel, eds), p. 141. Academic Press, London, 1983; M. Cole, *Drugs Future* **6**, 697 (1981).
5. A. G. Brown, D. Butterworth, M. Cole, G. Hanscomb, J. D. Hood, C. Reading, and G. N. Rolinson, *J. Antibiot.* **29**, 668 (1976).
6. C. Reading and M. Cole, *Antimicrob. Agents Chemother.* **11**, 852 (1977); T. T. Howarth, A. G. Brown, and T. J. King, *J. Chem. Soc., Chem. Commun.,* 266 (1976).
7. D. Brown, J. R. Evans, and R. A. Fletton, *J. Chem. Soc., Chem. Commun.,* 282 (1979); M. Wanning, H. Zähner, B. Krone, and A. Zeeck, *Tetrahedron Lett.* **22**, 2539 (1981); D. L. Preuss and M. Kellet, *J. Antibiot.* **36**, 208 (1983); R. H. Evans, Jr., H. Ax, A. Jacoby, T. H. Williams, E. Jenkins, and J. P. Scannell, *J. Antibiot.* **36**, 213 (1983); J.-C. Muller, V. Toome, D. L. Preuss, J. F. Blount, and M. Weigle, *J. Antibiot.* **36**, 217 (1983).
8. P. A. Hunter, K. Coleman, J. Fisher, and D. Taylor, *J. Antimicrob. Chemother.* **6**, 455 (1980); P. A. Hunter, C. Reading, and D. A. Witting, *Current Chemother. Proc. Int. Congr. Chemother., 10th, 1977* **1**, 478 (1978); P. A. Hunter, K. Coleman, J. Fisher, D. Taylor, and E. Taylor, *Future Trends Chemother., 4th, Proc. Int. Symp.* **5**, 1 (1979).

*Trademark of Beecham Group p.l.c.

9a. G. N. Rolinson and A. Watson, eds, "Augmentin." Excerpta Medica, Amsterdam, 1981.
9b. D. A. Leigh and O. P. W. Robinson, eds, "Augmentin." Excerpta Medica, Amsterdam, 1982.
10. A. G. Brown, J. Goodacre, J. B. Harbridge, T. T. Howarth, R. J. Ponsford, and I. Stirling, *in* "Recent Advances in the Chemistry of β-Lactam Antibiotics" (J. Elks, ed.), p. 295. Special Publication No. 28, The Chemical Society, London, 1977; A. G. Brown, D. F. Corbett, J. Goodacre, J. B. Harbridge, T. J. King, R. J. Ponsford, and I. Stirling, *J. Chem. Soc., Perkin Trans. 1,* 635 (1984); R. D. G. Cooper, *in* "Topics in Antibiotic Chemistry" (P. G. Sammes, ed.), Vol. 3, p. 39. Ellis Horwood Ltd., Chichester, 1980; C. E. Newall, *in* "Recent Advances in the Chemistry of β-Lactam Antibiotics" (G. I. Gregory, ed.), p. 151. Special Publication No. 38, The Chemical Society, London, 1981; C. E. Newall, *in* "β-Lactam Antibiotics; Mode of Action, New Developments and Future Prospects" (M. R. J. Salton and G. D. Shockman, eds), p. 287. Academic Press, New York, 1981.
11. M. L. Gilpin, J. B. Harbridge, T. T. Howarth, and T. J. King, *J. Chem. Soc., Chem. Commun.,* 929 (1981).
12. E. Hunt, *J. Chem. Res. (S)* **64,** 1981.
13. J. S. Davies, *Tetrahedron Lett.* **23,** 5089 (1982).
14. E. Hunt, *J. Chem. Soc., Perkin Trans. 1,* 1345 (1984).
15. P. H. Bentley, P. D. Berry, G. Brooks, M. L. Gilpin, E. Hunt, and I. I. Zomaya, *J. Chem. Soc., Chem. Commun.,* 748 (1977); P. H. Bentley, G. Brooks, M. L. Gilpin, and E. Hunt, *Tetrahedron Lett.,* 1889 (1979).
16a. A. G. Brown, *J. Antibiot. Chemother.* **7,** 15 (1981).
16b. P. A. Hunter, *Pharm. Weekbl.* **119,** 650 (1984).
17. C. Reading and T. Farmer, *Biochem. J.* **199,** 779 (1981); C. Reading and P. Hepburn, *Biochem. J.* **179,** 67 (1979); J. Fisher, J. G. Belasco, R. L. Charnas, S. Khosla, and J. R. Knowles, *Philos. Trans. R. Soc. London, Ser. B* **289,** 309 (1980).
18. A. R. English, *et al., Antimicrob. Agents Chemother.* **14,** 414 (1978).
19. B. A. Moore and K. W. Brammer, *Antimicrob. Agents Chemother.* **29,** 327 (1981); R. Wise, *et al., J. Antimicrob. Chemother.* **7,** 531 (1981); R. F. Pratt and M. J. Loosemore, *Proc. Natl. Acad. Sci. U.S.A.* **75,** 4145 (1978).
20. S. J. Cartwright and A. F. W. Coulson, *Nature (London)* **278,** 360 (1979).
21. W. J. Gottstein, *et al., J. Med. Chem.* **24,** 1531 (1981).
22. P. S. F. Mezes, *et al., J. Antibiot.* **35,** 918 (1982).
23. M. Arisawra and S. Adam, *Biochem. J.* **211,** 447 (1983).
24. A. G. Brown, D. F. Corbett, A. J. Eglington, and T. T. Howarth, *J. Chem. Soc., Chem. Commun.,* 523 (1977); D. F. Corbett, A. J. Eglington, and T. T. Howarth, *J. Chem. Soc., Chem. Commun,* 953 (1977); D. Butterworth, M. Cole, G. Hanscomb, and G. N. Rolinson, *J. Antibiot.* **32,** 287 (1979); J. D. Hood, S. J. Box, and M. S. Verrall, *J. Antibiot.* **32,** 295 (1979); A. G. Brown, D. F. Corbett, A. J. Eglington, and T. T. Howarth, *J. Antibiot.* **32,** 961 (1979); S. J. Box, J. D. Hood, and S. R. Spear, *J. Antibiot.* **32,** 1239 (1979).
25. J. S. Kahan, *et al., J. Antibiot.* **32,** 1 (1979); G. Albers-Schönberg, *et al., J. Am. Chem. Soc.* **100,** 6491 (1978); E. O. Stapley, *et al., J. Antibiot.* **34,** 628 (1981); P. J. Cassidy, *et al., J. Antibiot.* **34,** 637 (1981).
26. J. H. Bateson, A. J. G. Baxter, K. H. Dickinson, R. I. Hickling, R. J. Ponsford, P. M. Roberts, T. C. Smale, and R. Southgate, *in* "Recent Advances in the Chemistry of β-Lactam Antibiotics" (G. I. Gregory, ed.), p. 291. Special Publication No. 38, The Chemical Society, London, 1981; R. W. Ratcliffe and G. Albers-Schönberg *in* "Chemistry and Biology of β-Lactam Antibiotics" (R. B. Morin and M. Gorman, eds), Vol. 3, p. 227. Academic Press, New York, 1982; T. Kametani, *Heterocycles* **17,** 463 (1982).
27. M. J. Basker, R. J. Boon, and P. A. Hunter, *J. Antibiot.* **33,** 878 (1980).

28. H. Kropp, *et al.*, *Antimicrob. Agents Chemother.* **17,** 993 (1980).
29. H. Kropp, *et al.*, *Antimicrob. Agents Chemother.* **22,** 62 (1982); M. J. Basker, R. J. Boon, S. J. Box, E. A. Prestige, G. N. Smith, and S. R. Spear, *J. Antibiot.* **36,** 416 (1983).
30. S. R. Norrby, K. Alestig, B. Björnegard, L. A. Burman, F. Ferber, J. L. Huber, K. H. Jones, F. M. Kahan, J. S. Kahan, H. Kropp, M. P. Meisinger, and J. G. Sundelof, *Antimicrob. Agents Chemother.* **23,** 300 (1983).

CHAPTER 13

Ketoconazole and the Treatment of Fungal Diseases

J. HEERES
Department of Chemistry
Janssen Pharmaceutica
Beerse, Belgium

I. INTRODUCTION (*1–3*)

We are surrounded by fungi! Numerous fungi have their biological habitat in the soil. Some grow on trees, in grass and in woodlands: others inhabit the fur on our pets while still others grow on our skin and in our hair and beards. Some species, for example *Agaricus bisporus,* are excellent to eat with bacon and eggs!

For most of the time we co-exist quite happily with the fungi. However, it is possible for particular fungi to proliferate on and in the outermost layers of the skin causing irritation and unsightly growths. Mucous membranes (e.g., mouth, vagina) can be affected by overgrowths of fungi while systemic infection can give rise to deep-rooted fungi, and uncontrolled development of the latter condition can lead to a life-threatening situation.

Fungal diseases of humans are termed mycoses and in recent years there has been an increase in all types of mycoses. Cutaneous and subcutaneous infections spread as a result of community living; foot infections in coal miners, for instance, are a major problem of occupational health. Communal showering facilities, coupled with other working conditions which provide the environment for initiation of the infection, can lead to a rapid spread of the responsible organisms.

249

Some common human superficial mycoses are listed in Table I together with the causative organism(s); likewise some of the common deep mycoses are described in Table II.

Superficial infections caused by dermatophytes or yeasts are the most common form of fungal disease. Scalp ringworm, once common in school-children, has been controlled in large parts of the world thanks to the use of drugs such as griseofulvin (*vide infra*); however, in Africa the problem still remains, with dermatophytes such as *Microsporum audouinii* being the causative organisms. Sporadic outbreaks of scalp infections due to organisms such as *M. canis* (derived from the cat or dog) do occur locally. Pityriasis versicolor infections are believed to occur in up to half the population in some tropical countries. It is characterised by brown, red, or achromatic scaly patches which occur principally on the torso. *Candida albicans* is a normal inhabitant of the oral cavity, but in certain conditions a state of overgrowth develops with resulting oral infection. Candidal overgrowth is most likely to occur in aged people, in debilitated patients, and in persons receiving prolonged treatment with certain drugs, for example, corticosteroids. The dramatic rise in fungal infections of the vagina (principally due to *Candida albicans*) has been associated with a number of factors including the contraceptive pill and increased sexual activity.

The increase in incidence of serious systemic fungal infections is due, in part, to the increase in the number of immunocompromised patients and cancer patients, which can be associated with an increase in the consumption of immu-

TABLE I
Some Common Human Superficial Mycoses

Disease	Area affected	Most frequently found causative organism
Tinea capitis (scalp ringworm)	Head	Dermatophytes, e.g., *Microsporum* spp. and *Trichophyton* spp.
Tinea corporis	Body	Dermatophytes, e.g., *Trichophyton* spp. and *Microsporum* spp.
Other dermatomycoses	Body and folds of the skin	*Trichophyton* spp. and *Epidermophyton floccosum*
Tinea pedis (athlete's foot)	Foot	*Trichophyton* spp.
Onychomycosis	Nail	*Trichophyton* spp. and *Candida albicans* (yeast)
Perionychomycosis	Cuticles	Yeasts, especially *Candida* spp.
Pityriasis versicolor	Trunk and glabrous skin	*Malassezia furfur* (*Pityrosporon orbiculare* or *P. ovale*)
Oral thrush	Mouth	*Candida albicans*
Vaginal candidosis (vaginal thrush)	Vagina	*Candida albicans*, other *Candida* spp. and *Torulopsis glabrata*

TABLE II
Some Systemic Mycoses

Disease	Most frequently found causative organism
Systemic and mucocutaneous candidosis	*Candida albicans* and other *Candida* spp.
Cryptococcosis	*Cryptococcus neoformans*
Aspergillosis	*Aspergillus fumigatus* and other *Aspergillus* spp.
Mucormycosis (phycomycosis)	Various Zygomycetes, e.g., *Rhizopus, Mucor*
Paracoccidioidomycosis	*Paracoccidioides brasiliensis*
North American blastomycosis	*Blastomyces dermatitides*
Histoplasmosis	*Histoplasma capsulatum*
Coccidioidomycosis	*Coccidioides immitis*
Sporotrichosis	*Sporothrix schenckii*

nosuppressive agents. The most common pathogens identified are *Candida* species, *Cryptococcus neoformans, Aspergillus fumigatus* and *Mucor* species.

Paracoccidioidomycosis, by comparison, not only affects skin and the mucous membranes, but also affects the lungs and the other viscera. It is fairly common in South and Central America, and if untreated the disease generally follows a progressive, fatal course. Histoplasmosis is a systemic mycosis affecting the lungs, while coccidioidomycosis may occur as a chronic disseminated disease involving many organ systems including cutaneous and subcutaneous tissue and the bones. Aspergillosis, phycomycosis, and actinomycosis are relatively uncommon deep mycoses.

Because of the many similarities between human cells and fungal cells (both are eukaryotic and possess similar highly evolved metabolic processes; however, there is at least one major difference as explained in Section IV) the development of non-toxic antimycotics has been difficult and slow. (In contrast, prokaryotic bacteria and *Homo sapiens* differ appreciably, and hence safe anti-bacterial agents are relatively easy to design.)

Treatment of superficial mycoses can be achieved by topical application of an anti-fungal agent. Long-established remedies such as potassium iodide for the oral treatment of sporotrichosis and Whitfield's ointment (containing benzoic acid and salicylic acid) for the topical treatment of ringworm infections of the skin are still used today as anti-fungal therapies. The first potent anti-candidal anti-fungals were nystatin (**1**) and amphotericin B (**2**) (*1, 2*). The former compound is an effective anti-fungal agent, but systemic toxicity has restricted its use primarily to topical and mucosal *Candida* infections. Amphotericin B has been the mainstay of systemic anti-fungal chemotherapy for more than two decades. Unfortunately, it is poorly absorbed from the gastro-intestinal tract. Thus, in order to obtain appropriate serum levels the drug is given intravenously in the treatment of systemic mycoses such as candidiasis, cryptococcosis, coccidioidomycosis, histoplasmosis, mucormycosis, paracoccidioidomycosis, and

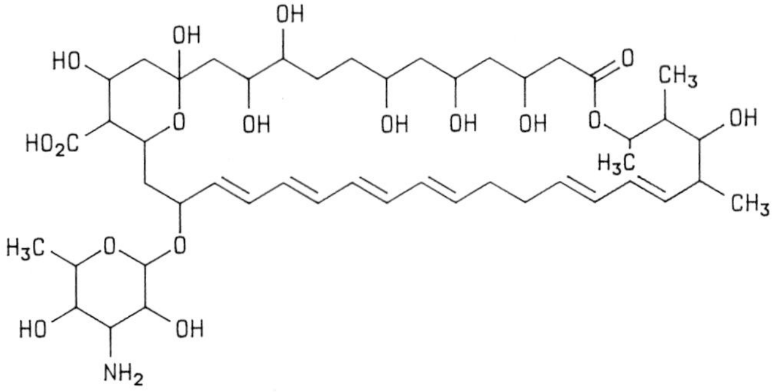

(1)

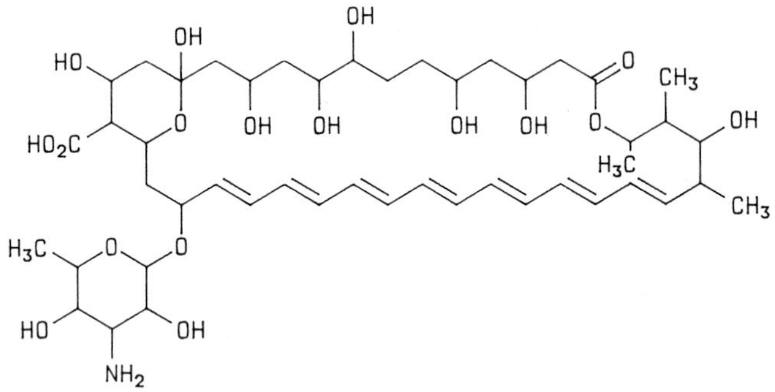

(2)

aspergillosis. Pronounced toxicity—for example, impairment of renal function—is a serious problem with this compound.

Griseofulvin (3) was introduced in the 1950s as the first potent oral anti-fungal
agent (it is not active when applied topically). Griseofulvin's fungistatic activity
is limited to actively growing dermatophytes and it has been used for many years
in the treatment of human (and animal) dermatophytoses that could not be cleared with topical therapy. Adverse effects are common but rarely serious, with
headache occurring most frequently.

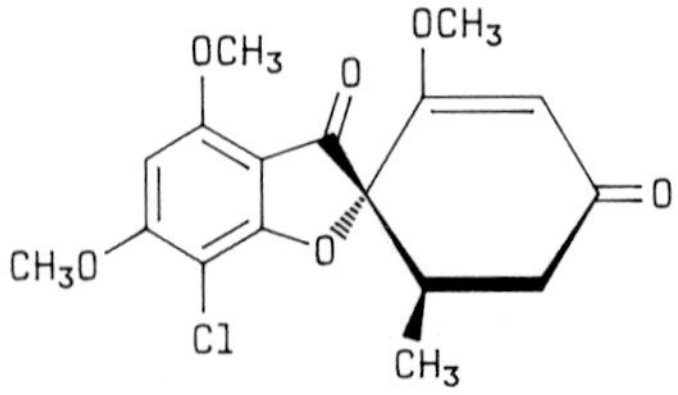

(3) Griseofulvin

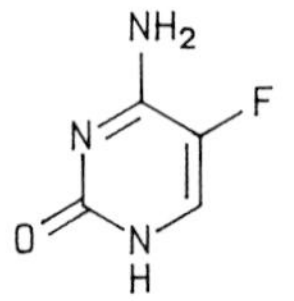

(4) 5-Fluorocytosine

More recently 5-fluorocytosine, a synthetic fluorinated pyrimidine derivative (**4**) having oral activity, has been shown to be clinically effective in the treatment of cryptococcosis, candidiasis, and probably aspergillosis (*2*). Because of the rapid development of *de novo* fungal resistance occurring during therapy with this agent, its use has been limited to (1) the treatment of candidal infection of the lower urinary tract where the drug achieves very high concentrations, and (2) combination therapy with amphotericin B and sometimes with miconazole in cryptococcal, candidal and aspergillus infection.

Miconazole, an imidazole derivative that is described in the next section, is a broad-spectrum anti-fungal agent, active against dermatophytes, *Candida* spp., *Cryptococcus neoformans, Coccidioides immitis, Histoplasma capsulatum, Paracoccidioides brasiliensis, Aspergillus fumigatus,* and other fungi. Applied as a topical agent, miconazole is effective against the majority of superficial fungal infections. It has also been administered intravenously in the treatment of systemic mycoses. Orally administered miconazole gives rise to low serum concentrations of the drug, hence the compound is not as effective when taken by mouth. Nevertheless on its introduction in the early 1970s the parenteral use of miconazole represented a real advance in the treatment of cutaneous and systemic mycoses. The promising results obtained with topical and intravenous miconazole encouraged us to continue with azole chemistry in order to find new antifungal agents with an improved oral activity against superficial and deep mycoses.

II.   CHEMISTRY AND STRUCTURE–ACTIVITY RELATIONSHIPS

Chemical exploration of the phenacylimidazoles (**5**) led to the discovery of substituted benzylamines (**6**), which display an *in vitro* activity against der-

		Y^1	Y^2
(**7**)	Miconazole	$2,4-Cl_2$	$2,4-Cl_2$
	Econazole	$2,4-Cl_2$	$4-Cl$
	Isoconazole	$2,4-Cl_2$	$2,6-Cl_2$

(8) Imazalil Y^1 = 2,4-Cl$_2$ (9)

matophytes. The real breakthrough came with the introduction of the benzyl ethers (7), of which miconazole (4, 5), econazole (4) and isoconazole (4) are the leading compounds. The importance of the imidazole nucleus is clearly illustrated by the fact that its replacement by other heterocyclic rings such as benzimidazole, piperazine or pyrazole generally resulted in less active or inactive compounds. Miconazole, econazole and isoconazole are broad-spectrum antifungal agents, active against dermatophytes, yeasts and moulds. *In vivo*, topical activity has been confirmed in experimental dermatomycosis in guinea-pigs and in vaginal candidosis in rats. Clinically these compounds constitute very useful contributions in the treatment of superficial mycoses, and intravenous miconazole is also effective in the treatment of systemic mycoses in man. The analogous alkyl and alkenyl ethers (8) were developed simultaneously, the selected compound being the allyl ether imazalil. This compound gives excellent therapeutic results in animal mycoses and is useful in veterinary medicine.

Another modification resulted from the ketalization of the phenacyl group, forming the ketals (9). *In vitro* most of these compounds are active against dermatophytes only at low concentrations. Analysis of the benzyl ether structure (7) and ketal structure (9) was translated into the synthesis of ketals with an aralkyl side-chain (6) (Fig. 1), resulting in compounds related very closely to the miconazole structure (n = 0). From the structure–activity point of view these ring structures can give us information concerning the influence of the spatial position of the aryl rings on antifungal activity. The relative disposition of the substituents on the dioxolane ring can give rise to cis and trans isomers (Fig. 1). *In vitro* some of these compounds were found to be active against dermatophytes, yeasts and other fungi, at a level comparable to miconazole. How-

(10)

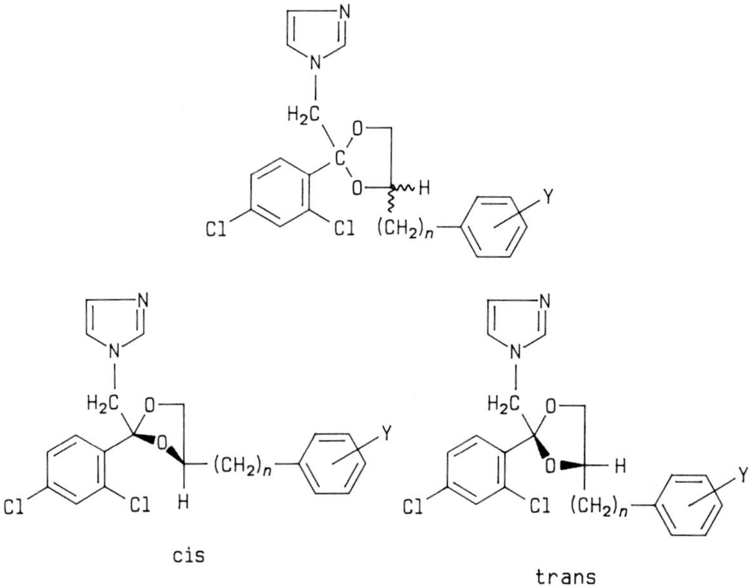

Fig. 1 1-{[2-(2,4-Dichlorophenyl)-4-(arylalkyl)-1,3-dioxolan-2-yl]methyl}-1*H* imidazole and its cis and trans isomers, respectively.

ever, *in vivo* some compounds were slightly superior to miconazole after oral administration in animals. The improved oral activity prompted further chemical modification, and this led to the synthesis of ketals in which a glycidyl ether fragment was incorporated. Glycidyl ethers were chosen since this fragment is present in a class of drugs of major importance, namely the β-blockers (see Chap. 5) and because one representative, chlorphenesin (**10**), is known to be an anti-fungal agent, displaying some activity against dermatophytes and *Candida* species (7). In this series of compounds (**11**) separation of cis/trans isomers

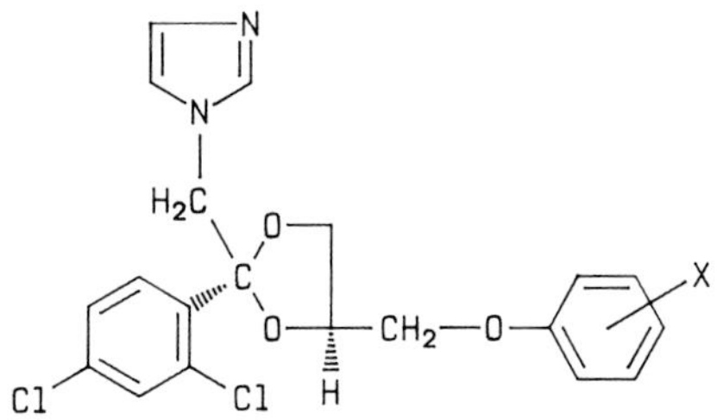

(**11**) Ketoconazole   X = 4-N⟨   ⟩N—C—CH$_3$

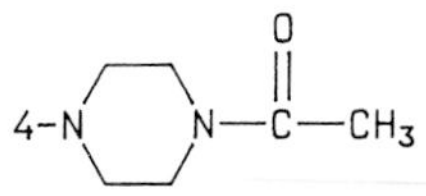

TABLE III

Anti-fungal Activity of Substituted 1-{[4-(Phenoxymethyl)-2-(2,4-dichlorophenyl)-1,3-dioxolan-2-yl]methyl}-1H-imidazoles[a]

(11)

X	Configuration	M. c.	T. m.	T. r.	Cr. n.	C. a.	A. f.	Skin candidosis guinea-pig[b]	Vaginal candidosis rat[b]
H	Cis	>+++	>+++	>+++	>+++	0	>+++	2/2[c]	2/2
2–Cl	Cis	>+++	>+++	>+++	>+++	+	>+++	1/2	1/2
3–Cl	Cis	>+++	>+++	>+++	>+++	0	>+++	0/2	—
4–Cl	Cis	>+++	>+++	>+++	>+++	0	++	0/2	0/2

Substituent	Configuration								
4-F	Cis	>++	>++	>++	>++	0	>++	1/2	2/2
4-Br*	Cis	++	>+++	>+++	>+++	0	>+++	2/2	1/2
4-CH₃O	Cis	>+++	>+++	>+++	>+++	0	++	2/2	1/2
2-Br	Cis	++	>++	>++	>++	0	++	0/2	—
4-CN	Cis	>+++	>++	>++	>++	0	++	0/2	1/2
4- (phenyl) *	Cis	0	+	0	+++	0	0	2/2	2/2
2- (phenyl)	Cis (40)/trans (60)	+	++	>+++	++	0	+	—	0/2
2,4-Cl₂	Cis	++	>+++	>+++	>+++	0	0	0/2	0/2
3,4-Cl₂	Cis	>+++	>+++	>+++	>+++	0	>+++	0/2	0/2
Miconazole		++	+++	+++	+++	++	++	4/13	0/2

[a] 0, inactive; +, 100% inhibition of growth at a concentration of 100 mg/litre after 14 days of incubation (in vitro); ++, 100% inhibition of growth at a concentration of 10 mg/litre after 14 days of incubation (in vitro); +++, 100% inhibition of growth at a concentration of 1 mg/litre after 14 days of incubation (in vitro). M. c., Microsporum canis; T. m., Trichophyton mentagrophytes; T. r., Trichophyton rubrum; Cr. n., Cryptococcus neoformans; C. a., Candida albicans; A. f., Aspergillus fumigatus.

[b] Dose 10 mg/kg/day p.o. for 14 consecutive days, treatment starting the day of infection.

[c] Ratio of cured animals versus total number of infected animals.

was realized, and their *in vitro* and *in vivo* activity was compared with that of miconazole (Table III). In this table the anti-fungal activity of the cis isomers is described with one exception (X = 2-Ph), which was tested as a cis/trans mixture. Although most of these compounds were highly active against dermatophytes, *Aspergillus fumigatus* and other organisms, and therefore comparable with miconazole, it was observed that one compound in particular (X = 4-Ph) was only active against *Cr. neoformans* under the test conditions; this may be attributed to its low solubility in the test medium. The *in vitro* activity improved considerably when the compound was dissolved in a suitable organic solvent. In this series of compounds only one representative (**11**, X = 2-Cl) showed some activity against *C. albicans*. Furthermore it was clearly demonstrated that the results obtained after oral treatment of either experimental skin candidosis in guinea-pigs or vaginal candidosis in rats were not consistent with *in vitro* activity against *C. albicans*.

Two compounds were selected and studied in more detail in other infection models. The first (**11**, X = 4-Br) was comparable to miconazole *in vitro* but superior in animals after oral administration. The second (**11**, X = 4-Ph), an even more potent compound in animals, was dropped for toxicity reasons. When comparing the *in vitro* and *in vivo* activity of the cis and trans analogues of some compounds (e.g., **11**, X = 4-Cl, 4-Br and 4-phenyl) it was shown that the *in vitro* activity of the cis isomers is greater than that of the corresponding trans analogues (Table IV). This effect has been confirmed in *in vivo* experiments with the compound **11** where X = 4-Ph, the cis isomer being highly active in vaginal candidosis and in skin candidosis at 10 mg/kg; the trans isomer is only marginally active in vaginal candidosis at the same dose.

It was hoped that the introduction of a heterocyclic ring instead of the second phenyl ring might decrease toxicity and enhance the bioavailability of the compound without loss of biological activity. This modification resulted in compounds which were highly active against *Trichophyton rubrum* and *Cr. neoformans*. Only one compound (**11**, X = 4-imidazole) displayed activity against *C. albicans* at a concentration of 100 mg/litre (Table V). Furthermore, this compound was highly active against *T. rubrum* and *Cr. neoformans* at a concentration of 1 mg/litre, moderately active against *M. canis* and *C. tropicalis* at 10 mg/litre and modestly active against *A. fumigatus* at 100 mg/litre. Substitution of the imidazole ring by other rings as depicted in table V gave compounds which showed no advantage in terms of *in vitro* activity. *In vivo* some of these compounds (X = imidazole, pyrimidine and oxadiazole) were highly active against experimental vaginal candidosis in rats, but only one compound (X = imidazole) was also active against skin candidosis in the guinea-pig and was consequently selected for further evaluation in various animal models. Unfortunately, this compound showed accumulation effects in dogs and caused severe side effects.

Despite this drawback it was hoped that equally active compounds with lower

TABLE IV

Comparison of the Anti-fungal Activities of Cis and Trans Isomers[a]

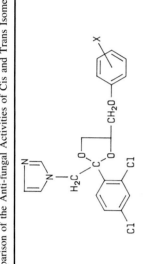

(11)

X	Configuration	M. c.	T. m.	T. r.	Cr. n.	C. a.	A. f.	Skin candidosis guinea-pig	Vaginal candidosis rat
4–Cl	Cis	>+++	>+++	>+++	>+++	0	++	0/2	0/2
4–Cl	Trans	++	>+++	>+++	++	0	++	0/2	0/2
4–Br	Cis	++	>+++	>+++	>+++	0	+++	2/2	1/2
4–Br	Trans	++	>+++	>+++	0	0	+	1/2	1/2
4–	Cis	0	+	0	>+++	0	0	2/2	2/2
4–	Trans	0	0	0	0	0	0	0/2	1/2

[a] Key and conditions as in Table III.

TABLE V

Influence of Heterocyclic Substituents on Anti-fungal Activity[a]

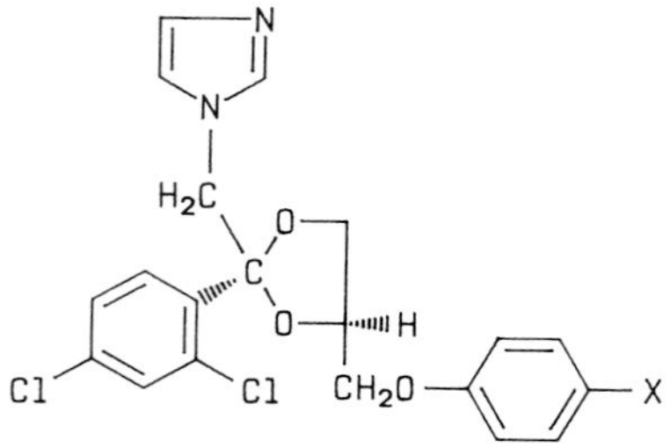

(11)

X	Anti-fungal activity								
	In vitro							In vivo	
								Skin candidosis guinea-pig	Vaginal candidosis
	M. c.	T. m.	T. r.	Cr. n.	C. tr.	C. a.	A. f.		
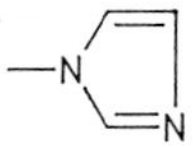	++	≥+++	≥+++	≥+++	++	+	+	5/6	7/8

(N-methylimidazole)	++	≥+++	≥+++	≥+++	+	0	0	0/2	3/6
(N-methylpyrrole)	+	≥+++	≥+++	≥+++	+	0	0	0/2	1/4
(N-methylpyrazole)	++	≥+++	++	≥+++	≥+++	0	+	0/2	4/6
(methylthiazole)	0	≥+++	≥+++	≥+++	0	0	0	0/2	0/2
(methylthiophene)	+	≥+++	++	≥+++	0	0	0	0/2	0/2
(methyloxazole)	+	≥+++	≥+++	≥+++	+	0	0	1/2	6/6
(methylpyrimidine)	+	≥++	≥++	≥++	≥++	0	0	—	3/4

[a] Key and conditions as in Table III, except C. tr., *Candida tropicalis*.

261

TABLE VI

In Vitro and in Vivo Anti-fungal Activity of Ketoconazole and Its Analogues

(12)

| Compound | | In vitro[a] | | | | | | | | | In vivo | |
X	Y	M. c.	T. m.	T. r.	Ph. v.	Cr. n.	C. tr.	C. a.	Muc.	A. f.	Microsporosis in guinea-pigs[c,d]	Vaginal candidosis in rats[b,c]
CH	H	—	—	—	—	—	—	—	—	—	0/2	0/2
CH	4-Cl	100	≤1	100	100	10	10	>100	>100	>100	0/2	0/2
CH	3-Cl	>100	10	100	100	100	>100	>100	>100	>100	—	0/2

CH	2-Cl	10	≤1	10	10	10	100	>100	>100	>100	0/2	0/2
CH	4 Br	100	≤1	100	100	10	100	100	>100	>100	0/2	0/2
CH	4-CH_3	—	—	—	—	—	—	—	—	—	0/2	0/2
CH	4-CH_3O	>100	100	>100	>100	100	>100	>100	>100	>100	0/2	0/2
CH	3-CH_3	100	10	100	100	>100	>100	>100	>100	>100	—	0/2
CH	2-Cl, 4-CH_3O	>100	10	100	100	10	>100	>100	>100	>100	0/2	0/2
CH	2-Cl, 4-CH_3	100	≤1	10	10	10	10	100	>100	100	0/2	0/2
CH	2-Cl, 4-F	100	≤1	≤1	10	≤1	10	>100	>100	100	0/2	0/2
CH	2-Cl, 4-Br	>100	≤1	10	100	10	≤1	>100	>100	>100	0/2	0/2
CH	2,4-Br_2	>100	≤1	≤1	100	≤1	≤1	>100	>100	>100	0/2	1/2
CH	2-Br, 4-Cl	100	≤1	≤1	10	10	10	100	>100	100	0/2	0/2
CH	2,3,4-Cl_3	>100	10	>100	>100	100	>100	>100	>100	>100	0/2	2/2
N	2,4-Cl_2	100	≤1	10	100	10	>100	>100	>100	>100	0/2[e]	0/2
CH	2,4-Cl_2	100	0.1	1	10	10	10	100	>100	100	4/34	2/8

[a] Complete or marked inhibition of growth after 14 days of incubation at the indicated concentration (mg/litre). Key: *M. c.*, *Microsporum canis*; *T. m.*, *Trichophyton mentagrophytes*; *T. r.*, *Trichophyton rubrum*; *Ph. v.*, *Phialophora verrucosa*; *Cr. n.*, *Cryptococcus neoformans*; *C. tr.*, *Candida tropicalis*; *C. a.*, *Candida albicans*; *Muc.*, *Mucor* species; *A. f.*, *Aspergillus fumigatus*.

[b] Therapeutic treatment for 3 consecutive days (dose 2.5 mg/kg, treatment starting 3 days post-infection).

[c] Ratio of cured animals versus total number of animals.

[d] Prophylactic treatment for 14 consecutive days (treatment starting the day prior to infection), with 10 mg/kg/day.

[e] Dose 20 mg/kg/day for 14 consecutive days.

toxicity could be synthesized, and it was decided that the aromatic heterocycles would be replaced with saturated nitrogen-containing heterocyclic rings, such as pyrrolidine, morpholine and piperazine. Finally, ketoconazole (**11**) (*8*) was prepared and proved to be equipotent with compound **11** when X = imidazole without being toxic or provoking side effects. In order to examine the influence of the acyl moiety on *in vitro* and *in vivo* activity, other acyl derivatives, carbamates, ureas and thioureas were synthesised (*9*), but no advantage was gained. As expected, the cis isomer of ketoconazole is clearly more active than the trans form both *in vivo* and *in vitro*. In a prophylactic treatment (starting on the day of infection), a daily oral dose of 5 mg/kg of ketoconazole for 14 consecutive days gave 100% protection in vaginal candidosis while with miconazole the same effect was obtained with 80 mg/kg.

Oral administration of ketoconazole prevented or cured experimental crop candidosis in turkeys, skin and systemic candidosis and dermatophytosis in guinea-pigs as well as vaginal candidosis in rats (*10*). The results obtained from animal models were confirmed in clinical trials (see later). Oral ketoconazole is also effective against superficial mycotic infections and deep-seated fungal infections, and it is already marketed in various countries for these indications. In order to examine substituent effects on biological activity, other compounds (**12**) were prepared possessing substituents other than 2,4-dichloro in the phenyl ring in the 2-position of the dioxolane ring (Table VI).

(**12**)

One compound (**12**, X = CH, Y = 2,4-Br$_2$) appeared to be highly active against *T. rubrum,* as well as against *Cr. neoformans* and *C. tropicalis,* at concentrations of 1 mg/litre or less. Both *in vitro* and *in vivo* ketoconazole is clearly more active than its triazole analogue (**12**, X = N, Y = 2,4-Cl$_2$). Only three compounds (ketoconazole, **12** where X = CH and Y = 2,4-Br$_2$ and **12** where X = CH, Y = 2,3,4-Cl$_3$) demonstrated activity against already established vaginal candidosis in rats at a low dose of 2.5 mg/kg. Against experimental microsporosis in the guinea-pig, ketoconazole showed some activity at 10 mg/kg, but all the other compounds were less potent. In an attempt to further optimize the structural requirements for the oral activity, alkylpiperazines were synthesised. However, in the imidazole as well as in the triazole derivatives the oral activity declined with this modification. In contrast to the disappointing oral activity, some of these compounds displayed a potent topical activity in experimental vaginal candidosis and dermatomycoses, and from this series of compounds terconazole (**13**) (*11*), a novel triazole derivative, was selected and developed for further clinical evaluation as a topical anti-mycotic.

(**13**) Terconazole

III. SUMMARY OF BIOLOGICAL ACTIVITY *IN VITRO* AND *IN VIVO*

The anti-fungal activity of ketoconazole qualitatively resembles that of miconazole. Ketoconazole is active against a wide variety of dermatophytes, yeasts and other pathogenic fungi. As with other antifungal imidazoles, the *in vitro* activity depends on factors such as inoculum size, pH, test medium and temperature (*12*). The pathogenic forms of *Paracoccidiodes brasiliensis* and *Histoplasma capsulatum* are very sensitive to ketoconazole (*15*).

Topically applied ketoconazole was highly active in the treatment of dermatophytic infections and of skin candidosis in guinea-pigs and vaginal candidosis in rats. Orally administered ketoconazole was highly effective both prophylactically (treatment starting the day of infection or the day prior to infection) and therapeutically (treatment starting 3 days after infection) against trichophytosis, microsporosis and skin candidosis in guinea-pigs and vaginal candidosis in rats. Oral ketoconazole was also highly active in the treatment of systemic candidosis and disseminated trychophytosis in guinea-pigs (*12*). In experimental cryptococcosis the life span of mice (infected intravenously) could be increased with oral ketoconazole (86 mg/kg/day for 16 days), but mortality was not prevented. However, after intraperitoneal infection the survival rate could be increased from 10% to nearly 50% with oral ketoconazole.

Ketoconazole effectively protected mice from death following infection with intravenous *H. capsulatum* (*1*).

IV.   MECHANISM OF ACTION OF THE IMIDAZOLE ANTI-FUNGALS

With N-substituted imidazole derivatives like clotrimazole, econazole, imazalil and miconazole, alterations of membrane permeability in susceptible yeast and fungal cells have been found. The membranes of most cells are composed of proteins, phospholipids and sterols. Both phospholipids and sterols play an important role in membrane structure and permeability. In mammalian cells cholesterol is the main sterol, but in yeasts and other fungal cells ergosterol is the main permeability regulating sterol. It has been found that ergosterol biosynthesis is inhibited by all antifungal imidazole and triazole derivatives investigated. Furthermore ketoconazole is a potent inhibitor of ergosterol biosynthesis in *C. albicans* grown in culture media (*13*).

The dose required to influence cholesterol synthesis in rat liver is at least six times that of inhibiting ergosterol synthesis in *C. albicans*. Similarly, cholesterol synthesis in a subcellular fraction of rat liver is about 20–70 times less sensitive to ketoconazole or miconazole than ergosterol synthesis in similar fractions obtained from *C. albicans* (*14*).

The inhibition of ergosterol synthesis in fungal cells coincides with an accumulation of 14α-methylsterols, indicative of an interaction of the drug with the 14α-methyldemethylase system. This is a carbon monoxide sensitive system indicating that a cytochrome *P*-450-dependent enzyme system is required to initiate oxidation of the 14α-methyl group of lanosterol, the precursor of ergosterol in yeast microsomes (Scheme 1). It has been shown that miconazole and ketoconazole affect cytochrome *P*-450 in yeast microsomes (*15*). Cytochrome *P*-450 of rat liver microsomes is much less sensitive, which correlates well with the lower sensitivity on cholesterol synthesis in mammalian cells. It has been suggested that the accumulation of 14α-methylsterols in the azole-treated yeast and fungal cells may lead to functional changes in cell membranes and to cell death.

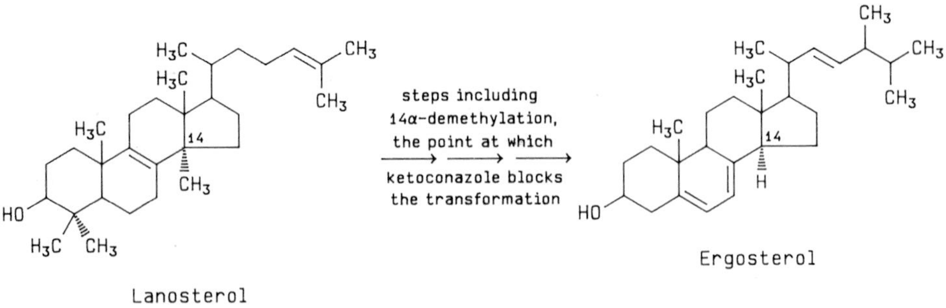

Scheme 1   Relationship of lanosterol and ergosterol.

V. PHARMACOKINETIC PROPERTIES AND METABOLISM OF KETOCONAZOLE

In contrast with miconazole, which is poorly absorbed after oral administration, ketoconazole is well taken up into the bloodstream after oral intake of the drug. In animal studies the tritiated drug was shown to be widely distributed in the body, including the fur of rats and guinea-pigs. Highest levels of radioactivity were observed in the liver and in the adrenals. Moderate levels occurred in the lung, kidney, bladder, bone marrow, teeth, myocardium and various glandular tissues, whereas low levels were found in the testis and brain (*1, 16*).

Ketoconazole is extensively metabolized into inactive metabolites. The main metabolic pathways in man are oxidation and subsequent scission of the oxidized imidazole ring, oxidative O-dealkylation, oxidation and degradation of the piperazine ring and hydrolysis of the dioxolane ring and of the amide moiety (*16*).

VI. CLINICAL STUDIES

Ketoconazole has been clinically evaluated and shown to be an effective treatment for a number of superficial mycoses, such as dermatomycoses, tinea capitis, pityriasis versicolor, oral thrush, vaginal candidosis, and onychomycosis. For the dermatomycoses the most frequently encountered susceptible organisms were the dermatophytes *T. rubrum, T. mentagrophytes, Epidermophyton floccosum, M. canis* and the yeasts *C. albicans* and *C. tropicalis* (*1, 17*).

The results obtained with ketoconazole in tinea capitis are very encouraging, but additional study is required to allow an accurate evaluation. The results obtained were significantly better when the fungus involved was of the "human type" (*M. audouini*) than when a fungus from animal sources (*M. canis*) was involved (*1*). Excellent rates of cure and remission were also observed for patients with oral candidosis, vaginal candidosis, onychomycosis, and perionyxis.

Ketoconazole has been shown to be effective in the treatment of deep-seated mycoses such as systemic candidosis, coccidioidomycosis, paracoccidioidomycosis and histoplasmosis. For example, the effect of orally administered ketoconazole was evaluated in patients with urinary tract candidosis, respiratory tract candidosis, candidal septicaemia, biliary candidosis, oesophageal candidosis and musculoskeletal candidosis. The median time to response was about 2 weeks: according to the degree and localisation of the infection, the response rate varied from 80% in septicaemia to 90% in respiratory tract infections (*1, 18*).

At the time of writing, well over 100 patients with coccidioidomycosis have been treated with oral ketoconazole (some of them remaining on therapy for up to 3.5 years) (*1, 2*). Remission or marked improvement of the disease was achieved very slowly with a median treatment time of 23 weeks. In only 13% of the total number of cases was remission shown, with an additional marked improvement in 22% more. Amphotericin B and miconazole do not perform well in the treatment of this disease state. Hence, it may be concluded that coccidioidomycosis is a very difficult disease to treat, and this is reflected by the relatively low remission rate compared with the results obtained in other fungal diseases after ketoconazole treatment. Nevertheless, the reported results are encouraging and indicate that ketoconazole may play an important role in the treatment of this disease (*19*).

More than 100 patients with paracoccidioidomycosis have been treated with oral ketoconazole (200–400 mg/day). Many of them had failed to respond to (or relapsed after) previous treatment with intravenous amphotericin B, or intravenous or oral miconazole (*1*). After a median treatment period of 10 weeks with ketoconazole, 79% of patients were in remission and 16% markedly improved. The results obtained in this study indicated that ketoconazole dramatically improved the prognosis of patients with paracoccidioidomycosis and might well become a first-line drug for the future treatment of this disease (*20*). Ketoconazole has been used in the treatment of histoplasmosis; in addition it has been used in the treatment of a small number of patients with cryptococcosis and aspergillosis, but the results obtained are of little predictive value.

In most patients ketoconazole was well tolerated. Nausea was the most frequently reported side effect (*17*). The estimated incidence of more serious symptomatic hepatic reactions is approximately 1 in 12,000 patients treated (*1*).

VII. CONCLUSIONS

Ketoconazole represents a significant step forward in the treatment of fungal disease. It is orally active and is effective at low concentrations against a wide range of organisms.

It appears that the selective destruction of fungal cells is due to a significant difference in the make-up of fungal cell walls when compared to the equivalent structures in human cells.

In the future, medicinal chemists should be able to use this information to design and produce more potent, less toxic anti-fungal agents.

REFERENCES

1. H. B. Levine, "Ketoconazole in the Management of Fungal Disease." ADIS, Balgowlah, Australia, 1982.

2. J. R. Graybill and P. C. Craven, *Drugs* **25**, 41 (1983).
3. D. C. E. Speller, "Antifungal Chemotherapy." Wiley, Chichester, 1980.
4. E. F. Godefroi, J. Heeres, J. Van Cutsem, and P. A. J. Janssen, *J. Med. Chem.* **12**, 784 (1969).
5. J. Van Cutsem and D. Thienpont, *Chemotherapy (Basel)* **17**, 392 (1972).
6. J. Heeres and J. Van Cutsem, *J. Med. Chem.* **24**, 1360 (1981).
7. P. F. D'Arcy and J. Scott, *in* "Progress in Drug Research" (E. Jucker, ed.), p. 93. Birkhauser, Basel, 1978.
8. J. Heeres, L. J. J. Backs, J. H. Mostmans, and J. Van Cutsem, *J. Med. Chem.* **22**, 1003 (1979).
9. J. Heeres, M. De Brabander, and H. Van den Bossche, *in* "Current Chemotherapy and Immunotherapy, Proceedings of the 12th International Congress of Chemotherapy, Florence 1981" (P. Periti and G. Grossi, eds), Vol. 2, p. 1007. Am. Soc. Microbiol., Washington, D.C., 1982.
10. D. Thienpont, J. Van Cutsem, F. Van Gerven, J. Heeres, and P. A. J. Janssen, *Experientia* **35**, 606 (1979).
11. J. Heeres, R. Hendricks, and J. Van Cutsem, *J. Med. Chem.* **26**, 611 (1983).
12. J. Van Cutsem, *Am. J. Med.* **74**–1B, 9 (1983).
13. M. Borgers, H. Van den Bossche, and M. De Brabander, *Am. J. Med.* **74**–1B, 2 (1983).
14. G. Willemsens, W. Cools, and H. Van den Bossche, *in* "The Host Invader Interplay" (H. Van den Bossche, ed.), p. 691. Elsevier, Amsterdam, 1980.
15. H. Van den Bossche and G. Willemsens, *Arch. Int. Physiol. Biochim.* **90**, B218 (1982).
16. M. Michiels, *in* "Chemotherapie von Oberflächen-, Organ- und Systemmykosen" (H. Seeliger and H. Hauck, eds), p. 36. Perimed Fachbuchverlagsgesellschaft, Erlangen, 1982.
17. J. Symoens, *in* "Chemotherapie von Oberflächen-, Organ- und Systemmykosen" (H. Seeliger and H. Hauck, eds), p. 134. Perimed Fachbuchverlagsgesellschaft, Erlangen, 1982.
18. J. Symoens and G. Cauwenbergh, *Mykosen* **24**, 70 (1981).
19. D. A. Stevens, R. L. Stiller, P. L. Williams, and A. M. Sugar, *Am. J. Med.* **74**–1B, 58 (1983).
20. A. M. Restrepo, I. Gomez, L. E. Cano, M. D. Arango, F. Gutiérrez, A. Sanin, and M. A. Robledo, *Am. J. Med.* **74**–1B, 48 (1983).

CHAPTER 14

Oxamniquine: A Drug for the Tropics

H. C. RICHARDS

Pfizer Central Research
Sandwich, England

I. INTRODUCTION: A DESCRIPTION OF THE DISEASE

It is probably not widely known that helminthiasis, a general term covering those infections caused by parasitic worms, is the most common disease in the world (*1*). One of the major human diseases of the tropics is of this type. The disease is called schistosomiasis (also known as bilharzia or bilharziasis), and an estimated 200 million people are afflicted although the number exposed to risk of infection is much higher, probably of the order of 500–600 million (*2*). Of the human parasitic diseases, schistosomiasis is second only to malaria in causing prolonged debilitating illness, and treatment and control of the disease present major challenges.

The causative parasite is called a schistosome [a small flatworm (trematode or fluke)], and to understand how the disease is contracted and transmitted one needs to consider the schistosome life-cycle shown in simplified form in Fig. 1. Schistosomes exist as separate male and female worms, pairs of which cling to the inside walls of certain blood vessels in the human host. The female parasite continually discharges large numbers of small eggs which are eventually ex-

271

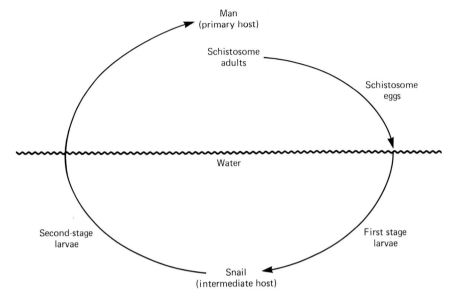

Fig. 1   Schistosomiasis life cycle.

creted in the urine or faeces of the infected person. On contact with water, the eggs hatch to produce small larvae (miracidia). These seek a species of snail that acts as an intermediate host and here develop into a large number of second-stage larvae (cercariae) which once liberated into water can rapidly penetrate human skin. During passage through the human body to the ultimate site of attachment, the larvae change form and develop into adult schistosomes, thereby completing the life-cycle. The particular blood vessels occupied depend on the species of parasite. The three principal species pathogenic to man are *Schistosoma mansoni*, *S. haematobium* and *S. japonicum*.

These three species produce distinctly different clinical effects which arise from inflammatory reactions caused by schistosome eggs becoming trapped in various tissues and organs of the body; the intestine, liver and spleen are primarily affected by *S. mansoni* and *S. japonicum* whereas *S. haematobium* mainly affects the bladder and urinogenital tract. Worms can survive up to 20 years in the host, and consequently schistosomiasis is a very debilitating and prolonged disease which in severe infestations can ultimately prove fatal. A great deal of suffering is experienced and children, because of their attraction to water in hot climates, are particularly susceptible to infection.

The disease is widespread, *S. mansoni* occurring extensively in Africa, South and Central America, *S. japonicum* in Asia and *S. haematobium* throughout Africa and the Middle East. Within these areas, the prevalence of schistosomiasis is increasing due to the spread of the snails' habitat associated with the introduction of new hydro-electric schemes and agricultural developments, thereby placing a greater burden on the economy by loss of working potential.

II. CHEMOTHERAPY IN THE 1960s

When the schistosomiasis project was established at the Pfizer U.K. laboratories in 1964, a clear need existed for a non-toxic, highly effective agent, ideally administered in a single oral dose, and of acceptable cost, which would be suitable in programmes of mass treatment and usable against all three species of schistosome. Two types of drug were in clinical use at that time but neither met the above criteria. These drugs were antimonials, typified by stibocaptate [astiban, sodium antimony-2,3-dimercaptosuccinate (**1**)], and lucanthone [miracil D, 1-(β-*N,N*-diethylaminoethylamino)-4-methylthiazanthone (**2**)]. The shortcomings of these drugs were as follows: each produced toxic side effects, repeated dosing was necessary and, in the case of stibocaptate, the drug was not effective orally but had to be given by intravenous or intramuscular injection. Lucanthone was effective only against *S. mansoni* and *S. haematobium.*

(**1**) Stibocaptate

(**2**) Lucanthone

During the period of our researches, three other drugs were described. One of these, a derivative of lucanthone (**2**), was of considerable significance to our research programme and is described in detail later in this chapter (Section VIII). The other two drugs were niridazole [Ambilhar (Ciba), 1-(5-nitro-2-thiazoyl)-2-imidazolidone (**3**)] and the organophosphorus compound metrifonate [Dipterex (Bayer), *O,O*-dimethyl 2,2,2-trichloro-1-hydroxyethylphosphonate (**4**)]. However, neither of these latter two drugs met our own objectives. Niridazole had to be given in multiple doses, and serious neuropsychiatric side effects have been observed. Metrifonate was active only against *S. haematobium* and needed to be given in divided doses, but as a treatment is effective and inexpensive. It is used extensively, particularly in Egypt.

In recent years, a further drug, praziquantel {Biltricide (Bayer), 2-cyclohexylcarbonyl-1,3,4,6,7,11b-hexahydro-2*H*-pyrazino[2,1a]isoquinolin-4-one (**5**)} has been described. Praziquantel displays high efficacy against all three species

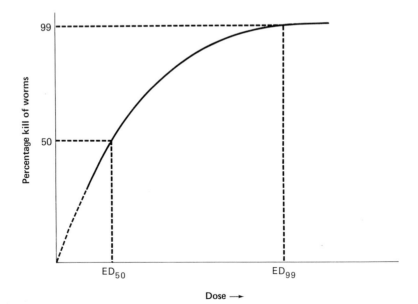

(3) Niridazole

(4) Metrifonate

(5) Praziquantel

of schistosome and seems to be well tolerated in patients although the cost of treatment is likely to limit its use.

III.   BIOLOGICAL ASSESSMENT

Compounds synthesised as potential schistosomicides were screened initially in laboratory mice harbouring a standard infection of *S. mansoni*. Test compounds were administered orally in one daily dose of 100 mg/kg for 4 consecutive days, and activity was measured as described by Foster *et al.* (*3*) by determining percentage kill of worms 24 hours after the final dose. Active

Fig. 2   Dose–response curve.

compounds were reassessed at lower concentrations, often as a single dose, and in some instances a dose–response curve was obtained to permit calculation of ED_{50} and ED_{99} figures—that is, the doses required to kill 50 or 99% of worms, respectively—in order to have comparative activity data. Figure 2 shows the shape of a typical dose–response curve and the relationship of ED_{50} and ED_{99} values.

Secondary evaluation of promising compounds was undertaken in *S. mansoni*-infected monkeys, and faecal egg output (initially 5000–10,000/24 hours) was determined daily before and after treatment by the method of Bell (*4*). Efficacy was judged by the reduction in egg load, and treatment was considered to be curative when the count fell to zero and remained so for several weeks.

Evaluation of compounds in the monkey was an essential step in the investigation since confirmation of schistosomicidal activity in this higher species would indicate possible efficacy in man, thereby justifying the subsequent very expensive development programme and clinical trials.

IV. CHEMICAL APPROACHES

In planning the chemical programme to meet the project objectives, we considered several approaches, and one of these concentrated on a series of compounds described some 8 years earlier by Mauss *et al.* (*5*), the mirasan series (*6*). These *p*-toluidine derivatives arose as simplified analogues of schistosomicidal xanthones and thiazanthones, the miracil series (*7*), of which lucanthone (*2*) was the most active representative (*6*). The common structural features in series **6** and **7** were (i) a methyl group para to the substituted β-aminoethylamino side-chain and (ii) an electronegative substituent ortho to the methyl group.

(**6**) Mirasan series   (**7**) Miracil series   (**8**) Mirasan

R^1 = H, alkyl; R^2 = alkyl;
R^3 = electronegative substituent; X = O, S

The parent member of series (**6**) was mirasan [2-chloro-4-β-*N*,*N*-diethyl-aminoethylaminotoluene (**8**)]. This compound was very active against schistosomiasis in laboratory mice but was ineffective in higher host species,

TABLE I
Activity[a] of Mirasan and Cyclic Analogues

	Structure	Host species		
		Mouse	Monkey	Man
8	Me —⟨ring⟩— NHCH$_2$CH$_2$NEt$_2$ Cl	+	−	−
9	Me —⟨ring⟩— N⟨piperazine⟩NH Cl	+ +	−	−
10	Me $\overset{5}{\underset{7}{}}$ Cl —⟨ring⟩N— CH$_2$CH$_2$NEt$_2$ Cl = 5 and 7	+	+	±

[a] Relative activity against *Schistosoma mansoni* infections.

namely, monkey and man. Several investigators have attempted to overcome the therapeutic deficiency of mirasan by modification of its structure, and two of these congeners are depicted in Table I, which shows activity in three species of host.

In mice, the cyclic analogue *N*-(3-chloro-4-methylphenyl)piperazine (**9**) was reported by Gönnert (7) to show high activity, approximately double that of mirasan (**8**). The potency of a drug depends on its pharmacodynamics, that is, the interaction of the drug molecule with cell receptors thereby eliciting the biological response, a process which is often stereospecific. In the case of the piperazine derivative (**9**) it can be argued that by stereochemical 'locking' of the aminoethylamino region of the molecule a favoured conformation is achieved which facilitates a drug–receptor interaction in the schistosome which is lethal to the parasite. However, no activity was demonstrated by the chlorodiamine (**9**) in monkey and man. Variation in drug efficacy in different animal species is frequently encountered—which can fascinate and at the same time frustrate the medicinal chemist!—and is explained in terms of pharmacokinetics, namely, rates of absorption, distribution and elimination of the drug, and its metabolism, that is, enzymic conversions in the liver and other tissues to biologically active or inactive derivatives.

As no pharmacokinetic studies for the chlorodiamines **8** and **9** had been reported, it was not possible for us to deduce what specific factor was responsible for lack of schistosomicidal action in primates, but, interestingly, a different pattern of activity was displayed by the cyclic analogues (**10**). As well as being active in the mouse screen, these compounds were effective against schistosomal infections in the monkey (Table I) although no convincing activity was demonstrated in man (5). It was evident that the particular conformational constraint in this class of compound, in which free rotation of the aminoethylamino portion of the molecule is prevented, dramatically influenced the pharmacokinetic properties compared with mirasan, but again in the absence of the relevant data it was not possible to tell in what precise manner this was achieved. Various chemical modifications of compounds **9** and **10** had been made: for example different substituents were introduced onto the distal nitrogen atom and the halogen atom was replaced by other electronegative substituents. These changes produced highly active schistosomicides, but none of the compounds displayed the desired efficacy in man.

Nevertheless, the variation in potency and the activity pattern of compounds of the same type as **8, 9** and **10** clearly established in our minds the importance of side-chain stereochemistry, and we were encouraged to consider other ways of introducing conformational constraint in anticipation of producing novel compounds which might achieve the required objective, namely, activity in man. The structures we proposed were **11–14**, in which ethylene linkages between the α-carbon atom of the mirasan side-chain and one of the ortho carbon positions of the aromatic ring, and additionally between the nitrogen atoms in the case of

(11)

(12)

(13)

(14)

R = electronegative substituent; R^1 = H, alkyl; R^2 = alkyl compounds of the same type as **13** and **14,** introduced a higher degree of confor-mational constraint than previously obtained.

We planned our programme to include a wide variety of substituents R, R^1 and R^2 into the basic structures. The overall aim was to identify a novel compound with high potency, which would be *selectively* toxic to the schistosome.

V. CHEMICAL SYNTHESIS

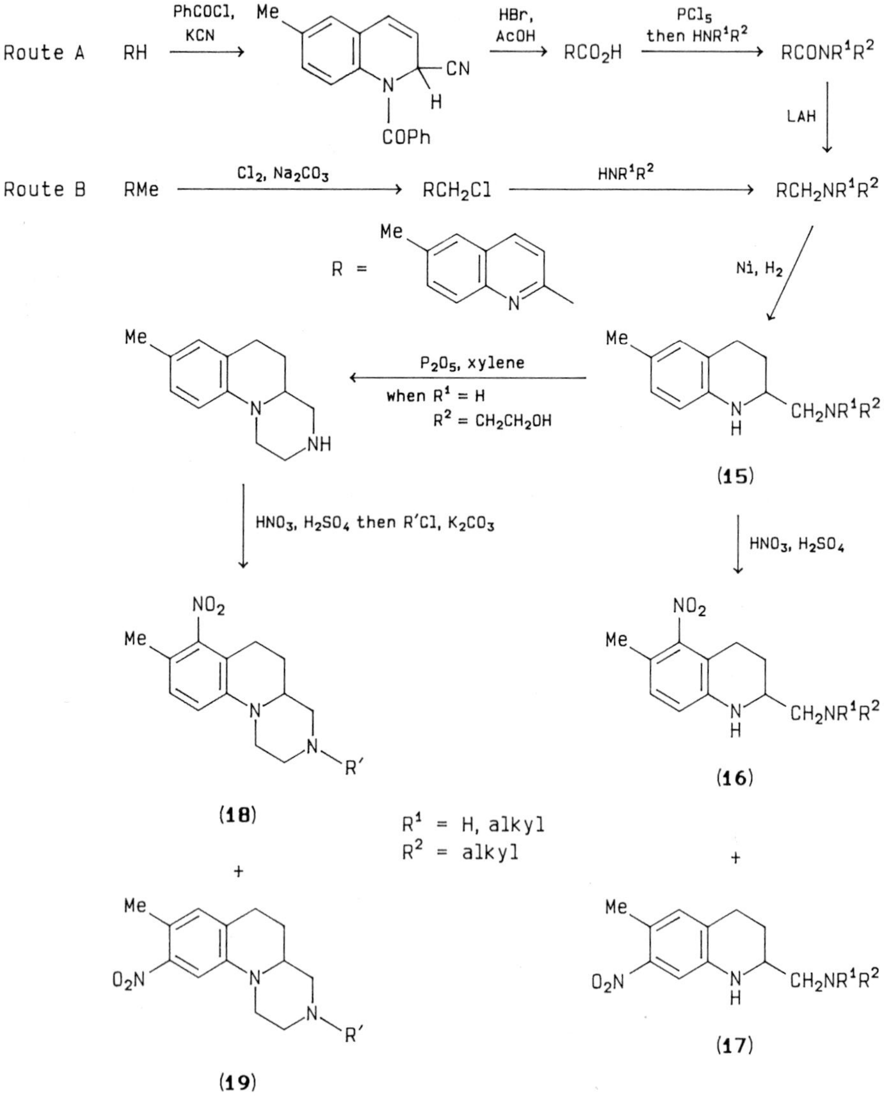

Scheme 1   Routes to nitro derivatives.

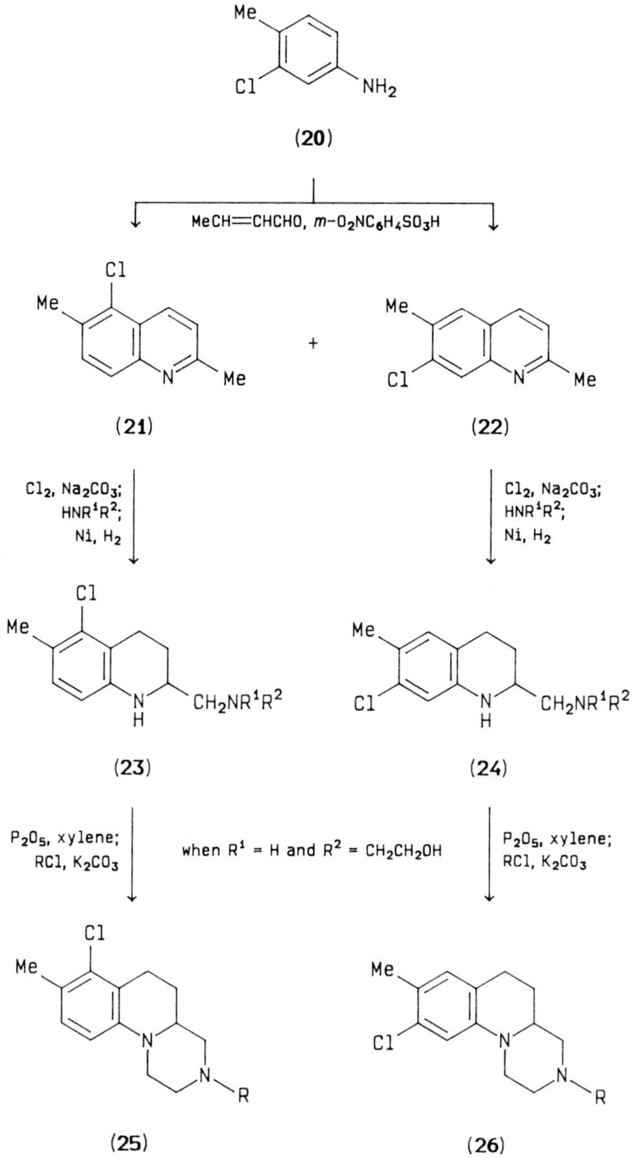

Scheme 2 Routes to chloro derivatives.

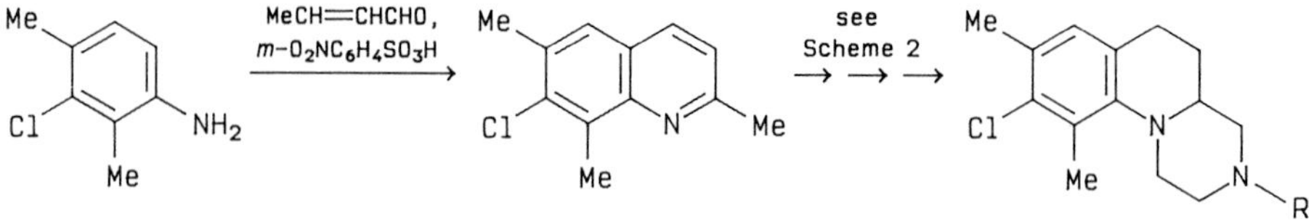

Scheme 3   9-Chloro-10-methyl tricyclic compounds.

The syntheses of the 1,2,3,4-tetrahydroquinoline series **11** and **12** and the 2,3,4,4a,5,6-hexahydro-1*H*-pyrazino[1,2a]quinoline series **13** and **14** have been described by Baxter and Richards (*9, 10*). The synthetic routes illustrated in Scheme 1 led to the key intermediate (**15**) and hence to the nitro isomers **16** plus **17** or **18** plus **19**, each pair of isomers being separated by fractional crystallisation. The chloro compounds **23** and **24** or **25** and **26** were derived from products **21** and **22** (separated by fractional distillation) obtained from a Doebner–Miller reaction on the chlorotoluidine (**20**) (Scheme 2). A series of 9-chloro-10-methyl tricyclic compounds (**27**) was also prepared, as shown in Scheme 3. Compounds were submitted for schistosomicidal screening either as the free base or, more usually, as the hydrochloride or maleate salt.

VI.   SCHISTOSOMICIDAL ACTIVITY IN MICE

A.   2-Aminomethyl-1,2,3,4-tetrahydroquinolines

Encouragingly, several compounds of type **11** displayed very high activity in the mouse screen (*9*).

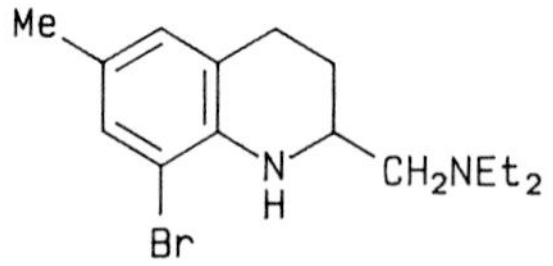

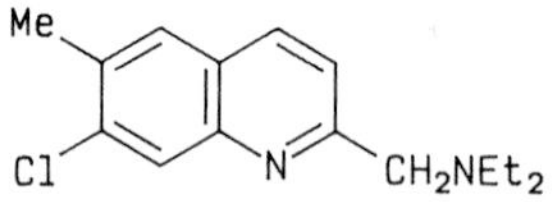

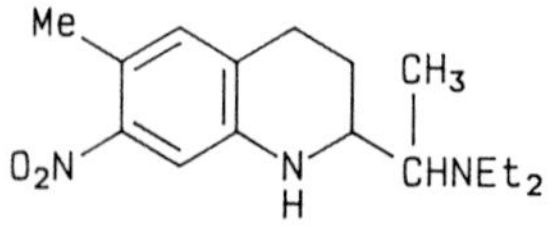

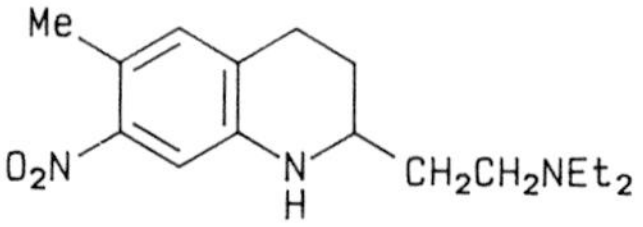

Compounds of type **12**, for example, **16** (Scheme 1) and **23** (Scheme 2), proved to be inactive, an unexpected result since the requirement of an electronegative substituent ortho to the methyl group (a necessary component of the molecule for biological activity in the mirasan series) had been met. Less surprising was the fact that compounds of type **28** (electronegative substituent meta to the methyl), type **29** (fully aromatised) and types **30** and **31** (side-chain branched or extended, respectively) showed markedly reduced or nil activity.

The features which were found to be essential for display of activity are depicted in the structure below. Particularly important was the need to have R^1 as a methyl group and both nitrogen atoms basic, that is, nonacylated.

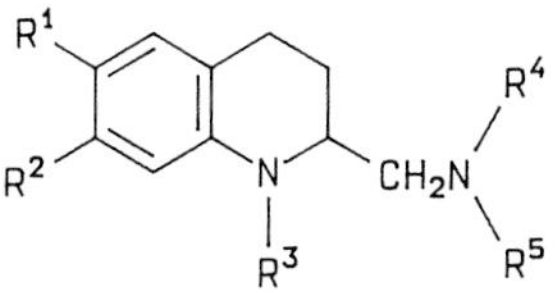

	Active compounds	Inactive compounds
R^1	Me	H, Et
R^2	Electronegative substituent, order of decreasing activity $NO_2 > CN > F > Cl > Br$	H
R^3	H, Me, Et	Higher alkyl, acyl
R^4	H, lower alkyl (up to C_4)	Acyl, higher alkyl
R^5	Lower alkyl (up to C_4)	Acyl, higher alkyl

In summary, the most active compounds were those of the 7-nitro series. The effect on schistosomicidal activity of different substituents on the terminal nitrogen atom was investigated and it was shown that isopropyl-NH > *tert*-butyl-NH > ethyl-NH ≫ primary amine ≈ tertiary amines ≈ other secondary amines. Thus compound **32** was most effective, and indeed this compound was shown to be

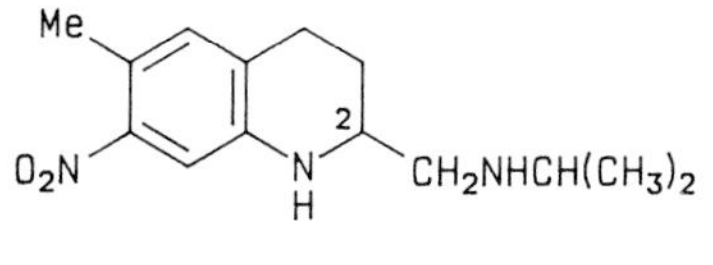

(32)

significantly more active than the standard schistosomicidal agents when administered in single or multiple doses (Table II); of particular interest to us was the realisation that molecular constraint imposed upon the flexible side-chain of the original mirasan series had brought about the desired enhancement of activity.

Compounds in the series were tested in their racemic form (optical isomerism

TABLE II
Activity against S. *mansoni* in Mice

| | Dosage (mg/kg) | | | |
| | Multiple ($\times$ 5) | | Single | |
Compound	ED_{50}	ED_{99}	ED_{50}	ED_{99}
32	8.7	17	22	65
Mirasan (**8**)	10	56	20	163
Lucanthone (**2**)	68	189	110	525
Niridazole (**3**)	105	278	740	4650

arising from chirality at position 2 of the molecule), but in a few instances optical resolution was carried out using d-α-bromocamphor-π-sulphonic acid. It was found that the dextro isomer was the more active form, an observation which emphasised the stereochemical importance of the side-chain in influencing activity. In the case of the nitro compound (**32**) there was a severalfold difference in activity between the two enantiomers.

B.   2,3,4,4a,5,6-HEXAHYDRO-1*H*-PYRAZINO[1,2a]QUINOLINES

Again, high schistosomicidal activity in the mouse screen was displayed by several members of this structural class. General activity was of a higher order than that of 2-aminomethyltetrahydroquinolines. This was in keeping with our ideas on conformational constraint. However, two interesting differences emerged between the bicyclic and tricyclic series in terms of structure–activity relationships.

Firstly, compounds of type **14** with a 7-nitro or 7-chloro substituent, [e.g., **18** (Scheme 1) and **25** (Scheme 2)] as well as the isomeric 9-substituted compounds **13** [e.g., **19** (Scheme 1) and **26** (Scheme 2)] were active: that is, in the tricyclic class, the electronegative substituent could be on *either* side of the methyl group.

Secondly, chloro compounds were more active than the corresponding nitro analogues which is the case for the mirasan series but is reversed for the 2-aminomethyltetrahydroquinolines (*vide supra*). These results highlight the difficulties in predicting the influence of structural modification upon biological activity and demonstrate that several factors operate to determine the eventual response.

The effect of introducing a substituent onto the 3-nitrogen position was usually diminished or destroyed activity, particularly in the chloro series. A potency enhancement was obtained when a methyl group was present in the 10-position,

(**33**)

and this has been ascribed to the twisting of the fused piperazine ring out of plane with the quinolino portion of the molecule (*10*). The compound with the highest intrinsic activity was the diamine (**33**). In the mouse screen, the curative single oral dose of the tricyclic compound **33** was 20 mg/kg, that is, the compound is about three times more active than the bicyclic compound (**32**) (Table III).

VII. SCHISTOSOMICIDAL ACTIVITY IN THE MONKEY

As explained earlier, an important step in the evaluation programme was to demonstrate schistosomicidal activity of our bicyclic and tricyclic compounds in

TABLE III
Efficacy in Mouse and Monkey

	Structure	Dose (mg/kg)[a]	
		Mouse (ED_{99})	Monkey (curative)
8		163	Inactive
32		65	50
33		20	70

[a] Doses are quoted as base equivalents; compound **8** was given as hydrochloride, **32** as maleate and **33** as free base.

the monkey. Reassuringly, high efficacy was demonstrated for several compounds, often in single oral doses, and structure–activity patterns roughly paralleled those observed in mice (11). The two compounds of particular interest were the amines **32** and **33,** which effected complete cures in monkey on administration of single oral doses of 50 and 70 mg/kg, respectively (Table III).

In view of this promising display of high potency, more detailed assessment of each compound was undertaken and on the basis of extended biological evaluation, preliminary toxicity studies, and projected cost of synthesis, the compound **32** was selected as a candidate for full development. We considered evaluation of the more active dextro isomer (*vide supra*), but the optical resolution step on a production scale would have added significantly to cost and the option was not pursued.

The decision was taken to develop the tetrahydroquinoline derivative (**32**), even without evidence of efficacy against *S. haematobium* and *S. japonicum,* because no completely suitable agent was available to treat *S. mansoni,* and this species afflicts an estimated 70 million sufferers.

VIII.   ACTIVE METABOLITES

During our investigations, a disclosure was made by Rosi *et al.* (12), from the Sterling-Winthrop Research Institute concerning lucanthone (**2**). It had been suspected for some time that the schistosomicidal effect of lucanthone was not due to the compound itself but to a derivative formed by metabolism within the host. A number of workers had reported unsuccessful attempts to identify the suspected metabolite by examination of the urine from lucanthone-treated animals, including man. The Sterling-Winthrop group approached the problem from a different standpoint. They subjected lucanthone to the action of a range of moulds in the expectation that one of these microorganisms would duplicate the metabolic effect of host enzymes. It was found that *Aspergillus sclerotiorum* converted lucanthone to a mixture of three products, the major one of which was the 4-hydroxymethyl derivative (**34**), subsequently named hycanthone, together with amounts of the corresponding aldehyde (**35**) and acid (**36**), as shown in Scheme 4.

Hycanthone proved to be highly schistosomicidal and more potent than lucanthone in several animal species. Chemical investigation showed hycanthone to be acid-labile, and by avoiding the acid treatment adopted by earlier investigators, it was possible to extract hycanthone from the urine of animals dosed with lucanthone (12, 13). This, and other evidence, suggested that hycanthone was the elusive active metabolite (14).

Hycanthone, prepared by the oxidative fermentation process, became commercially available as the methane sulphonate salt [Etrenol (Winthrop)] and is

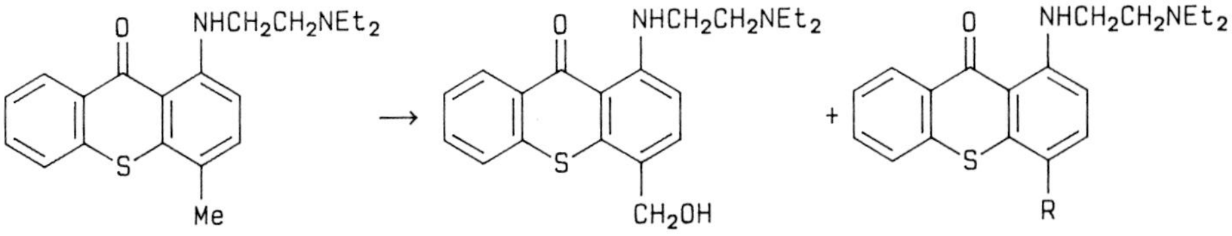

O   NHCH$_2$CH$_2$NEt$_2$ O   NHCH$_2$CH$_2$NEt$_2$ O   NHCH$_2$CH$_2$NEt$_2$

→   +

Me   CH$_2$OH   R

(2) Lucanthone   (34) Hycanthone   (35) R = CHO
(36) R = CO$_2$H

Scheme 4   Microbiological oxidation of lucanthone.

effective against *S. mansoni* and *S. haematobium* when administered as a single intramuscular injection. However, treatment is associated with nausea and vomiting; liver damage and other serious toxicity problems have also been encountered, and these shortcomings have limited the use of the drug.

The investigations described for lucanthone were extended to mirasan (8), and it was demonstrated that the corresponding hydroxymethyl compound (37) was formed in mice (8, 15). Significantly, this transformation did not occur in monkey, in which species mirasan, it will be recalled, is ineffective. It was shown that the diamine (37), prepared by oxidative fermentation or by chemical synthesis, displayed high activity in the mouse screen.

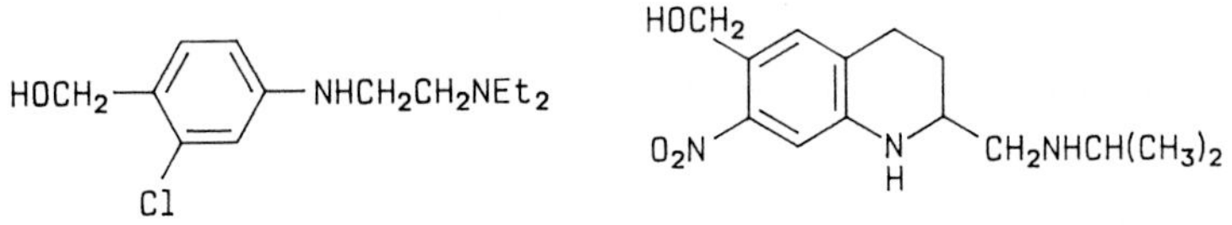

HOCH$_2$—⟨ ⟩—NHCH$_2$CH$_2$NEt$_2$ HOCH$_2$
Cl   O$_2$N   N   CH$_2$NHCH(CH$_3$)$_2$
                                                              H

(37)   (38) Oxamniquine

These studies demonstrated why the presence of a methyl group in the molecule was so necessary for activity in mirasan and lucanthone, and we decided to study this aspect in our own compounds (9, 10). A strain of *A. sclerotiorum* Huber (No. 549.65), obtained from the Centraalbureau voor Schimmelcultures, Baarn, Holland, was used in a series of fermentation studies in which members of the bicyclic and tricyclic series were incorporated as substrates. By means of preparative thin-layer chromatography and nuclear magnetic resonance (NMR) studies of the separated fractions, we were able to demonstrate that microbiological oxidation did occur to produce hydroxymethyl derivatives. Scale-up and optimisation of the conditions gave sufficient material for biological evaluation. High schistosomicidal activity was demonstrated for these derivatives in mice, and the potency was invariably higher than that of the parent methyl compound.

A derivative of particular interest to us was that obtained from the tetrahydroquinoline (32) previously selected as a development compound. This product

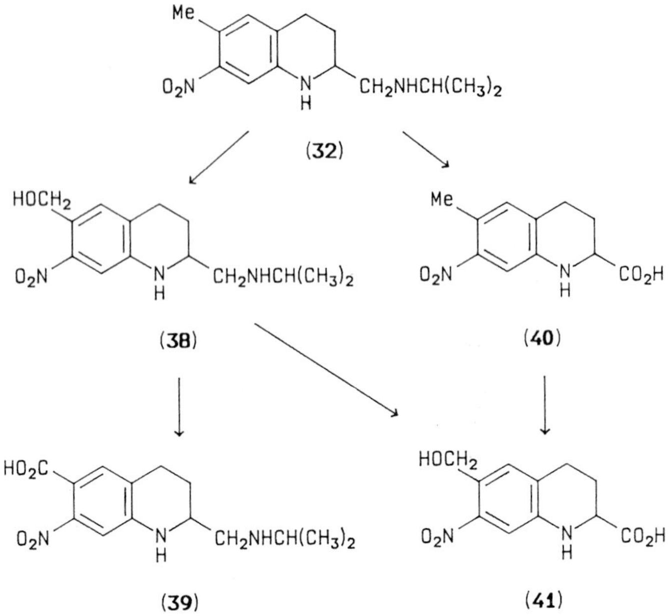

Scheme 5   Metabolism pathway of compound **32.**

(**38**) was shown to be very effective in the mouse screen in single oral doses and proved to be about three times more potent than hycanthone (**34**) in this species (*16*). Monkeys were cleared of *S. mansoni* infections following treatment with single intramuscular doses of 5.0–7.5 mg/kg or single oral doses of 15–20 mg/kg, thus demonstrating that the hydroxymethyl compound (**38**) was more potent than the parent compound (see Table III) (*17*).

8-Hydroxymethyl derivatives of the tricyclic series, prepared by the fermentation route, also proved to be highly active but, in preliminary safety evaluation, were also more toxic than compounds in the bicyclic series. For this reason, the diamine (**38**) was selected as the best representative for development, replacing the 'parent compound' (**32**). The generic name oxamniquine (derived from 6-hydroxymethyl-2-*N*-isopropylaminomethyl-7-nitro-1, 2, 3, 4-tetrahydroquinoline) was given to compound **38.**

Metabolism studies confirmed that the methyl compound (**32**) was converted into the hydroxymethyl compound (**38**) in mouse, monkey, rat and rabbit; various other (biologically inactive) metabolites were also detected, for example, the 6-carboxylic derivative (**39**) and/or the 2-carboxylic acid derivatives (**40** and **41**), the amounts depending on the species of host (Scheme 5).

Oxamniquine (**38**) was shown to be lethal towards schistosomes *in vitro*, which contrasts with the inactivity of the parent compound (**32**) (*18*). This fact, taken in conjunction with the metabolism studies described above, strongly suggested that derivatives of type **38** are the active metabolites of the original series and are formed in mice and, importantly, monkeys. The inactivity of mirasan in the latter species allowed the conclusion to be drawn that the consequence of conformational constraint in compounds of type **32** was to facilitate the essential hydroxylation step. Whether such a metabolic process would have occurred for the amine (**32**) in man was an intriguing question which was to remain unanswered in view of the decision to turn all attention to the hydroxylated derivative, oxamniquine (**38**).

IX. CLINICAL TRIALS WITH OXAMNIQUINE

Extensive pre-clinical toxicology in several animal speices was undertaken with oxamniquine prior to studying the safety of the compound in healthy human volunteers who were carefully monitored during administration of gradually increasing doses up to anticipated therapeutic levels. Following the successful outcome of these studies, extensive clinical trials were arranged to establish the safety, tolerance and efficacy of oxamniquine in patients harbouring natural infections of *S. mansoni*. In South America and Africa it was shown that oxamniquine was effective either after a single intramuscular dose or when given orally.

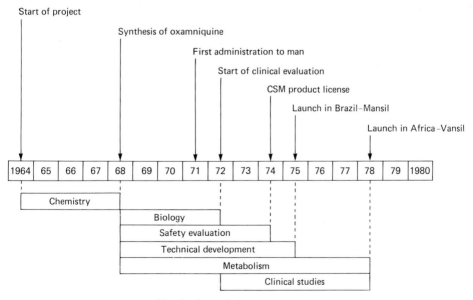

Fig. 3   Oxamniquine programme.

Pharmacokinetic investigations were undertaken to establish that after a single dose, high blood levels of drug were attained and persisted for several hours, during which time the schistosomes were exposed to its action.

As a result of satisfactory efficacy and no untoward adverse reactions in patients, oxamniquine was launched in Brazil in 1975 as Mansil (Pfizer) and during 1978 was marketed in Africa as Vansil (Pfizer) and is now available in over 20 countries in that continent.

A summary of the development programme for oxamniquine is shown in Fig. 3, and it can be seen that the time taken from its first preparation in 1968 to initial launch was 7 years, and to launch in Africa, 10 years. Such time-spans are quite usual for new pharmaceutical products.

X.   CLINICAL EXPERIENCE WITH OXAMNIQUINE

Soon after its introduction, oxamniquine became the drug of choice for treatment of human *S. mansoni* infections, and the position remains unchanged today. The compound is particularly effective in Brazil, cures being achieved with single oral doses in adults and with two doses, taken a few hours apart, in children. In some parts of Africa the strain of schistosome is more resistant to treatment and, depending on the geographical location, a higher total dosage taken over 1–3 days is required. Well over 100 publications to date refer to clinical efficacy of oxamniquine throughout the world, for example, South America (*19*), Saudi Arabia (*20*), Egypt and other parts of Africa (*21*) and the Carribean (*22*). Results show that the compound gives high cure rates, is well tolerated and is effective in all stages of infection, including the early acute and later chronic and complicated phases (*1*).

As a consequence of its efficacy, safety and convenience of treatment, oxamniquine can be administered by paramedical personnel under field conditions and became the first schistosomicide suitable for mass administration. It thus made a major contribution towards the control and treatment of *S. mansoni* infections and, very satisfyingly for those associated with its discovery and development, oxamniquine is listed in a report of the World Health Organization, "The Selection of Essential Drugs" (*23*).

The oxamniquine story has not quite finished. Recent work shows that oxamniquine in combination with the earlier-mentioned drug praziquantel (**5**) exerts a synergistic effect against *S. mansoni* infections in laboratory mice, that is, the efficacy of the drug combination is markedly superior to a simple additive effect of the components (*24*). It has now been confirmed in a clinical trial in Africa that simultaneous administration of oxamniquine and praziquantel produces efficacy at doses considerably lower than for either drug alone; of great interest was the observation of a synergistic effect against *S. haematobium* as well as *S. mansoni* (25).

ACKNOWLEDGEMENTS

The author wishes to acknowledge scientific colleagues and collaborators—too many to mention individually—for their invaluable contributions to the oxamniquine programme in all its phases.

REFERENCES

1. I. M. Rollo, *in* "The Pharmacological Basis of Therapeutics" (L. S. Goodman and A. Gilman, eds), 6th Edition, p. 1013. 1980.
2. G. Webbe, *Br. Med. J.* **283,** 1104 (1981).
3. R. Foster, B. L. Cheetham, and E. T. Mesmer, *J. Trop. Med. Hyg.* **71,** 139 (1968).
4. D. R. Bell, *Bull. W.H.O.* **29,** 525 (1963).
5. H. Mauss, H. Kolling, and R. Gönnert, *Med. Chem. Abhandle. Med. Chem. Forschungsstaetten Farbenfabriken, Bayer* **5,** 185 (1956).
6. W. Kikuth, R. Gönnert, and H. Mauss, *Naturwissenschaften* **33,** 253 (1946).
7. R. Gönnert, *Bull. W.H.O.* **25,** 702 (1961).
8. D. A. Berberian, E. W. Dennis, H. Freele, D. Rosi, T. R. Lewis, R. Lorenz, and S. Archer, *J. Med. Chem.* **12,** 607 (1969).
9. C. A. R. Baxter and H. C. Richards, *J. Med. Chem.* **14,** 1033 (1971).
10. C. A. R. Baxter and H. C. Richards, *J. Med. Chem.* **15,** 341 (1972).
11. R. Foster, B. Cheetham, D. F. King, and E. T. Mesmer, *Ann. Trop. Med. Parasitol.* **65,** 59 (1971).
12. D. Rosi, G. Peruzzotti, E. W. Dennis, D. A. Berberian, H. Freele, and S. Archer, *Nature (London)* **208,** 1005 (1965).
13. D. Rosi, G. Peruzzotti, E. W. Dennis, D. A. Berberian, H. Freele, B. F. Tullar, and S. Archer, *J. Med. Chem.* **10,** 867 (1967).
14. S. Archer and A. Yarinsky, *in* "Progress in Drug Research" (E. Jucker, ed.), Vol. 16, pp. 11–66. Birkhäuser, Basel, 1972.
15. D. Rosi, T. R. Lewis, R. Lorenz, H. Freele, D. A. Berberian, and S. Archer, *J. Med. Chem.* **10,** 877 (1967).
16. R. Foster and B. L. Cheetham, *Trans. R. Soc. Trop. Med. Hyg.* **67,** 674 (1973).
17. R. Foster, B. L. Cheetham, and D. F. King, *Trans. R. Soc. Trop. Med. Hyg.* **67,** 685 (1973).
18. N. M. Woolhouse and B. Kaye, *Parasitology* **75,** 111 (1977).
19. A. C. Sleigh, K. E. Mott, J. T. Franca Silva, T. M. Muniz, E. A. Mota, M. L. Barreto, R. Hoff, J. H. Maguire, J. S. Lehman, and I. Sherlock, *Trans. R. Soc. Trop. Med. Hyg.* **75,** 234 (1981).
20. M. B. El-Mallah, *J. Egypt. Med. Assoc.* **63,** 255 (1980).
21. P. O. Pehrson and E. Bengtsson, *Trans. R. Soc. Trop. Med. Hyg.* **77,** 282 (1983).
22. P. Jordan, *Am. J. Trop. Med. Hyg.* **26,** 877 (1977).
23. W.H.O., "The Selection of Essential Drugs," Tech. Rep. Ser. 165. World Health Organisation, Geneva, 1977.
24. J. R. Shaw and K. W. Brammer, *Trans. R. Soc. Trop. Med. Hyg.* **77,** 39 (1983).
25. R. N. H. Pugh and C. H. Teesdale, *Br. Med. J.* **287,** 877 (1983).

Index

H

6-Halopenicillanic acid, 243, 244
Heart rate, control, 11, 13, 51, 70, 71
Hecogenin, 169–171
Helminthiasis, 271
Heroin, 120, 121
2,3,4,4a,5,6-Hexahydro-1*H*-
  pyrazino[1,2a]quinoline derivative, 277
  biological activity, 282–284
  synthesis, 278–280
Histamine, 14, 50, 95
Histamine receptor, 13, 14, 97–99
  H_1-receptor, 99
  H_2-receptor
    antagonist, 99–117
    partial agonist, 102
Hofmann elimination, 152, 153, 158
Hormone, 6
Hycanthone, 284, 285
Hydrophobic bonding, 16

I

Imazalil, 254
Imidazole tautomerism, 106–111
Insulin, 45
Intrinsic activity, 21
Ion channel, opening, control, 5, 144
Isoconazole, 253, 254
Isoenzyme, 29
Isoetharine, 51
Isoprenaline, 50, 52, 71

K

Ketoconazole, 255, 264
  analogues, 255–264
    biological activity, 256–265
  biological activity, 262–265
  clinical studies, 267, 268
  mechanism of action, 266
  metabolism, 267

L

Lanosterol, 266
Leucocyte, 1
Levorphanol, 125
Lucanthone, 273
  biological activity, 273, 282

  metabolism, 284
  microbiological oxidation, 285
Luteinising hormone, 199
Lynestrenol, 193, 194, 198, 202, 204

M

Mansil, *see* Oxamniquine
McKenzie assay, 176
Medroxyprogesterone acetate, 204, 205
Meperidine, *see* Pethidine
Mepyramine, 98
Mestranol, 191–193, 202
Methadone, 124
Methicillin, 210, 229
Methotrexate, 40
Metiamide, 107, 110
Metocurine, 148, 149
Metoprolol, 80, 81
Metrifonate, 273, 274
Miconazole, 253–255, 266, 267
  analogues, 254, 255
Migraine, 89
Miracil, *see* Lucanthone
Mirasan, 275
  analogues, 276, 277
  biological activity, 276, 282, 283
  metabolism, 285
Morphinan, 125, 126
Morphine, 12, 120–127
  analogues, 123–127
    biological activity, 129–138
    receptor theory, 131, 132
    stereochemistry, 130–132
  antagonist, 126, 132–140
    test procedure, 133, 138
Muscarinic receptor, *see* Acetylcholine
  receptor
Muscle relaxant, 143–164
Mycosis, 249–251
Myocardial infarction, 89

N

Nadolol, 74
Nafcillin, 229
Nalorphine, 12, 126, 135
Narcotine, 120
Neoantergan, *see* Mepyramine
Neostigmine, 144, 160
Nerve cell, structure, 3